Biological Relatives

WITHDRAWN

EXPERIMENTAL FUTURES: *Technological Lives, Scientific Arts, Anthropological Voices*
A series edited by Michael M. J. Fischer and Joseph Dumit

SARAH FRANKLIN Biological Relatives

IVF, Stem Cells,

and the

Future of Kinship

Duke University Press   Durham and London   2013

© 2013 Duke University Press
All rights reserved
Printed in the United States of America on acid-free paper ♾
Cover designed by Amy Ruth Buchanan. Interior by Courtney Leigh Baker
Typeset in Whitman and Din by Tseng Information Systems, Inc.

Library of Congress Cataloging-in-Publication Data
Franklin, Sarah, 1960–
Biological relatives : IVF, stem cells, and the future of kinship / Sarah Franklin.
pages cm—(Experimental futures)
Includes bibliographical references and index.
ISBN 978-0-8223-5485-7 (cloth : alk. paper)
ISBN 978-0-8223-5499-4 (pbk. : alk. paper)
1. Fertilization in vitro, Human—Social aspects. 2. Kinship—Philosophy.
3. Feminist anthropology. I. Title. II. Series: Experimental futures.
RG135.F74 2013
618.1′780599—dc23   2013018962

To Pat Spallone, who stayed

with the rouble, and has always

found the words.

CONTENTS

ACKNOWLEDGMENTS

Funding for the research conducted in the book was generously provided by the Economic and Social Research Council (Stem Cell Initiative) and the Wellcome Trust (Medical Humanities). Without the long-standing support and encouragement of Professor Peter Braude, none of the fieldwork for this project could have been undertaken in the new labs at Guy's Hospital in London. Dr. Dusko Ilic, the current head of the iPS cell core facility at Guy's, and Dr. Emma Stephenson, who is responsible for the design, setup, and running of the stem cell laboratory at Guy's, were both generous with their time and patient with their explanations of the work they do. Glenda Cornwell, Dr. Yacoub Khalef, Dr. Alison Lashwood, and Dr. Victoria Wood have been unfailingly helpful over many years as my research migrated from PGD to stem cells. In particular I would like to thank the artist Gina Glover for not only providing a thoughtful and inspiring account of her installation project, *The Art of A.R.T.*, in the Guy's Assisted Conception Unit, but also for allowing the images to be reproduced in this volume, courtesy of both www.ginaglover.com and www.artinhospitals. I am indebted to the many individuals who read parts of this manuscript, including Karin Lesnik-Oberstein, Nick Hopwood, Christina Brandt, Donna Haraway, Stevienna De Saille, Barbara Orland, and Zeynep Gurtin, and to all of the audiences who heard parts of it presented, in places too numerous to list. In addition to the three external reviewers who read the manuscript in its entirety, and gave detailed and helpful feedback, I am especially grateful to Sara Ahmed and Marilyn Strathern, who read the complete manuscript-in-progress and offered essential encouragement as well as constructive advice for revision at critical points in the development of *Biological Relatives*. Thanks to Emily Martin, Mary Poovey, and Troy Duster, who hosted me in the Institute for the History of the Production of Knowledge during my research leave in 2008–2009 at NYU. Throughout the writing of this manuscript I have had the benefit of working closely with Professor Martin Johnson and Dr. Nick Hopwood of Cambridge University on our project concerning the history of mammalian developmental biology in the U.K., in partnership with the Generation to Reproduction project at Cambridge. Having moved to Cambridge myself during the completion of *Biological Relatives*, I have been able to benefit from the unique concentration of "reproductive studies" there in more ways than would be possible to describe adequately here, and it is my hope that this book will strengthen the contribution from social science to this richly interdisciplinary endeavor. Like all major writing projects, this one had many ups and downs, and I am deeply indebted to my partner Sara Ahmed for her support, encouragement, and advice. As ever, the Duke team has been unfailingly professional, friendly, enthusiastic, and rigorous in their stewardship of the manuscript into print. Special thanks to Ken Wissoker, Jade Brooks, Liz Smith, and Amy Buchanan for always being responsive and never letting the reins slip. It is both a pleasure and privilege to be part of the Duke list, and this book could not have found a better home. Finally, I would like to thank my very dear friend Pat Spallone, who has been with me on the journey this book describes since the beginning.

INTRODUCTION Relatively Biological

Thirty-five years after its initial success as a form of technologically assisted human reproduction, and five million miracle babies later, in vitro fertilization (IVF) confronts us with a paradoxical legacy. Since its controversial clinical debut in 1978, IVF has rapidly become more routine and familiar, while at the same time also becoming, as Alice might have said, "curiouser and curiouser." Conception in vitro is now a normal fact of life, yet having passed through the looking glass of IVF, neither human reproduction nor reproductive biology look quite the same. Among other things, human conception can now be looked at—and not only through the microscope. The moment of conception can be viewed on the Internet; it is depicted in films and advertisements, and shown on the evening news. It can be downloaded in 3D from YouTube. This technologization of reproduction is both ordinary and curious. These images reflect the desire to know and understand that is conveyed in the normal meaning of "curious," but it is equally curious in the sense of surprising and unusual, that such images are ordinary at all. What does it mean that IVF has become a looking glass through which we see ourselves? What kind of view is on offer in the technological reproduction of human conception as a public spectacle? What species of technology is IVF? After all, it is not just a means of looking, or a spectacle—the point of IVF is to produce a new human being.

In reflecting upon the meaning of life after IVF, we must also consider the life of IVF—a technology that has had a complex evolution out of the study of natural history and the life sciences into clinical practice, and which is now intimately interrelated with the horizon industries of regenerative medicine and stem cell science. From an experimental research technique used in embryology, IVF has evolved into a global technological platform, used for a wide variety of applications, from genetic diagnosis and livestock breeding to cloning and stem cell research. One way to view the history of IVF is as a basic technique that has circulated through science, medicine, and agriculture as part of an increasingly complex tool kit for the control of mammalian reproduction. From this point of view, the history of IVF is that of a stem technology that has become ever more thickly imbricated in the remaking of the biological that so distinctly characterized the twentieth century—a model technique for remaking life.

As such, IVF is also a lens or window onto the history of the process Evelyn Fox Keller (2002) describes as "making sense of life"—a process that, like IVF, has also become "curiouser and curiouser" over time. As Jane Maienschein (2003) argues, IVF has changed scientific understandings of what life is—a question that never had a particularly clear answer to begin with. Some of the earliest attempts to induce fertilization in glass, such as those carried out in the late nineteenth century by Jacques Loeb in sea urchins, were precisely designed not only to control life, but to redefine it. Loeb's discovery that eggs could be experimentally activated without sperm, by chemically inducing development in vitro, was explicitly intended to confirm a new definition of life as mechanical, and thus reengineerable. As Maienschein points out, for Loeb, his manipulations were life, and thus "called into question what we mean by a life" (2003: 79). And as Evelyn Fox Keller similarly observes, this process has continued to dissolve its object precisely through the attempt to clarify its particularity, to define its principles, and to characterize its specificity. As Keller notes, the effort to define what life is began only two centuries ago with Jean-Baptiste Lamarck's call for a "true definition of life" that did not rely upon classifying things that are alive, but could determine what life is, or its "essence." As Keller notes, "By far the most interesting feature of the quest for the defining essence of life, and surely its greatest peculiarity, is that even while focussing attention on the boundary between living and nonliving, emphasizing both the clarity and importance of that divide, this quest for life's essence simultaneously works toward its dissolution" (2002: 292). As Keller argues further, the "peculiar" process of defining life in the twenty-first century has cycled right back around to its pre-Lamarckian, late eighteenth-century form in the context of projects such as synthetic biology, which are aimed to demonstrate that the border between life and nonlife is entirely porous—and that life can be built from scratch from inorganic compounds. In a sense, this has already occurred in the form of synthetic chemistry, also known as organic synthesis, through which organic compounds are manufactured out of inorganic components. The meaning of the word "synthesize" to describe "making" derives from chemistry, and has equally significant implications for the meaning of "organic" in biology today.

The "greatest peculiarity," as Keller (2002) describes it, in the history of defining life is precisely replicated by IVF, which has been one of the key research techniques involved in the characterization of life's defining properties in the past, and continues to shake them up in the present. Like Loeb in the nineteenth century, Shinya Yamanaka and his team in Kyoto discovered a means of chemically reactivating cellular potency using only four transcription factors to force differentiated mammalian cells back into their pre-differentiated state—a process that is akin to making a viable developing embryo without either sperm or egg. They succeeded in mice in 2006 and in human cells in 2007, and this cell type—induced pluripotent stem (iPS) cells—has itself now become a new technological platform for basic research into the precise mechanisms of cellular development (Takahashi and Yamanaka 2006). This "going forward by going backward" biology is typical of the twentieth-century discoveries that employed in vitro models and techniques to explore the process of biological development only to "dissolve," as Keller puts it, the very concepts being explored (such as cellular differentiation).

Another peculiarity of this process involves the use of tools to remake biology—also a boundary that has been repeatedly breached in the attempt to define what life is, especially now that biology is itself increasingly understood as a technology—and thus as something that can be made. That biology has become a technology is not a metaphoric description: to make iPS cells, viruses are used to transport the required genes, and the genes, or factors, themselves become tools in the process of forcing a cell to reorganize itself. Indeed, the use of biological bits and pieces as tools to reengineer other biological systems is so ubiquitous in biology it is completely normal to think of biology as a technology in this sense.[1] But here too we come to another "curiouser and curiouser" moment, as this also means that technology is becoming more "biologized." And what might be considered particularly peculiar about IVF is that it not only models this process, and reproduces it, but makes new human beings too—and perfectly normal ones, at that. In vitro fertilization is at once a technique, a model, an imitation of a biological process, a synthetic process, a scientific research method, an agricultural tool, and a means of human reproduction—of making life. It is an experimental model system with more than one life of its own. Consequently, one way to think about IVF is that it is less easy to understand than it may seem—or that it makes a very curious kind of sense.

This thought is the basis for this book, which does not so much track the history of IVF, or analyze its present, as attempt to make a different kind of sense of this technique both in and of itself and as part of a wider process through which the biological has become a more explicitly relative condition. I describe this as the emergence of biological relativity, which is explored in this book from the point of view of IVF, using this technique as a lens to consider what it means not only to understand biology as a technology, but technology as biological. I suggest that the dissolution of the biological and the technical has implications that go far beyond the questions raised by IVF itself, but that IVF offers a unique perspective from which some of these implications can be observed—a looking glass, of sorts (figure Intro.1). My aim in this book is to focus this looking glass not so much by following IVF around as by holding it still—using it as a dish model of itself, changing the filters, the depth of field, and the background light.

In vitro fertilization both recapitulates and personalizes a wider process through which biology is not only denaturalized but "cultured up." While continuing to function as an experimental tool, IVF technology is embedded in a naturalized and normalized logic of kinship, parenthood, and reproduction: it is pursued in the hope of alleviating childlessness. It has come to be viewed as normal and natural in the same way that most technologies that become highly popular and successful are quickly taken for granted (indeed, this is how revolutionary technologies are now defined).[2] But this too is a curious process—the way technology becomes, in Raymond Williams's terms, a cultural form—often associated with new social and institutional norms, and thus routinized. Williams urges us to read technological change neither as an inevitable process of historical invention nor as a response to human needs, but "in terms of its place in an existing social formation" (1990: 12)—taking into account both the intentions that produced it and its changing role as it evolves over time. In this way he challenges the "sterile" opposition between the view of technology as either determined by human intention, or determining it—as either a cause or an effect. Instead he urges us to understand both the causes and the effects of technologies as component parts of larger wholes, within which technology is not, in his words, "isolated" as a "self-acting force" (Williams 1990: 6) but belongs to a "complex" of a specific kind (25).

In this book, I try to read IVF in this way—as a complex or matrix of a particular kind. My concern is not only to read IVF as a technologization of biology, or as a biological technology, but as a case study that asks us to consider in more depth how this particular technology works, exactly. The first thesis of this book is that IVF constitutes a most unusual technology that works in a

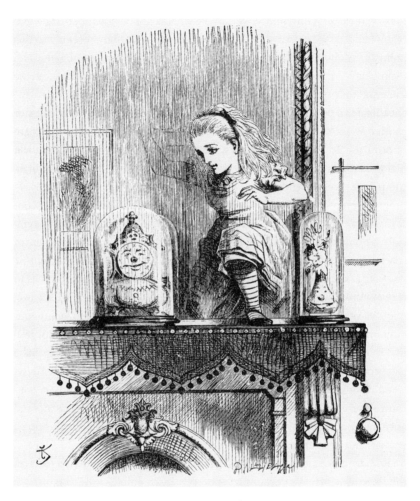

FIGURE INTRO.1. Sir John Tenniel's illustration of Alice's looking glass, or speculum: "Then she began looking about, and noticed that what could be seen from the old room was quite common and uninteresting, but that all the rest was as different as possible. For instance, the pictures on the wall next to the fire seemed to be alive." Lewis Carroll, *Through the Looking Glass* (1871).

most unusual way—so much so that its own workings reveal a looking-glass view on both biology and technology in general, as well as the evolving relationship between them. The second thesis of this book is that it is the very obviousness of how IVF works that makes it a useful case study, because by looking through it differently, we can see what is not obvious about its workings at all. And in this way, we can perhaps arrive at a different set of starting points to ask questions about the evolving relationship between biology and technology—and more specifically between reproductive technology and the future of kinship.

Williams's point returns us to the question of how IVF has become more routine, more naturalized and normalized, more regular and even quotidian or ordinary. To begin with, IVF is a technique that replicates a well-known biological process, namely fertilization, and confirms the ability to simulate this process technologically. It is thus doubly reproductive: it successfully reproduces reproduction, and its reproductive success biologically is what confirms, or proves, that it works technologically. Representations of IVF typically reproduce, and condense, familiar narratives—from the naturalness of reproduction and the universal desire for parenthood to the value of scientific progress and the benefits of medical assistance—and the success of IVF is in turn offered as proof, or evidence, of how these logics fit together. As Foucault might have observed, IVF is normal because it already belongs to techniques of normalization—including, among others, those of marriage, kinship, gender, scientific progress, experimental embryology, livestock breeding, baby showers, consumer culture, and medical technology, not to mention Hollywood cinema, *Sex and the City*, Brangelina, and Mumsnet.com. But as Foucault also might have noted, this is what is useful about IVF as the condensed epistemic point of the many intersecting strands that make its logic seem so obvious and normal.

Primary among the norms IVF reproduces is a dominant kinship pattern, the logic of which IVF recapitulates exactly in its emphasis on the biological fertilization of two gametes in glass. However, this marriage of cells now exists in two forms as a result of IVF—the one occurring in vivo, and the other in glass. In vitro fertilization thus allows a new method of conception to be slotted in, as it were, to an older pattern by "marrying up" a biological model of sexual reproduction with a biologically based system of descent and family formation. The normalization of IVF, as Charis Thompson points out, is a "hybrid culturing" (2005: 115) that allows new technology to coevolve with existing sexual, gender, and kinship norms, adding a degree of flexibility to the reproduction of reproduction, while largely keeping the structure of bilateral, biological kinship norms intact. Yet it is because this logic is recursive, in the sense of the "strange folding" of repetition, or the "turning back" of meanings onto themselves, that this reproduction is not exact, but rather, as I am calling it here, curious.

The manner in which IVF is embedded in, and is seemingly evidence for, the normalizing systems it both relies upon for its success and reproduces through its workings, is precisely where we encounter the curiouser side of IVF. Indeed, these two sides of IVF—how it is both normal and not—help to explain why the experience of undergoing it remains so paradoxical and ambivalent, despite the apparent obviousness of why IVF came into being to begin with. The more peculiar aspects of IVF very quickly become obvious to anyone commencing an IVF program, or entering what many women I interviewed for my first book on IVF described as the "intense" and "traumatic" world of IVF treatment (Franklin 1997: 11). Once inside this topsy-turvy world, a very different logic of IVF becomes visible, which is neither as normal nor as self-evident as that available from the other side of the door into the assisted conception clinic. Here, as for Alice, nothing is normal at all. In vitro fertilization is not a simple process of steps leading to potential success—it is a confusing and stressful world of disjointed temporalities, jangled emotions, difficult decisions, unfamiliar procedures, medical jargon, and metabolic chaos. You have to believe you will succeed even though you will probably fail, and the terms on which you reach either end point to treatment are constantly changing. As in the context of amniocentesis, another form of high-tech reproductive roulette, where negative results are positive, the experience of IVF is full of ironies. It is a complex and daunting medical procedure that requires a high level of compliance and commitment, as well as time and resources. Even people who succeed in the effort to achieve a take-home baby are often left disoriented and changed by their experience of undergoing IVF. Some will wish they never attempted it to begin with, and others will try again and again until they either succeed or give up (Throsby 2004). Few people go through IVF, in other words, without experiencing, either temporarily or permanently, and to a greater or lesser extent, a degree of ambivalence about this procedure—a view that is widely shared by IVF clinicians and nurses, who know better than anyone the potentially high costs of IVF. This ambivalence indexes the difference between the norms that IVF belongs to, and the extent to which it also challenges or contradicts these very same conventions.

The ambivalence that characterizes the IVF encounter, while specific in its form to IVF treatment, is also more generic, and I refer to it throughout this book as "technological ambivalence," arguing that it is a constitutive component of biological relativity. As many social theorists have noted, such as Ulrich Beck (1992), ambivalence is one of the defining characteristics of the modern relationship to technology—be it television or e-mail, robotics or biotechnology, electric kettles or plastic bags. In vitro fertilization offers a useful perspective on this ambivalence because it is generated out of a context that, like IVF itself, is becoming much more routine—namely that of managing our biological relations to technology in the context of remaking life. This is why IVF provides a useful lens on the wider condition I am describing as biological relativity—because IVF is not only typical, but arguably prototypical of this condition and its corresponding ambivalences. The topsy-turvy world of IVF, in all its both obvious and not-so-obvious complexity, and precisely in its normality, thus offers us a looking-glass into a looking-glass world, a model system of a model system, and a vivid picture of the retooling of reproductive substance. The very recursion that makes IVF confusing—that it both is and is not like what it imitates—is what makes it a useful hermeneutical apparatus for understanding "the age of biology."

However, I also argue that the ambivalence so profoundly associated with the technique of IVF, while derivative in part of its role as a modern, synthetic, high-tech procedure, also references older questions of sex, gender, and kinship—which IVF may help us to appreciate more explicitly. In other words, IVF not only offers a perspective on the ambivalence associated with modern technology, such as that described by Beck, but on older structures of sociality, including marriage and kinship. The fact that the normalization of IVF has not diminished the ambivalence felt by many who undergo it arguably tells us something about norms and norming themselves—namely that these too are reproductive technologies that engender deeply contradictory feelings. As Michael Peletz notes in his insightful discussion of ambivalence ("the simultaneous experience of powerful, contradictory emotions or attitudes toward a single phenomenon," as he defines it), anthropologists "have devoted scant attention not only to the myriad sources of ambivalence but also to their implications for an understanding of structure and agency as well as critically important processes of sociality, domination, and resistance" (2001: 414). This book takes up Peletz's challenge to examine "ambivalence as such" as a point of "frequently overlooked continuity between the old and new kinship studies" (2001: 414) in the context of being "after IVF."

This is also why this book attempts to integrate several different kinds of thinking about biology and technology into a conversation about IVF that may at times appear to stray rather far from its object. As noted above, to understand the workings of IVF not only as a technology, but as a complex or cultural form—including its past, its coming into being, the history of its recent present, and its evolution and dissemination, as well as its future—requires an account of how it works in and through other systems. This includes other technologies—such as technologies of kinship as well as clinical equipment, and technologies of sex as well as the medium of the Internet. Similarly, such a conversation has to ask what "technology" means, as well as what it means to have become "biologically relative." There is obviously a limit to how far such a project can go in a single volume, so in truth this book only outlines one way to approach these questions. However, insofar as it successfully describes and illustrates the recognizable outlines of a problematic, it will have succeeded at the very least in its aim of opening a door to a different kind of conversation, not only about IVF but about "the question concerning technology" and its new kinship with "the question concerning biology." These questions centrally concern the embodiment of technology, and the ambivalence that accompanies its normalization.

This is a conversation that has already been very substantially developed in some areas of social theory, for example in the anthropological debate about technologies of kinship, and in the feminist debate about technologies of gender, as well as in the responses to Foucault's account of sex as a technology. I also draw attention to the extent to which Marx's and Engels's models of technology were suffused with analogies to organicism and biology, and to their account of the relation between hand and tool. This book is an attempt to retheorize reproduction, as well as reproductive technology, and I have given prominence to feminist debates on both of these topics, as well as to feminist science studies, drawing in particular on the work of Donna Haraway (1976, 1997). Returning to the idiom of the frontier that I explored in my previous book on cloning, *Dolly Mixtures* (Franklin 2007b), I attempt to examine the role of "pioneering" in the context of experimental embryology, and to contrast this to the model of "moral pioneering" developed by Rayna Rapp (1999) in the context of contemporary reproductive biomedicine. I explore the ambivalence of the frontier—a place of oscillation, fluctuation, and instability— toward the close of the book in relation to the artwork of a photographer in residence in the assisted conception unit (ACU) where I have worked for the past ten years, as a way of returning to the question of embodying technology that I argue IVF poses in a distinctly equivocal manner.

As in my previous work, this book relies on close collaboration with scientists and clinicians working in the fields of IVF, stem cell research, and regenerative medicine, as well as patients undergoing various procedures, or active in patient support groups. Although this book is not traditionally ethnographic, it draws on fieldwork in clinics and labs, and the expertise of scientists who took the time to introduce me to their technical working methods. The analysis I offer of the visual cultures of IVF, human embryonic stem cell derivation methods, and micromanipulation of embryos has benefited from the enormous ease with which it is now possible to record fieldwork exchanges using a handheld video camera. In turn, this allows for a much richer analysis of biology in the making, some examples of which I have included in this book, particularly concerning the precise techniques of culturing and passaging human embryonic cell lines.[3]

As a result of its own somewhat eccentric "passaging techniques," this book is composed of a series of loosely interconnected chapters that attempt to make sense of the social, cultural, and technological legacies of IVF through a series of interpretive frames that both overlap and diverge. Throughout, I analyze IVF as a bridge to both new life and new kinds of life, and as a lens through which to depict changes in the meaning of biology, technology, and kinship. To do this I analyze reproductive substance as technology, but also technology as a reproductive substance, and more broadly the merging of the biological and the technical that are substantialized in, through, and as IVF. The mixing together of these perspectives in this book—a bit like the fusion of biology and technology it describes—is less a properly developed narrative analysis than a thought experiment in the form of a mosaic. The aim is to characterize the condition of being after IVF.

That mosaics are also embryonic tools ("fusion embryos"[4]) is apt because a major question this book asks is what it means that IVF has enabled a retooling of human reproductive substance. Ordinarily, technology might be imagined as something humans make in order to achieve desired ends: it is traditionally defined as the application of science. However, many of the most influential theorists of technology have argued that technological equipment and agency are a form of inheritance—indeed of inherited substance—as much as a means of altering the conditions of human existence in the present or the future. This is a similar, though inverted, form of the argument from kinship theory that institutions such as monarchies are technologies—indeed reproductive technologies—aimed at the controlled passaging of human substance over time and controlling the order of succession. The lineages of technology bequeathed from the past are far more numerous and formative than are the novel contemporary technologies most prominently associated with contemporary social change or impact—such as those associated with stem cell science, cloning, or reproductive biomedicine. If we consider the technologies of agriculture or domestication, for example, not to mention electricity or antibiotics (and this list could be rather long), we can see that they are already so much a part of who we are that we often do not even notice them, their pervasive structuring effects as invisible as grammar (language also being among the most important human technologies). Heidegger, for example, in *The Question Concerning Technology*, employed the Greek meaning of the word *techne* as a form of exposition or demonstration: "It is as revealing, and not as manufacturing, that *techne* is a bringing-forth" (1993: 319). Similarly, in "Building, Dwelling, Thinking," Heidegger argues that tools and technologies are the means by which the world becomes "enframed" for its inhabitants, shaping the "basic character" of Being or existence (1993: 350). This equipment, with and in which we live, is both inherited and formative, shaping both how we know and "do" the world. Jacques Derrida (1974), following the paleoethnologist André Leroi-Gourhan, more radically describes "man" or "anthropos" as rooted in an "originary technicity"—a position recently interpreted by Vicki Kirby (2011) as one that might also allow for a view of "life itself" as technics. Bruno Latour (1993) has described all identities as conjunctions, hybrids, and assemblages—as consubstantial "devices." Or, as Donna Haraway puts it more vividly, "chimeras of humans and nonhumans, machines and organisms, subjects and objects, are the obligatory passage points, the embodiments and articulations, through which travelers must pass to get much of anywhere in the world" (1997: 43). We do not need cellular technologies to evince for us that technology is cellular. How we have coevolved with technology is both an obvious and an unfolding question: as Williams (1990) so wisely noted, it is the very obviousness of this question that makes it so difficult to analyze.

As well as reframing technology, this book also seeks to reframe some of the arguments concerning "technological reproduction" from within the history of social theory. For example, with the benefit of hindsight, I argue it is possible to read Marx's accounts of machines and technology as more "morphogenetic" than perhaps even he intended. Marx repeatedly argued that the origins of modern technology are not to be found in the engineering genius of great inventors such as James Watt, whose name is now enshrined on every lightbulb for the eponymous energy source by which you may be reading this book. Although Marx's endorsement of the value of modern technology is often opposed to Heidegger's concern with its dehumanizing legacies, the chief argument of much of Marx's work is that technological innovation is the product of history, not its material progenitor. The equipment of the Industrial Revolution, he argues, comes into being as a result of political and economic conditions, not the other way around. He situates the evolution of machines such as the self-acting mule jenny in the context of the social apparatus that provided the conditions of their production, or brought them into existence, such as the division of labor and the fetishization of commodities. In both Marx's and Engels's writings, the actual equipment used in industries such as agriculture is not only an inherited condition of human existence, but a crucial force in molding the human species being.

As Marx wrote in Volume 1 of *Capital*, the human body itself is a product as much as a means of the labor process: "Labour is, in the first place, a process in which both man and Nature participate, and in which man of his own accord starts, regulates, and controls the material re-actions between himself and Nature. He opposes himself to Nature as one of her own forces, setting in motion arms and leg, head and hands, the natural forces of his body, in order to appropriate Nature's productions in a form adapted to his own wants. By thus acting on the external world and changing it, he at the same time changes his own nature" (MECW, Vol. 35, *Capital*, Vol. 1, Book 1, C 7, section 1). Marx understood the history of both technology and the division of labor not only in terms of how people used their bodies to do things, but in how they adapted themselves to the physical conditions of production and were transformed by them. He also emphasized the sociality of bodies—their crucial interconnections with other bodies, and not only human ones. Both animals and tools were understood as crucial components of a systematic mode of production that was, in the case of industrial production, highly organized, and even to a certain extent symbiotic (e.g., clover = nitrogen = fodder = cattle = proletariat = surplus value = commodity = finance, etc.). As this book suggests, Marx's model of the human-tool-machine relation was vividly biological. His picture of human thought and action is of a process of *substantialization* through which the human is molded not only by the inherited, "given" (or "standing," as Heidegger would have it) conditions of equipment of any historical moment but by being continually reconditioned by the evolution of this equipment, much as, for example, the laborer must continually adapt to new mechanical conditions of production. His depiction of the evolution of machine technology is deeply infused with the conceptual apparatus of organicism and biological development that became increasingly prominent during his lifetime.

The evolution of technological equipment is complemented by Marx and Engels's view of the human as technological. This too presupposed a merging of biology and tool, and is described in Bernard Stiegler's (1998) reading of Marx as a new theory of life as much as of technology. The evolution of the human hand into tools, and later into technological systems, such as factory production, is central to Marx's dialectical theory of machines and mechanization, often invoking Darwin's model of natural history (despite Marx's and Engels's critiques of Darwin as an apologist for industrial capitalism, they borrowed from his models of selection and adaptation to describe technology). Similarly, Marx and Engels depicted the natural and physical world as a tool kit made available for human use, and transformed by these uses into a "second nature" (Smith and O'Keefe 1980). To his tool kit, Marx added the legal, economic, and bureaucratic technologies through which the mode of production is organized and maintained. These too, he argued, provided the essential devices and mechanisms necessary for the machinery of industrial capitalism to develop, to grow, and to reproduce itself.

From this point of view, the traditional definition of a tool as a means, or device, that is given purpose by its user is not fully adequate—because, as both Marx and Engels argued, the significance of tools cannot be measured by their function alone. Tools, and the evolution of technology, must be understood as both inherited equipment and as the molding conditions of human existence, constantly reshaping what the human is by what it can do, in a dialectical process that extends beyond historical time into the mists of human species emergence. More than this, tools are never merely instrumental: as Heidegger insisted, they belong to the history of thought, and as Marx also argued, tools are the offspring of imagined worlds as much as actual ones. Tools are substantialized concepts.

As Donna Haraway (1997: 52) has argued, the context of contemporary biotechnological production is not only one that is defined by fusions of tools, concepts, and biological substances in the form of "living tools," but one in which biological relations are "corporealized" as both a conversion of nature into technique and an implosion of material and semiotic technologies as new kinships and kinds. The transgenic mouse model, she argues, is the product of a "recursive miming" that positions humans and nonhumans as biotechnological kin to one another—the materiality of their genomes "simultaneously semiotic, institutional, machinic, organic, and biochemical" (Haraway 1997: 99). The mouse model is an "instrument built to be engaged, inhabited, lived . . . and so building particular worlds rather than others" (135–136), and thus part of "the circulatory systems that constitute kinship—replete with all of its transhybridities" (134). To the extent that molecular biology is premised on the trope of rewriting biology, its genealogy simultaneously reconfigures the future of "biological" kinship as a set of relationships not only to, and through, but of, technology.

This brings us back to our central question, which is how to evaluate the significance of the fact that humans are now making tools out of reproductive substance, including our own. A question raised by the rapid evolution of IVF technology over the past half century, and in particular its new interface with stem cell research, is what it means to consider not only reproductive substance as a technology, but technology as a reproductive substance, as new biological relations and relativities are literally being made by hand, often using handmade tools. Arguably we are not particularly well prepared to address this question by either Marx or Heidegger, or many other theorists of technology, who have not provided many theoretical resources for analyzing either reproduction or reproductive substance. Indeed it could be said we need some new conceptual tools to describe the human conceptus as a tool.

Conventionally, reproduction has been understood in two distinct senses — as a process of social replacement (as in the reproduction of labor power), and as a biological process (as in sexual reproduction). Somewhat confusingly, reproduction is itself a term derived from manufacturing to refer to copying. This is the exact opposite of what it has meant in the context of biology, where sexual reproduction is precisely not the same thing as copying, or asexual reproduction, also known as cloning. This confusion is compounded by others, and also by a general neglect of the importance of what Marx called the "mode of reproduction" or the sexual division of labor. Indeed, throughout Marx's work the former is imagined to be largely explained by the latter. However, from the late twentieth century onward it has been increasingly evident that not only is sexual reproduction a process that can be dramatically reshaped by technology (which is what the phrase "artificial reproduction" means), but that it can be used as a technology (e.g., to produce new life forms, such as transgenic organisms). What IVF very publicly introduces is a form of technological transfer, or passaging, by which the technologization of biological substance becomes a mode of reproduction — including (and often uniting) not only sexual but also animal, human, digital, informatic, virtual, and mechanical reproduction. Put bluntly, the increasing control of biological reproduction "artificially" is one of the major technological advances of the twentieth century, and yet one that has only recently begun to be theorized (particularly in the work of Haraway). In vitro fertilization is the means by which this new form of technological control has been transferred into the human, thus confirming not only a new means of establishing a pregnancy but a new role for technology in making life.

One of the most helpful models for addressing the contemporary "engineering ideal" of biology (Pauly 1987), or the process of "culturing life" (Landecker 2007), is that described in Adele Clarke's (1998) account of "disciplining reproduction." As Clarke notes, "the reproductive sciences have themselves been marginalized, and their centrality to the overall project of controlling life has thereby been comparatively ignored," despite the fact, as she was among the first to point out, that it is "the reproductive sciences that have to date facilitated not only control over reproduction but control over heredity, and hence over life itself" (1998: 276).[5] The control of reproductive substance through technologies of selective breeding is, after all, as old as agriculture while also more central than ever today to the production, for example, of new cell factories. During the nineteenth century, modern agricultural methods of selective breeding began to be introduced by figures such as Robert Bakewell, who carefully "disciplined" the reproductive substance of his livestock in order to increase their economic value, using methods such as in-and-in breeding among close biological relatives to "fix" desirable traits—a process that relied, as Harriet Ritvo (1987) has shown, on new forms of standardizing animals, as well as new means of calculating their fitness, documenting their reproductive performance, and devising new financial instruments to market their "genetic capital." Lineages of breed records, as well as still-existing Bakewell breeds (such as the Dishley Leicester sheep) continue this instrumental legacy (and have themselves now become valuable commodities). Selective breeding, which substantializes a concept in the form of a technique applied to animal reproduction (i.e., in-and-in mate selection to concentrate desirable traits), relies on a fusion of biology and technique to achieve the "disciplining" of reproduction (Clarke 1998). The same basic principle applies today at the most advanced levels of cellular reengineering, where both conceptualities and conceptions are being reconceived, remixed, and rewritten.

A different technology was invented in the nineteenth century to describe the organization of human reproductive substance—and the disciplining of reproductive outcomes—namely, the concept of kinship. In the work of Darwin, as both Gillian Beer (1983) and Marilyn Strathern (1992a) have shown, the idiom of kinship performed a function of translation—importing the aristocratic technology of pedigree into natural history to ground a new theory of the biological relatedness of all organic life through shared descent—that is, through shared reproductive substance. It was by this very means, Foucault argues, that a new definition of life, as a natural system, acquired an organic and conceptual unity and gave rise to the modern scientific discipline of biology (Foucault 1973). Once it became lawlike and systemic, Foucault argues, biology also came to be understood as a new apparatus of social and political control, at both the individual and the species level—inaugurating what Foucault describes as biopower. This is the same "reproductive model" that gave birth to human IVF—just over a century after Darwin's reinvention of natural history (via kinship) as a system of interrelated, metamorphic, biological relations (evolution). Like Darwin's model of evolution, IVF models kin connections in a double sense: it introduces new kinds of biological relatives, as well as new models of biological relatedness.[6] This doubling effect of IVF is one of the main themes to which this book returns because it replicates a wider process I describe as "biological relativity," through which biology now exists as a more explicitly contingent, or relative, condition. One of the most striking features of IVF is how quickly and thoroughly the explicit technologization of reproductive substance it makes so graphically visible, and the radical new models of biological relativity it introduces, have been naturalized and commercialized.

One reason for the rapid adoption of IVF technology is, of course, that biological relativity is not so new. As Bruno Latour argues, the critical power of moderns is the ability to reverse their principles without acknowledging contradiction. How convenient it is, he notes, that "in spite of its transcendence, Nature remains mobilizable, humanizable, socializable" (Latour 1993: 37). The same is true of beliefs about biology, kinship, and shared reproductive substance—all of which are characterized by enormous flexibility in spite of often being tied to deterministic models. As Janet Carsten has argued, the term "substance" has an enormous and varied range of meanings, covering a full three pages in the *Oxford English Dictionary*. She reduces these to four broad categories: "vital part or essence; separate distinct thing; that which underlies phenomena; and corporeal matter" (Carsten 2001: 29). While on the one hand, Carsten surmises, the highly varied meanings of "substance" may be one of the reasons it is "good to think with," this breadth has also introduced analytic confusion. For example, a "blood tie" is imagined to be at once a physical and a symbolic connection. That blood is one of the only substances that does not perfuse through the placental membrane, and in that sense is never "shared," has not inhibited its widespread use as an idiom of consanguinity—or blood relatedness. But what are blood relations? Traditionally, and in a Euro-American context, these would be described as kinship relations that are defined not only in terms of what they "are" but what they "code for" in the form of conduct, obligations, and roles (Schneider 1968). As Carsten notes, however, such a definition both confuses and conflates two very different meanings of substance—as symbol and essence. This conflation is also evident in Mary Douglas's description of blood as a "natural symbol," used in "social systems in which the image of the body is used in different ways to reflect and enhance each person's experience of society" (1970: 10). A very different perspective on blood is introduced by Annemarie Mol (2002), who argues it is instrumentally conceptualized in ways that give this substance different meanings in terms of how it is "done" through various techniques—for example, in the context of disease. In her view, blood does not "code" as a unified corporeal matter but as a multiple one: it is neither an essential substance nor an essentialized sign, but rather comes into existence as "a separate distinct thing" entirely in relation to its specific sociotechnical milieu.

For the purposes of this book, substantialization is used much the same way as it has been in psychoanalysis, science studies, or anthropology, where similar concepts such as "sedimentation," "concretization," "somatization," or "materialization" have been employed to describe the relationships between embodiment, sociality, identity, material objects, and technology. It is the inextricability of these interwoven forces that the breadth of definitions of the word "substance" usefully both expresses and confirms. At the same time, this term is also useful for this book because it has a much more specific meaning in the context of reproduction, where the term "reproductive substance" would normally refer to gametes and embryos. Arguably, one of the most important contemporary changes in this "specific" definition of reproductive substance is that it has been vastly widened by the development of methods to cultivate the regenerative potential of almost any living cell. As the iPS cell discussed earlier confirms, regenerativity and reproductivity are increasingly blurred in the context of stem cell science (which is also what the Dolly experiment confirmed). This returns us to IVF, which today must be seen as an evolving technological platform, serving as a base for an expanding variety of human cell cultivation methods, which are in turn linked to the prospect of improved human cellular replacement and repair. Human embryonic stem cell research is a direct offspring of the evolution of the IVF platform: it was derived from the same research on early mammalian development that enabled IVF to be used in humans, and is dependent on human IVF for the supply of research embryos necessary to the refinement of its clinical applications.[7]

Both the change in the meaning of "reproductive substance" brought about through stem cell research (so that even a skin cell can become a gamete) and the future translation of new cellular potentials into applications increasingly rely on IVF in complex ways. Much of my research preceding this book was conducted in a new generation of U.K. laboratories that have been designed, built, and custom engineered to facilitate a more efficient interface between IVF and stem cell research. The axis of these labs, both architecturally and conceptually, is a hole in the wall, or hatch, connecting them to an adjacent ACU. The direct transfer of reproductive substance — gametes and embryos — can thus be more reliably, or "cleanly," facilitated from one context to another, that is, from an IVF unit to a stem cell lab (and back and forth; see Franklin 2010b). This book begins and ends in the leading U.K. lab dedicated to the facilitation of this novel transfer of reproductive substance, at Guy's Hospital in London, where the IVF–stem cell interface offers yet another window onto the question of what kinship futures are being engendered in the context of new reproductive technologies.

The new labs connecting IVF clinics to stem cell research substantialize what it means to be after IVF not only in their architecture but through the division of labor that occurs on both sides of the hole in the wall. On one side are patients attending ACUS for a variety of procedures, including IVF. These patients may be seeking a specific reproductive goal — namely, biological off-spring — but their presence in an ACU is conditioned by many other factors, and will have additional outcomes, including a potential change in what they understand by "biological reproduction." In the same way the textile industry cannot be explained by a desire for clothing, IVF is not simply a response to a desire to have children. In vitro fertilization is indexical of its modern heritage, a combined apparatus of family and gender norms, scientific research programs, legal instruments, bureaucratic procedures, technical skills, and ethical codes (and so on). Now an expanding global service sector, the IVF industry has in turn become a generative matrix for new technologies, procedures, products, and markets.[8] This matrix is also the source of new biological relations and relativities that exceed the frame of existing concepts and understandings, much as they also both rely upon and extend familiar models of biology, technology, and kinship.

These new relations and products are what are being developed through the hole in the wall (figure Intro.2), linking the stem cell lab to the ACU, through a complex series of embryo transfers (Franklin 2006a, 2006b, 2006c, 2008, 2010b; Franklin and Kaftantzi 2008). In the lab, behind air-lock doors, the complex and delicate effort to take reproductive substance "in hand" is being laboriously pursued by dedicated research teams who are attempting to translate stem cell science into new applications, such as tissue engineering, regenerative medicine, and diagnostics. Here, the sophisticated handiwork of top-notch embryologists is not only yielding new life lines of cleanly cultivated cells for a wide variety of uses, but new templates for semiautomated production of cellular products as this field scales up toward biomanufacturing. Similarly, at the UK Stem Cell Bank, which is the hub of a national network of stem cell researchers, the basic guidelines and standards for cultivation, storage, transport, handling, and banking of human embryonic stem cells are being refined, along with the code of practice governing their legal and ethical status (Franklin et al. 2008; Franklin and Kaufman 2009). These new standards comprise the most elaborate quality management protocols ever written for reproductive substance. They are the equivalent in the contemporary biological sciences of Greenwich Mean Time.

The hole in the wall thus offers a window onto a new mode of reproduction, or perhaps a two-way mirror (figure Intro.3). Through it, human reproductive substance is being "shared" in a way that enables an IVF embryo to become a tool that is embedded in a new set of codes for conduct. These codes of practice govern not only what happens to embryos, but the relationships that are established through them, thus establishing a novel system based on the exchange of reproductive substance. This new system of embryo transfer and human cell-based translation is an essential part of the equipment used to transform reproductive substance and to make it become differently productive — that is, to become pluripotent in order to be able to redirect cells to new commercial and therapeutic purposes. It is thus also here, in the interstices of codes and substance, that the meaning of "biological relations," and indeed of "biological relatives," is newly problematized, and it is this contemporary matrix that is the subject of this book.

Technologies of Sex

A crucial resource in the effort to understand the retooling of the human embryo is another twentieth-century invention, namely the analysis of sex as a technology. The phrase "technologies of sex" was introduced by Michel Foucault at more or less the same time human IVF was perfected in the 1970s.[9] Like Marx, however, Foucault used a relatively narrow model of reproduction in his highly influential work on both the history of the human sciences and the birth of biopower through the technologization of sex. His work provided crucial new understandings of what is meant by technology, primarily through his discussions of the relationship between knowledge and power as a technological one. As he pointed out, the discourses of sex with which he was concerned composed a "strangely muddled zone" with only a "fictitious" relation to reproductive physiology (Foucault 1990: 54–55).[10]

The significance of technologies of sex for understanding both reproduc-

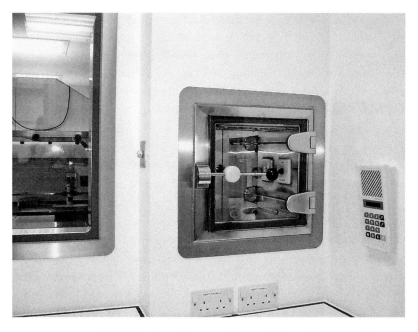

FIGURE INTRO.2. The hole in the wall between the IVF clinic and the stem cell laboratory enables the passage, or transfer, of eggs and embryos back and forth between two contexts of "remaking life." Photo by the author, published with permission of the Guy's stem cell team.

tion and reproductive technology was pursued more directly within feminist scholarship in the 1980s. Building both on Marxist approaches and on the work of earlier feminists, such as Simone de Beauvoir, Ruth Herschberger, and Shulamith Firestone, the phrase "technologies of sex" took on new meanings, in particular through the work of Teresa de Lauretis (1987) and Judith Butler (1990). New models of sex, gender, and reproduction began to emerge from within feminist anthropology, elaborating Gayle Rubin's (1975) concept of "the sex/gender system" or what Shulamith Firestone (1972) before her had called "the political economy of sex." The critique of the categories "woman" and "female" repositioned the global biologism of a naturalized, a priori presumption of an automatic sexual "base" to human social arrangements as itself an artifact of the system it allegedly explained.

Anthropologists such as Marilyn Strathern were among the first to begin to apply these insights specifically to IVF. Somewhat ironically, Strathern (1992a, 1992b) pointed out, IVF explicitly artificialized the very facts of life that were formerly imagined to ground the natural origins of gender and sex: these facts

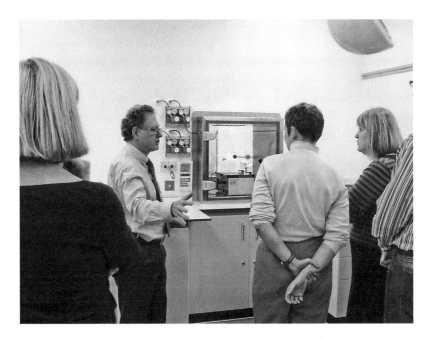

FIGURE INTRO.3. A view of the IVF interface where the director of the Assisted Conception Clinic, Professor Peter Braude, explains the way that eggs will travel from a "dirty" IVF surgery into a clean room. Photo by the author, published with permission of the Guy's stem cell team.

were rendered contingent, or relativized, by the very technology developed to "assist" them. By replicating "natural" conception, IVF itself became a new technology of sex—oddly and exactly paralleling the feminist argument that it is technologies of sex and gender that produce the effect of naturalized origins, rather than biology. For the same reason, the new assisted conception techniques "born" of the union of reproductive substance and technological innovation not only produced a new kind of biological relative but revealed a new condition of biological relativity, through which nature and artifice became interchangeable. Intended to enable a couple to reproduce biological offspring, IVF and its ilk paradoxically denaturalized biological reproduction by imitating it, or "taking it in hand." The fertilization these techniques substantialized in the form of new offspring was not only that between egg and sperm, but that between technology and biology. This fecund coupling has quickly been translated into the twenty-first-century ethos of biological engineering that now defines the fields of both genomics and synthetic biology. This is how IVF was transformed from "a bridge to new life" into a bridge to new kinds of life. In sum, the bridge became a platform, a stage, and a launch pad by means of a translational imaginary that was animated by the prospect of future kinships not only between parent and child, but between technology and offspring. The evolving relationship between IVF and the wider context of biotechnological innovation of which it is a crucial part thus today poses new questions about the meanings of both biology and technology, as well as their relationships to both old and new technologies of gender, reproduction, and sex—all of which have become somewhat more curious.

The rapid expansion of IVF not only as a form of infertility treatment but as a technological platform, and now a vector to the biotechnology industry, is thus investigated in this book by means of the pair of related questions described at the outset of this introduction. First, how might we think about reproductive substance as a technology, and technology as a reproductive substance? And second, how can these related questions be analyzed together? As noted above, the animating technology of this book is experimental. *Biological Relatives* is organized as a series of close readings of texts and examples to offer a recursive perspective on the question of being after IVF. It is less a series of chapters than a mosaic, or complex of frames. Reading across several disciplines, I focus on the intersecting mechanics that enable the emergence of biology as a technology in the context of IVF, and I read IVF as both a model and a manifestation of this process. It is thus the role of IVF as both a working model and a model system that is at the heart of the thought experiment this book offers—which by definition is highly speculative rather than conclusive.

A result of this method and focus is that each chapter makes most sense in relation to the larger whole that emerges from their collective accumulation. While this is always true of any book, it is particularly true of this one. Much is left to the reader to infer across the chapters, which together attempt a serial reframing of a matrix that is still only barely sketched across all of them. Other books have provided much more coherent histories of IVF, including Robin Marantz Henig's (2004) *Pandora's Baby*, or Robert Edwards and Patrick Steptoe's (1980) *A Matter of Life*. Similarly, there are much better historical accounts of reproductive biology, including Adele Clarke's (1998) *Disciplining Reproduction* and Jane Maienschein's (2003) *Whose View of Life?* Neither is a contemporary portrait of IVF provided in these chapters, such as that on offer in Debora Spar's (2006) *The Baby Business*, and my aim is not to debate the ethical implications of new reproductive and genetic technologies, as has been done by Jürgen Habermas (2003), Francis Fukuyama (2002), and many others. In the long list of things this book does not do should also be mentioned that it takes a highly selective approach even to the topics it does discuss in depth, such as the feminist debate over new reproductive technologies, the anthropology of new reproductive technologies, and the feminist literature on technologies of gender and sex. In sum, while drawing on a wide range of sources and many divergent avenues of scholarly debate, there are inevitably many obvious exclusions and oversights in the chapters that follow, and indeed within the book as a whole. It works best as an invitation to travel a particular journey in the effort to think through a particular problem, and to the extent that it achieves this aim in part by stimulating readers to identify significant resources or arguments that are inadequately presented here, I hope they will be motivated to contribute further to the general sociological problem *Biological Relatives* attempts to analyze.

This book also attempts to synthesize some of the ongoing themes in my own previous work, as I have sought to both document and theorize the emergence of new reproductive technologies including IVF (1997), embryo research (1999), preimplantation genetic diagnosis (Franklin and Roberts 2006), and cloning (2007b), as well as visual cultures of reproduction (1991, 1995, 2000). For example, it extends the analysis I developed with Celia Lury and Jackie Stacey (2000) in *Global Nature, Global Culture* of what we called "the traffic in nature," and it is a contribution to the "reconfiguration" of kinship (Franklin and McKinnon 2001) and the "remaking of life and death" (Franklin and Lock 2003b) in conference-based anthologies developed and coedited with Susan McKinnon and Margaret Lock. In places, I have returned to themes developed in these and other previous publications, such as the concept of "thick genealogies" introduced in *Dolly Mixtures* (2007) and the depiction of IVF as a "hope technology" in *Embodied Progress* (1997). Some of the ideas in this book first took shape in *Reproducing Reproduction* (Franklin and Ragoné 1999) and in *Technologies of Procreation* (Edwards et al. 1993), as well as *The Sociology of Gender* (1996). In the context of the contemporary attention to the development of IVF occasioning the award of the Nobel Prize in Physiology or Medicine to Robert Edwards in 2010, the question of how to understand its legacies has become more prominent, and *Biological Relatives* is also a contribution to that effort, organized in part as a reprise on my own long-standing interest in this technology since the mid-1980s, and more recently through collaborative work with Martin Johnson and Nick Hopwood on the British culture of mammalian developmental biology in the postwar period (Johnson et al. 2010).

To the extent that *Biological Relatives* revisits themes that were first introduced in these earlier, and ongoing, projects, some material will already be familiar to some readers, especially where certain problems have been reread and re-presented in order to develop the analysis further. The emphasis on close readings of key texts throughout this book is also a reproductive technology of sorts, manifesting the premise that reproduction is never an exact process, and that repetition is itself a generative mechanism. The pluricentric thought experiment that grounds this project is reflected in this book's format, which is more like a series of essays than a traditional (or even untraditional) ethnographic monograph. As noted in the afterword, a subtheme of the generative relations interconnecting practices of rereading and re-producing permeates much of the argument presented here, at the level of both substance and style.

Chapter 1, "Miracle Babies," examines IVF as a way of thinking and seeing reproduction, as well as of "taking reproductive substance in hand." It reviews, among other things, the emergence of the IVF–stem cell interface in the form of a new generation of purpose-built labs in the United Kingdom, and the public and parliamentary debate that has accompanied the introduction of a new generation of embryonic tools, most recently "human-admixed embryos," legalized in 2010. In addition, this chapter explores the condition of being after IVF and attempts to characterize how it has "become genealogical." The embeddedness of the logic of IVF in the pattern set by an earlier Industrial Revolution, also begun in the northwest of England, is combined with rereadings of both Marx and Foucault that build on those introduced above.

Chapter 2, "Living Tools," reframes the overall project of *Biological Relatives* by drawing on the work of Donna Haraway and Shulamith Firestone, as well as by visiting one of the new stem cell derivation labs that is annexed to an IVF clinic. Here we encounter stem cell science close up as it moves from being a still quasi-artisanal craft into a more mechanized and industrialized mode of reproduction. We also travel through the hole in the wall, following IVF eggs as they are "taken in hand" to become either potential offspring or living human tools. Drawing again on Marx's analysis of machines, this chapter both develops the theoretical models outlined in chapter 1 and introduces more empirical material to exemplify the general problems being examined in this book.

Chapter 3, "Embryo Pioneers," contains an episodic tour of some of the instructive scenes in the history of experimental embryology that I suggest are helpful in appreciating the long lineage of technique that is ancestral to human IVF — and to understanding the effort to "mechanize" reproductive substance, or "put it to work." In addition to extending the emphasis on technique that structures chapter 2, it provides some technical background to the birth of human IVF. The aim of this chapter is also to explore the combined use of embryo transfer, artificial fertilization, and tissue culture in the making of what has come to be known as the "reproductive frontier" and to further explore this term. As a result, chapter 3 introduces a consideration of the work of the frontier idiom in the context of biology as technology (a theme that is developed further in chapter 7). Drawing on many of the historians who have addressed this topic far more cogently than I have, including Hannah Landecker, Scott Gilbert, and Nick Hopwood, I try to situate the history of human IVF in relation to the technological experiments and imaginaries that preceded it, conceiving of this exercise as a potted tour of various instrumental orientations that become relevant in different ways in various other places throughout this book.

Chapter 4, "Reproductive Technologies," contrasts the history of "making sex" in the context of experimental embryology and developmental biology with the "exact mechanisms" of sex and gender technologies as they began to be theorized within feminist debates in the 1980s, and in particular within feminist anthropology. This chapter offers close readings of the work of both Gayle Rubin and Marilyn Strathern, while also rereading the emergence of a model of gender as a technology. The goal of rehearsing such well-trodden ground is a "mechanical" comparison between the technologies of kinship, gender, and sex, and those discussed in chapter 3 — an exercise that activates the mosaic, recursive, comparative structure of the book as a means to reflect on how IVF "works." Here, as elsewhere, the effort is not only to reread earlier work on kinship and gender in the light of being several decades after the birth of the first test-tube baby, but to emphasize how the logics of IVF both model and transform the structures of gender and kinship — thus potentially enabling us to think differently about their future manifestations.

Chapter 5, "Living IVF," also revisits a famous feminist history, namely the feminist debate over new reproductive technologies in the 1980s. Again, with the benefit of so many excellent and insightful accounts of this history available, this rereading brings a specific question into focus, namely the turn to understanding the experience of women undergoing IVF — arguably one of the earliest empirical investigations of human reproductive biology as technology, and of assisted conception as a means of "doing gender" as well as "making kinship." I argue that the early feminist analysis of women's experience of IVF deserves to be explored in greater depth — anticipating as it does many of the ways in which ambivalent relationships to biological technologies have been theorized since the 1980s. This chapter more explicitly engages with the ways in which the actual nuts and bolts of IVF parallel feminist accounts of gender and sex as "technologies" — and indeed as reproductive technologies. It revisits IVF not only as a technology of living substance, but as a biological technology that is lived as "a way of life," arguing that this pattern is now normative in ways that remain more curious than they may initially appear.

Importantly, this argument has already been made very elegantly by Charis Thompson (2005) in her pivotal study of IVF as a technology of gender, aptly titled *Making Parents*. Drawing on Thompson's work in chapter 6 ("IVF Live"), I explore the question of what IVF is reproducing in addition to, or at times in lieu of, biological offspring. This chapter poses another variation of the question of what IVF is "after." How has it become such a popular technological convention worldwide, and what kind of new norm is IVF? To explore these questions in a somewhat different way, I turn in the second half of chapter 6 to the role of IVF technology as a sign, an iconic technology that now not only remakes biological substance but makes visually explicit a new form of technological substance as biology. In order to understand not only the logic of IVF but its "call" and reach, a visual analysis is offered of the literal window IVF technology provides into the remaking of life, by enabling the translation of the retooling of reproductive substance into a circulating, public, interfaced, mainstream, and iconic image that is now widely and popularly legible as a primal (screen) scene of biological relativity.

This book closes in the ethnographic site where it began. Chapter 7, "Frontier Culture," returns to the hole in the wall, this time from within the ACU, opposite the lab, where the British artist Gina Glover has inhabited the "lens" of IVF as a photographer in residence. Looking through Glover's images enables the question of IVF as a "way of life" to be expanded into a broader question of how biotechnology is composed, domesticated, and familiarized. Here, the question of the future of biology is explored more explicitly as the future of kinship, and the future of kinship is explored from the point of view of how technology itself has become a form of shared reproductive substance. This question is once again reframed in this chapter through a consideration of technological progress as a frontier, and IVF as a site of both ambivalent and embodied progress. Looking back once again at the historical imaginaries that both preceded and engendered it, the question of being after IVF is explored both visually and experientially as a site of recrafted identity and women's work.

The overall themes of the book are briefly summarized in the afterword by rereading Derrida's understanding of the relationship between technics and life through the lens of IVF. Drawing also on the work of Hannah Arendt, the question concerning technology is here posed as one of dialogue: what are the kinds of conversations we might have about the future of technology as biology, or the future of biology as technology—or the future of kinship in relation to both of these questions? By reviewing the main arguments of *Biological Relatives* in this final section, I make the case for why the history of reproduction—and in particular the retooling of reproductive substance in the context of IVF—provides an important window onto the ambivalent process of remaking life. What resources would we need for the remaking of life to become more dialogic in the future? Might IVF be a context in which this model of "originary technics" could be productively explored?

By combining an account of the various kinds of mechanisms that are the necessary preconditions for a human embryo to become a tool, my overall aim is to offer an account of IVF that extends our ability to engage more thoughtfully with the questions posed by the future of bioscience, biomedicine, and biotechnology. As set out in this introduction, the aim is to provide a different set of starting points for addressing the relation between the technological and the biological as one that is lived as the remaking of life. In particular, the aim is to challenge the isolating models of technological impact that presume what Habermas (1971: 58) has critically described as the automatic model of technological progress. By attempting to use models from kinship and gender theory to explore what it means to be after IVF, *Biological Relatives* provides an account of IVF and stem cell research that resists approaching these phenomena as embedded in a social context, or even as molded or shaped by social forces. As is so readily evident in the common phrases "science and society" or the "social consequences of technology," an implicit separation between the domain of the social and the scientific or technological is difficult to avoid. Yet this separation is fundamentally misleading: science and technology are never outside the social, just as IVF did not invent itself, and stem cell lines did not exist before they were cultivated or forced into existence.

Of the many reasons why it has proven difficult to integrate social and scientific, or cultural and material, visual and biological, or textual and physiological perspectives on IVF, one of the most prominent is the difficulty of integrating the models of technology that correspond to contexts as diverse as embryology, anthropology, historiography, feminist theory, continental philosophy, or biopolitics. This problem is compounded by the question of what is meant by "technological." Hence, for example, we might describe an automobile or the Internet as a technology, but be less likely to use this word to describe a newspaper, a child's imaginative game, a song, or a dinner party. However, on second thought, we can see how all of these cultural forms are thoroughly technological—they depend on prior technicity, and we engage them through complex techniques that include not only know-how but understandings of who we are, what we can do, and how we want to live. Kinship, gaming, and cuisine, not to mention play, child rearing, and sharing meals are the outcome of an accumulation of highly skilled practices and technical systems, such as language, writing, and cooking, that have been developed and passed on for millennia. Indeed, these are some of the oldest human technologies, and are often imagined as the technologies that make us human.

It might be claimed from this point of view that everything is technological. And it is worth asking what our definition of humanity would be if it were denaturalized in this way. For one thing, such a thought experiment would require that we become both more and less precise in what we mean when we use the words "technology," "technique," and "tool"—in part by observing them close at hand, in specific contexts, and also over time, as they develop, change, fail, cease to exist, or expand. *Techne* is the Greek term for arts, whereas "technics" is often more narrowly used to describe methods or rules. "Technique" is used to describe skilled practices, whereas "technology" is often associated either with the application of science, or with systems of mechanical techniques, as in the context of industrialization. While we do not conventionally associate technology with gender identity or marriage, these too are, of course, highly organized activities that rely on prior art. Technology is derived from the Greek word *tekhnologia*—systematic knowledge of the arts, including both manual arts and skills and knowledge practices. From an anthropological point of view, all of human culture is composed of technics, techniques, and technologies—a marriage ceremony is no less technological than a windmill.

One reason, however, that it is not conventional to interpret marriage as a technology is that it is not seen as the application of science so much as an automatic reaction to the natural facts of reproductive biology, in essence merely socializing them as identity, ritual, and natural fact. In vitro fertilization is used as a case study in this book to explore not only what it means for an embryo to become a biological tool, or for our understanding of technology to become "more biological," but for these two perspectives to be combined in the form of a thought experiment through which our understandings of both biology and technology are both deepened and reconfigured. I argue that IVF reveals our biological relativity in the form of a technology employed to create biological relatives, thus changing how we understand the adjective "biological." Through IVF technology, reproduction becomes relatively biological—indeed, the contingency of biology achieved through the technique of

IVF is its raison d'être: "failed" biology can be made to work, or repaired, by being "taken in hand." The origin of IVF lies precisely in the effort to mechanize biological substance, while this impetus has also been described as the origin of kinship—commonly interpreted as the effort to organize, facilitate, and activate human reproductivity, and also commonly presumed to be one of the oldest and "elementary" human technologies. So in another sense, these two technologies—IVF and kinship—are already biologically related. They not only share the same form but serve the same purpose: they are kindred technologies in the making of kin and the kinding of life. The point of this book is to explore this connection—one that IVF makes highly explicit, but in such a densely compacted form as to appear at once miraculous and ordinary, recognizable and unfamiliar, routine and exceptional—a curious new norm of civilized existence. These paradoxes are among many that make IVF "good to think with" anthropologically. The project of this book is to do just that. If it is successful, neither biology nor technology will look quite the same again after we have reexamined them through the looking glass of IVF, and the curiouser and curiouser window its transfer "into man" has opened.

ONE Miracle Babies

When I began my PhD research on IVF in 1986, I could not have imagined that a quarter of a century later I would still be writing about this technology, nor that I would be witnessing a whole-scale redefinition of biology as technology for which IVF provides one of the most well-known case studies. Yet the transformation expressed in the title of bioeconomics consultant Rob Carlson's (2010) book *Biology Is Technology* could be described as a direct translation of the logic of IVF and its role as a foundational model for the biosociety. Since the mid-1980s when I was a graduate student researching IVF in Birmingham — the second-largest city in Britain — the IVF procedure has rapidly evolved from what was then still known as the "test-tube baby" method into a major global platform for the health sector and emergent bio-industries. Now defined as a reproductive biotechnology, IVF was a pioneering technique inaugurating what Edward Yoxen calls "the change in our relation to nature that biotechnology embodies" (1986: 9) despite the fact that he, like many other early commentators on the late twentieth-century explosion of the biosciences, was largely concerned with the field of molecular genetics.

The crucial importance of reproductive technologies to an understanding of biology as technology, now defined as much through cellular as genetic models, is due not only to the fact that IVF has expanded dramatically in both its scale and scope, becoming a platform, or stem technology, for myriad human and animal applications, from fertility treatment and livestock improvement to genetic screening and the production of cloned cell lines. In vitro fertilization is distinctive because this technology, and the model of reproduction it relies upon, have become ubiquitous and commonsensical. Unlike the Human Genome Project, IVF did not derive its celebrity from high-profile molecular genetic innovations such as polymerase chain reaction or gene-sequencing robotics, but from the narratives and hopes of couples seeking children—indeed from a technology that quickly became a new norm of family life. In addition to establishing a new method of sexual reproduction, and a powerful new window into the mechanisms of biological development, IVF has played a leading role in the establishment of new technologies of remaking life as a normal, familiar, and even naturalized part of human reproduction. Indeed, IVF is arguably the preeminent example of how a living human tool—a cultured ex vivo embryo—has substantialized an ordinary and intimate understanding of biology as technology. We could simply say that after IVF we had a new kind of biological kinship with technology.

Ironically, what has disguised the more radical implications of IVF's rapid routinization is precisely the fact that it establishes a biological relation: IVF is a technology that substantializes scientific progress in the form of biological parenthood. Carlson's (2010) book does not mention IVF, or even reproduction. And yet the transformation from which he derives his title is rooted in the technologization of reproductive substance, and in particular the effort to take the regenerative and productive powers of reproduction "in hand." As noted earlier, reproduction has been almost entirely absent from the study of economics, technology, and political philosophy, so in some ways it is not surprising that it is also absent from many discussions of biotechnology. Even within sociology and anthropology, reproduction has largely been treated as a self-evident domain of natural fact—or, as Annette Weiner (1978) described it, "mere biology." Feminist scholars have done the most to analyze the social organization of biological reproduction, in particular as it is shaped through the division of labor and political economy. These are what can also be described as technologies of gender and sex.

Today, IVF is a kind of matrix uniting these different technologies, and transforming them, while also doing so in a context that is highly publicly celebrated and acclaimed. One reason it is no longer possible to envisage reproduction as "mere biology" is because if matters were so simple IVF would not be necessary. In vitro fertilization exists because mere biology is not enough: in the context of IVF the phrase becomes nonsensical.[1] This is another way to describe the transformation in meanings and perceptions of the biological that IVF models as a "working up" of biological substance, and thus as both a tool-sign, and a "culture medium," manifest as a new technology of sex. In vitro fertilization is one of the most prominent and highly publicized examples of how biology has become increasingly technologized through two processes that are essentially interlinked. On the one hand, biological mechanisms have been broken down into cellular and biochemical components and replicated technologically in vitro—which is the process IVF performs, or stages. Indeed, clinical IVF confirms the viability of this synthetic trajectory "in man": it produces human offspring as its "proof" who embody its artifice. On the other hand, IVF also functions as a means of substantializing biology as technology—bringing into being a new human reproductive mechanism, which has since become established as a desirable and legitimate social norm. In vitro fertilization thus models what it means to claim that biology is technology not only by providing a working model, or model system, but through its rapid evolution into an established form of parenthood. The profoundly intimate artifice of IVF, now a standard medical procedure, confirms the viability of a new technological ground state, or norm, of human existence and renewal. After IVF, in the context of new reproductive technologies, reproduction has become a matter of technique, and mere biology has become an oxymoron.

This is not the argument being made by Robert Carlson (2010: 1) in *Biology Is Technology*, in which he claims that "biology is the oldest technology" and that even cells are essentially technological. Carlson's concern with the "explicit 'hands-on' molecular manipulation of genomes" and their implications for "the human condition" (4–5) makes no reference to human reproductive technologies at all. However, the importance of IVF as a template for the transformation Carlson describes has been noted by other, similarly minded biotechnology commentators such as the eco-futurist Stewart Brand. Indeed, for Brand (2010) it is assisted conception that most powerfully confirms the link between the old and new version of biology as technology precisely because IVF has grounded their union in family life. In vitro fertilization, Brand argues, has made the connection between new and old models of biology as technology more familiar, ordinary, and normal—indeed, "IVF is the big example" of this transformation, he claims. "I remember when [IVF] was an abomination in the face of God's will. As soon as people met a few of the children, they realised that they were just as good as the 'regular' ones" (quoted in Honigman 2010).

The implication of Brand's claim is that the reason IVF offspring are "just as good" as the so-called regular ones is because they are just like them. And of course, as anyone who has met an IVF child can easily testify, they are indeed just like the regular ones. But here again we reencounter the IVF paradox—since it is at once just like the real thing, and also not. In fact, IVF is not at all like regular conception—as anyone who has undergone it can confirm. This part of the condition of being after IVF—the way in which the expression "biology is technology" can be experienced as both familiar and strange—is also a ground state, or social norm, of being after IVF that remains to be fully characterized. In contrast to the analogies employed by Carlson (2010: 47) to equate basic cellular functionality with synthetic biology, and the "short DNA handles" used to redesign biological components with unassisted cellular signaling, the concept of "biological relativity" describes something else, namely what is not only similar, but also different, about biology that has been "handled." In vitro fertilization is the "big example" not only of how this transformation has become more "regular," but, equally important, how it has not. It is to the two sides of this process that "biological relativity" refers—a problematic for which I suggest IVF is indeed the big example, despite rarely being mentioned in the context of most debates about new biotechnologies, and for reasons that are somewhat different from those cited by Brand.[2]

These two sides of IVF are the source of its ambivalence, and thus of its complexity. Within the expression "biology is technology" lie both a metaphoric equation and an assertion that this equation is beyond metaphoric. This is a double message that IVF repeats in its promise of delivering children who are "just like" other offspring, but through a process of mimicry that is not quite the same as the original process on which it based. This ambivalence of mimicry lies at the heart of the paradox IVF presents, and is the source of the biological relativity this technique substantializes as both norm and novelty, and thus as both a confirmation of the norms it relies upon and a disruption to their authority and authenticity.[3]

When I was a PhD student in Birmingham researching IVF, I was not alone in failing to predict, or even to imagine, that within the space of a single human generation approximately five million miracle babies would be born worldwide from this technique, nor that IVF would be responsible for as much as 5 percent of the birthrate in some countries. I could not have known then that its own technological offspring would greatly amplify the historical importance of this technique's success "in man," while making its social or anthropological significance even harder to interpret. The transformations in understandings of heredity, development, and reproduction that have accompanied the rapid worldwide spread of IVF in the postwar period have become so taken for granted that it can be difficult even to point them out. This is why it is important to emphasize that this process of transformation is not only obvious, but also curious, and in ways that deserve much fuller exploration.

In order to examine how being after IVF has become both more regular and curiouser, this chapter considers the emergence of IVF in the double sense of "genealogical." It considers how we inherit the effects of routine IVF in direct, or proximate, historical time, while also analyzing how its logics have been regularized in the Foucauldian sense of tracking the sedimentation of new norms.[4] From these two points of view, the emergence of IVF can be analyzed as a continuous but dialectical history of biotechnical innovation that derives from deliberate human intentions, and responds to specific desires and hopes, while simultaneously transforming the terms through which new aspirations are imagined, and changing the meaning of the biological connections such interventions are aimed to make, alter, or improve. This is the process the concept of biological relativity is designed to characterize by charting both the ambivalent genealogies of IVF and the normative paradox they continue to reproduce.

Revisiting IVF

The award of the Nobel Prize in Physiology or Medicine to Robert Edwards in 2010 offered a very public occasion to revisit the recent present of IVF, and to reflect on its significance. According to the press release from the Nobel Assembly at the Karolinska Institute in Stockholm, the award recognized Edwards's contribution to the development of IVF for the treatment of infertility. As Dr. Ruth Edwards described the prize at the award ceremony that her husband was too unwell to attend: "The award was given for the successful development of techniques by which human oocytes were fertilized in vitro and then successfully returned to the mother's womb." And as Professor Martin Johnson, one of Edwards's first PhD students and his long-standing Cambridge colleague, noted in his Nobel lecture describing Edwards's achievements (Johnson 2010), the development of these techniques required an unusually interdisciplinary tool kit, reflecting both Edwards's wide-ranging scientific interests and his itinerant career path.[5]

As Johnson relates in his lecture, Robert Edwards was born into a working-class family in Batley, Yorkshire, to parents who worked in traditional northern industrial occupations—his father on the Settle-to-Carlisle railway and his mother in a manufacturing mill (Johnson 2010, 2011). During the period Edwards received his secondary education, the family resided in his mother's home town of Manchester—famously the birthplace of the Industrial Revolution in the eighteenth and nineteenth centuries, due to the rich crossbreeding between agriculture, engineering, mercantile innovation, and trade, served by a dense transportation infrastructure comprising roads, canals, shipping ports, and railways. These influences strongly shaped Edwards's own biography, spending summers as he did on Yorkshire farms in the Dales, near his father's engineering works, where he developed an early interest in the mechanics of animal reproduction. Following a period in the army during World War II, Edwards initially pursued agricultural studies at Bangor University in Wales, followed by a PhD from the Animal Genetics Institute in Edinburgh, where the director, Conrad Hal Waddington, had cultivated an exceptionally vibrant and creative research culture combining developmental biology with modern genetics.

It was from a background of basic research in mammalian reproductive systems (Edwards's model organism, like that of many of his British contemporaries, was the mouse), mixed with an unusual (for the early 1950s) amount of genetic science, that the basic problems of mammalian IVF were initially envisaged by Edwards midcentury. Human IVF was not his initial focus, although technical means of manipulating fertilized mammalian eggs in order to evaluate, and alter, their genetic capacities were the subject of Edwards's PhD dissertation. By his own account, the road to human IVF was "bumpy" (Edwards 2001)—and Edwards has written extensively, and often personally, on this history, including its ethical dimensions, in numerous publications throughout his career (Edwards 1989; and see Johnson 2011). From these accounts, and the work of many other scholars on the history of reproductive biomedicine, it is evident that the turn to human clinical IVF was neither straightforward in its aims nor simple in its origin. As with all successful scientific projects, the road to IVF was built using tools that had been developed over centuries, by generations of investigators, across a wide range of disciplines, and with disparate practical and theoretical goals in mind. Like other frontiers, the landscape in which human IVF was pioneered was shaped by broad historical forces, such as international concern about population growth, as well as distinctive local and regional circumstances, including the comparative freedom Patrick Steptoe enjoyed as a provincial consultant in a small northern hospital (Pfeffer 1993). Like other transformative technological innovations before it, the lengthy history of IVF tells us a great deal about what we can expect from its future.

The IVF Platform

Over the course of its development through invertebrates to amphibians, reptiles, fish, and eventually mammals, the IVF technique gradually evolved from an experimental scientific method into a variety of clinical and agricultural applications.[6] In the 1960s mouse IVF was used to create new models of early mammalian development for research purposes, including mosaics, chimeras, and hybrids. In the 1970s it took its now-famous human turn into clini-

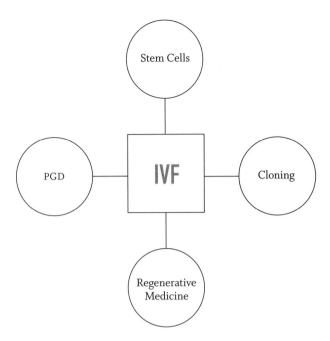

FIGURE 1.1. Schematic illustration of the expansion of the IVF platform as it becomes the base, or stem technology, for a range of other human applications including preimplantation genetic diagnosis (PGD), somatic cell nuclear transfer, human embryonic stem cell derivation, and regenerative medicine. In vitro fertilization has also been used in agricultural applications, and basic scientific research on mammalian development and reproductive biology. Author's diagram.

cal applications. In the 1980s it produced a new generation of miracle babies and the embryo transfer industry in livestock, while in the 1990s it provided the basic platform for transgenesis, cell reprogramming, and the cloning of Dolly the sheep. In the twenty-first century, IVF has provided the core techniques for the creation of savior siblings, admixed human chimeras, and new cellular tools, such as induced pluripotent stem cells. In sum, for more than a century IVF has been the crucible for new means of reconstructing reproduction, manipulating development, and retooling embryology (figure 1.1). Since its successful clinical translation in 1978, IVF has continued to undergo a rapid evolution as a technological platform, yielding newer mechanisms to facilitate human reproduction, such as aneuploidy screening, as well as new means of harnessing the regenerative properties of embryos, such as stem cell derivation.

The vast scale of human IVF now undertaken worldwide, combined with the ease of cryopreservation, storage, and transport of fertilized eggs, embryos, and blastocysts, has facilitated the mining of cellular plasticity, linking IVF to the futures of tissue engineering and regenerative medicine. Now a crucial vector for these emergent bioindustries, clinical IVF generates a supply of research embryos in the same way this technique was used in the 1950s to generate model "dish" systems to explore the basic mechanisms of mammalian conception, heredity, and development. Without IVF, human embryonic stem cell (hES) research would be impossible, and basic cellular processes, such as regulation and transcription, could not be studied ("in man") during the crucial early embryonic stages of development when they are most accessible experimentally (in vitro). These biotranslational fields are, like IVF, driven not only by research priorities but by economics. Retaining a lead at the bioknowledge horizons of new human cell-based applications is a major economic priority of governments around the world, as well as an expanding market for large and small corporate enterprises. This too is how the legacy of IVF is translated into new kinds of biological relations—such as our connections to the now-vast standing reserve of carefully banked and stewarded biomaterials and soon-to-be-marketed bioproducts on the much-vaunted horizon of biotherapies designed to repair everything from macular degeneration to global warming. Some of these products are "purely" human; others are from every species imaginable, but most of them are of mixed genealogical and technological ancestry, and they are all forms of what Latour and Woolgar (1979) have named "laboratory life."

Tools in the Age of Machines

The question of how these new living technologies have come into being is a central question of this book, as is the question of how they coevolve with each other, as well as with their makers and their milieux. An obvious comparison for addressing the "reproductive revolution" that began in Manchester in 1978, and one that was invoked by the film and theater director Danny Boyle in the opening ceremony to the 2012 Olympics in London, is the earlier Industrial Revolution that also began in the northwest of England two centuries before the birth of Louise Brown, where tools were also powerful signs as well as means. On trend, as ever, Boyle's highly praised didactic parable transformed machinery into legacy, and the eruption of industrial technology into a source of rebirth, symbolized by a giant baby surrounded by National Health Service workers. Crucial to his vision was the steam engine's enduring popularity as an iconic technology. On a morning off from writing this chapter, in the spring of 2011, I visited London's cavernous Science Museum on Exhibition Road to see a new exhibit featuring a reconstruction of James Watt's eighteenth-century engineering workshop. Watt (1736–1819) was the mechanical engineer who worked with Matthew Boulton in the Soho Foundry in Birmingham to make fundamental improvements to one of the most influential species of machine ever invented (Watt's high-pressure steam engine was patented in 1769). To follow the spreading paths of these engines on a map of Britain is to watch the Industrial Revolution unfold and to observe its circulatory system, connecting mines to mechanical workshops, manufacturing mills to waterways, and later animating the crucial railway and shipping systems. Watt, originally trained as an instrument maker, greatly increased the efficiency of steam engines by doubling their piston action, for which timely ingenuity he is widely hailed as one of the heroes of the Industrial Revolution.[7]

Among the 8,434 items assembled at the Science Museum for the Watt exhibit are the ten instruments he took when he left home at the age of eighteen for his first apprenticeship in London. These include a hand plane, two saws, a former, two files, and four chisels. As if in testament to the technological fecundity of this period in mechanical history, this original font of hand tools is now situated at the center of a sprawling network of kindred instruments, including everything from reconstructed industrial giants such as "Old Bess," the vast pumping engine that looms overhead, to the finely wrought coin-minting collar for stamping pennies, and the obscure collection of punches, counters, molds, dyes, condensers, and scale models, now displayed as hand-made testimonials to the dawn of the machine age.

Of course, it was not only tools that made tools, or indeed machines, money, or models in Watt's workshop. As the British industrial historian L. T. C. Rolt (1967) records in his account of the rapid mechanical progress that defined the "age of the machine," Watt and Boulton's workshop "attracted a galaxy of talent" including numerous energetic polymaths such as Erasmus Darwin, Joseph Banks, William Hershel, Joseph Priestley, Josiah Wedgewood, and Samuel Galton. Meeting on full-moon nights, in order to make their travel more efficient, these members of the Lunar Circle (or as they called themselves, the Lunarticks) belonged to an informal learned society based in Birmingham, often meeting at each other's houses to exchange ideas. "In this way," claims Rolt, "minds trained in the study, the laboratory, the business office, and the engineer's workshop met and pooled their knowledge to their mutual profit" (1967: 10). Out of this "rich ferment," he claims, "the modern world was born," adding that it was no coincidence that this society was mechanical in origin, given that "the most ingenious invention must be stillborn unless the tools and the techniques are available to make it" (10).

This was, after all, the era in which mechanical progress appeared to mark a watershed in the history of technology, during which tools and machines appeared to acquire a life of their own.[8] It was also an age of mixed emotions toward new tools, new tool-making techniques, new machines, and the corresponding transformation of human society — epitomized by the rapid growth of cities such as Birmingham and Manchester. By 1861, forty years after Watt's death, William Fairburn, speaking at a meeting of the British Association in Manchester, could describe the evolution from hand tool to "self-acting machine tool" as complete:

> When I first entered this city the whole of the machinery was executed by hand. There were neither planing, slotting nor shaping machines; and, with the exception of very imperfect lathes and a few drills, the preparatory operations of construction were effected entirely by the hands of the workmen. Now, everything is done by machine tools with a degree of accuracy which the unaided hand could never accomplish. The automaton or self-acting machine tool has within itself an almost creative power; in fact, so great are its powers of adaptation that there is no operation of the human hand that it does not imitate. (in Rolt 1967: 13)

The depiction in this passage of the "creative power" of the "self-acting machine tool" is echoed in more explicitly evolutionary language by Karl Marx in the *Economic Manuscripts of 1861*, written in the same year as Fairburn's speech, and indeed in the same city. Tellingly, as *The Origin of Species* had been published only shortly before, in 1859, Marx cites Darwin at the outset of his analysis of the mechanical workshop, introducing natural selection as an analogy for the evolution of tools and machines:

> By a low level of organization I mean a *low degree of differentiation of the organs* for different particular operations; for *as long as one and the same organ has to perform diversified* work the reason for its variability may probably be seen in the fact that natural selection preserves or suppresses every little deviation of form less carefully than *when the organ has to serve for one special purpose alone*. In the same way that knives intended to cut all kinds of things may be of more or less the same shape,

whilst a tool intended solely for some particular use must have a different shape for every particular use. (Darwin [*On the Origin of Species by
Means of Natural Selection, or the Preservation of Favoured Races in the
Struggle for Life*, London, 1859, 149], cited in MECW, Vol. 33: 387, original emphasis)[9]

Marx is evoking several analogies here to explain what he, like Fairburn, describes as the "interposition" between machine and hand that defines indus-
trialism, and the vast network of "self-acting" machines and tools that took
on the Spencerian qualities of a social organism. In his writings on technologies, the evolution of the hand tool to become part of the machine (one of
its organs, as it were) is crucial to Marx's model not only of machines and
manufacturing, but of the division of labor in society. The two crucial processes for which Marx relies on Darwin's model of natural selection in this
section are specialization and differentiation, thus implying that part of the
"creative power" of machines is their capacity to evolve. Although like Rolt,
Marx was concerned with how machines evolve, it was not his argument that
machines made history, nor even that men like Watt invented better steam
engines, but that history molded the machinery and the mechanic together
with their milieu.

Marx's emphasis on specialization and differentiation in the "organs" of
machinery corresponds to his description of the Industrial Revolution as occurring in two primary phases. The pivot of this analysis is the relation between machine and human "organs," and in the first instance between machine and hand. Thus in the first stage, there is a "conversion of movement":
the hand's power, and even its grip, is assumed by the machine, much the way
a handheld tool can be given a longer handle to gain greater leverage. "The
industrial revolution *first affects* the part of the machine which does the work.
The motive force here is at first still man himself. But operations such as
previously needed the virtuoso to play upon the instrument, *are now brought
about by the conversion* of the movement directly effected by the simplest mechanical impulse (turning the crank, treading the wheel) of human origin into
the refined movements of a working machine" (MECW, Vol. 33: 390, emphasis added). For Marx, the introduction of the "working machine" itself does
not necessarily comprise a revolutionary change—because its principles are
evident in the very oldest technologies, such as weaving or hand milling. Indeed, in his view, it is the simple harnessing of movement to tools that comprises "the first great industrial revolution": "From the moment when direct
human participation in production was reduced to the provision of simple

power, the principle of work by machinery was given. The mechanism was there; the motive force itself could later be replaced by water, steam, etc." (MECW, Vol. 33: 390).

This first (mechanical) revolution, which belongs to antiquity as much as the present, is greatly superseded in importance, Marx claims, by the second (motive power)—a truly revolutionary transformation that can be summed up in the simple word "steam."[10] After this first great industrial revolution, whereby the hands doing the work were replaced by the (mechanical) action of the tool (which replicates the work of hands), but humans (or animals) still supplied the "simple power," the employment of the steam engine as a machine for producing movement was the second revolution—producing a power source that was no longer anthropomorphic in any way. Characteristically, as in his work on both agriculture and finance, scale is the crucial factor for Marx. The second great revolution, in his view, was one not of kind but of degree. It was the steam engine that could enable not one knife but a thousand knives to function in a specialized manner simultaneously, thus amplifying one worker into a thousand hands. The machine that made superior products, more efficiently, at lower cost, and in less time was almost inevitably (and still today often indirectly) driven by steam.

Thus, although Marx would agree with Rolt, and with all of those who describe Watt as the hero of the Industrial Revolution (figure 1.2), by pointing to steam power as the preeminent industrial force ushering in the modern technological era, he adds a crucial element to the heroic histories that posit either mechanical engineering or mechanical genius as the driving force of social change. For Marx, it is very much the other way around, for it is the social technology of the division of labor associated with capitalist production that is necessary for the machine age to be born, and with it a new form of social evolution driven by the historical dialectic of humans and "self-acting" machines.

Marx argues his points most explicitly concerning human-tool-machine relations in his notes on the evolution of the mechanics workshop, which later become part of chapter 15 of Volume 1 of *Capital*. Using the direct analogy to Darwin's theory of natural selection cited above, Marx argues that in earlier periods of human history the differentiation and specialization of tools and techniques arose "spontaneously" through direct experience of using them, and "without any need for a prior insight into the laws of mechanics" (just as Darwin argues organs "naturally" evolve in response to specific adaptations), so that the evolution of tools was essentially unified with the division of labor. As ever, his preferred example is of mills and milling, which are gradually im-

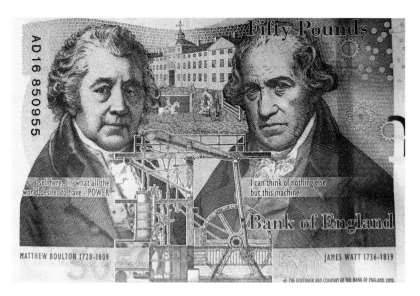

FIGURE 1.2. Matthew Boulton and James Watt are paired on the back of the British fifty-pound note, where Watt is accompanied by the caption "I can think of nothing else but this machine."

proved across millennia, and comprise a classic example of specialized labor "combined" with specialized tools and "spontaneously" adapted to a specific milieu. The turning point in this process—its axis—is not mechanical, according to Marx, but historical, in the form of the great economic transformation to the capitalist mode of production and accumulation. It was, he argues, again a change of scale that supplies the driving transformational force: "[It was] only after the manufacture of commodities by machinery had attained a certain extent [that] the need to produce the machinery itself by machines [made] itself felt" (MECW, Vol. 33: 390).

From this point of view, it is not so much the interposition of the hand and tool that is crucial for Marx but a new scale of motive power driving an increasingly specialized and differentiated machine apparatus that enables a new form of production—industrial capitalism. This occurs, according to Marx, by the replacement of the hand, tool, and worker by machines—linked to a more efficient (better adapted) system of production on a new scale powered by engines (such as Watt's). These new engines are grouped together in such a way as to produce enormous and continuous power—a power that is superhuman—which is in turn mechanically organized to enable continuous and superior factory production of commodities. Coincident with colonization and the opening up of world markets, it is the result-ing commodity economy and its new division of labor — not only between workers and owners, but between machines and tools — that marks a defini-tive historical change. Marx describes this as the birth of the "automatic work-shop," which becomes the centerpiece of production, driven by a "great prime mover" such as a "reunion" of Watt's double-action engines. "Here we have the correct view" of the machine-tool relation, argues Marx: "The tools with which the human being worked reappear in the machinery, but now they are the tools with which the machine works. Its mechanism brings about the movement of the tools (previously performed by the human being) required to treat the material in the manner desired or to accomplish the purpose desired. It is no longer the human being but a mechanism made by human beings, which handles the tools. And the human being supervises the action, corrects accidental errors, etc." (MECW, Vol. 33: 431).[11] As later commentators have noted, such as the philosopher of technology Bernard Stiegler (1998), although Marx is critical of the technological determinism that equates steam power with historical progress, he nonetheless provides a compelling and em-pirically persuasive account of the evolution of technology driven by steam. Precisely in order to chart the social consequences of technological change (while always seeking to argue these were the result not of manifest destiny but of commodity fetishism), Marx sought to locate, identify, and character-ize the exact mechanisms by which machines coevolved with each other his-torically. How these machines evolved "hand in hand" with the divisions of labor, and how their specialization and differentiation in turn reshaped the laboring and owning classes alike, were the focus of Marx's effort to produce a new theory of technology.

The Age of Biology

Marx's observations take on many new dimensions in "the age of biology," in which a defining feature of human tool use is the increasing prominence of biological entities, such as embryos, which are, as we shall see throughout this book, hand tools that are already in the process of amplification and con-version into cell-based production systems (mechanics) capable of harness-ing new forms of biological potential ("motive power"). Made by hand in the craftsman-like interiors of specialist workshops, and supported by congeries of national legislation, public and private investment, and financial specu-lation similar to those that were required to encourage an expanding com-modity economy in the nineteenth century, the carefully derived and passaged human stem cell colony is today, like IVF, a bridge to a new life, a hope technology, a symbol, and a new kind of mechanism or device of bioindustrialization. These cell constructs not only model biological processes, enabling them to be taken in hand, harnessed, explored, or rebuilt, but manifest what Charis Thompson (2005) has described as the promissory future of biocapitalism. Thompson argues that this future will be organized around reproduction as "the predominant focus of value":

> Social theorists typically focus on production, whether in the service of the state or the market or both, to understand the social order and the motors of history. Even social anthropologists, who have made kinship central to their understandings of societies' economies, have theorized kinship as a system of production and exchange rather than of reproduction. Critics have pointed out that production also involves reproduction. For example, the Marxist tradition . . . has been excoriated by feminists for ignoring the labor of reproduction and the reproduction of labor. . . . In economies and social worlds that are organized around certain biomedical conditions, including ARTS, I suggest that reproduction is becoming the predominant focus of value, exchange, emancipation, and oppression. (2005: 252)

Like previous machine-tool-human relations, the cell construct in the embryology lab is brought into being through complex divisions of labor, which are variously professional, international, sexual, and now also reproductive. Indeed, to the extent that IVF makes visible a new reproductive division of labor, it is an overdue complement to Marxist approaches, in which both reproductive labor and reproductive substance are famously undertheorized. The meaning of "the labor of reproduction and the reproduction of labor" have today taken on new dimensions, as have the implications of Marx's emphasis on scale and mechanization.

Thompson's model of "the biotech mode of (re)production" responds to a growing sense of the need to acknowledge the changing meanings of capital, production, labor, value, and distribution in the context of biotechnology shared by many scholars—but her account is particularly relevant to the annexation of the assisted conception workshop to the larger scene of biotechnical innovation in the life sciences.[12] The importance of a specifically reproductive model to the project of theorizing biocapital is a theme Margaret Lock and I explored in our coedited volume *Remaking Life and Death*, in which we suggested that the mode of generating reproduction not only as labor, but as value, "is driven by a form of extraction that involves isolating and mobilizing the primary reproductive agency of specific body parts, particularly cells, in a manner not dissimilar to that by which, as Marx described it, soil plays the 'principal' role in agriculture" (Franklin and Lock 2003b: 8).

As Lock and I emphasized in our description of what an anthropological approach to such shifts in the meaning of reproduction might involve, "it is inadequate to speak about changes or transformations simply in terms of their following 'after' developments in biotechnology and the biosciences" or to "bookmark a space for dealing with the consequences of this technology [as if] society and sociality [are] after the fact of technological innovation" (Franklin and Lock 2003b: 4). In order, then, to ensure we do not fall into the habit of representing "technological innovation as the root of scientific progress" but instead "emphasize ways in which technology is socially informed and demonstrate how specifically desired ends are built into the knowledge and techniques associated with biomedicine, the biosciences, and biotechnology" (4–5), it is necessary to turn, as Marx did, to the social forces shaping the composition of technological assemblages, and the structural forms determining not only the division of labor but the principles and values that are often (mistakenly) imagined to inhere "automatically" in such forms.[13] We thus need to turn to a different division of labor, which rests precisely on such an unexamined principle of value, namely that of sex. As we shall see, the effort to extract reproductive value from sex in the context of biotechnology has an exact precursor in the presumption of sex as principled, or divided, along the lines of its corresponding reproductive outcome — a formulation that relies in the first instance upon the presumption of an automatic sexual mechanism (that is reproductive), to which the social order is a response. In the following section, then, it is useful to introduce a counterpoint to this perspective in the form of the proposal that sex itself is not so much automatic as organized. I pick up this theme in much more depth in chapter 4, but begin by turning briefly to it here.

Technologies of Sex

The loss of sexual decency and propriety (and thus polarity) among the working poor, and the converse accentuation of femininity (the "cult of true womanhood") to disguise the labor of social reproduction among the bourgeois elite described by Marx in his account of nineteenth-century industrial society give a backhanded acknowledgment of industrial capitalism's dependence on what are now called technologies of gender or technologies of sex. But neither Marx nor Engels investigated this machinery in anything like the detail provided for other instruments of capitalism, including the division of labor by class. Both Marx's passing references to gender roles as a mark of class distinctions in *Capital* and Engels's more elaborate reconstruction of "the world historic defeat of the female sex" as a result of the discovery of physical paternity ([1884] 2010) root the origins of the sexual division of labor in a naturalized reproductive — or biologically automatic — one. Reproduction, in sum, is the prior naturalized basis from which the principle of sexual division in society is presumed to have arisen "automatically."

Yet throughout their discussions of both agriculture and livestock production both Marx and Engels imply a more complex relation between the sexual division of labor and sexual reproduction: that is, they imply that sex was "worked" or even "made," and to a certain degree, then, that fertility is a product or even a sign. Darwin (1874) also theorized this sexual work of reproduction explicitly in his lengthy discussion of sexual selection in *The Descent of Man*, in which he argues that courtship work is as important as adaptation to the mechanics of natural selection.[14] However, the machinery of gender and sex necessary to the production of either fertility or successful reproduction awaited more explicit theorization in the work of later, largely feminist, authors (as we shall see in subsequent chapters). As noted in the introduction, the advent of not only assisted conception but the larger effort to mechanize reproductive substance associated with biotechnology is an effort that more explicitly reveals the relationship of both sex to reproduction, and reproduction to sex, as contingent and partial — indeed as variable and plastic, and thus significantly capable of being reworked, reengineered, and indeed remade.

It is, for example, precisely the "reengineerable" dimensions of the sexual division of labor, fertility, and reproduction in the nineteenth century that are the objects of Foucault's account of the history of sexuality, which is among the first efforts to divorce sexuality from biological reproduction — and to explicitly theorize sex as a technology. Whereas for Marx and Engels, following Morgan, the evolution of modern society could be tracked through distinctive stages identified with progressively evolving structures of kinship and marriage, this model is rejected by Foucault, who postulates for "the modern forms of society" a set of sexual arrangements that is *not governed by reproduction*," but is manifest instead as "an intensification of the body — with its exploitation as an object of knowledge and an element in relations of power" (1990: 107, emphasis added). This new apparatus for the production of sex did not replace the older system based on kinship and alliance, argues Foucault, but, rather like the changed relationship of machine and tool described by Marx, it adds a crucially transformative layer to them. Foucault describes this interposition as a new apparatus or machinery—namely a specific "technology of sex."

Foucault argues that in the nineteenth century a new technology of sex— what he calls sexuality—does not so much displace the "relations of sex" established through marriage and kinship rules as alter its mechanisms by adding new ones. Specifically, he claims that the "new apparatus which was superimposed" on the deployment of alliance "connects up with the circuit of sexual partners . . . in a completely different way" (1990: 106) along a different set of principles. I examine in more detail in subsequent chapters what both the "deployment of alliance" and the "circuit of sexual partners" refer to—especially insofar as they have been theorized (for example, by Lévi-Strauss) explicitly as mechanisms. Indeed, as we see in chapter 4, these "exact mechanisms" are precisely what Gayle Rubin (1975) and a generation of feminist anthropologists have analyzed in the effort to disentangle reproduction from sex, gender, sexuality, and kinship—as well as all of these from biology.

The important question from Foucault, however, is how technologies of sex are linked to what he describes as "the birth of biopower." For it is here that the substantial disconnect, or interposition, Foucault proposes between structures of sex and of sexuality acquires importance in relation to what he elsewhere describes as "technologies of self"—or more simply, identities. For Foucault, the important feature of kinship systems is their stability, predictability, and constraint. These technologies of sex (which could also be called reproductive technologies) are "built around a system of rules defining the permitted and the forbidden, the licit and the illicit" (or what Lévi-Strauss defines as the "law" of exogamy that provides the "elementary structure" of kinship). Foucault's technologies of sex comprise "a system of marriage and fixation" combined with "mechanisms of constraint"—the "chief objective" of which is "to reproduce the interplay of relations and maintain the law that governs them. . . . In a word, the deployment of alliance is attuned to a homeostasis of the social body, which it has the function of maintaining; whence its privileged link to the law; whence too the fact that the important phase for it is 'reproduction'" (1990: 107). Here, Foucault uses the word "reproduction" to mean what is often understood instead as replication—the maintenance of the same, also the sense of "reproduction" often used in accounts of social reproduction, such as those of Marx and Engels. This traffic—the switching back and forth between reproducing something that is the same, or identical, and reproducing something different—is a constant feature of the discussion of reproductive technologies in this book. Indeed, the traffic between mimesis and alteration is epitomized by IVF—at once intended to be just like the real thing and not.[15] In the context of both Foucault's biopolitics and Marx's and Engels's accounts of social reproduction, the ambivalence of reproduction—its ability to both imitate and transform—is part of its strategic value, or even "magical" power, while at the same time this duality can act as camouflage, mixing together what is novel with established norms.[16]

In contrast to the reproductive function of alliance described by Foucault, namely the maintenance of rules that ensure the predictable transmission of status and goods over time through a fixed apparatus of kinship, the modern family, he argues, is based on the reverse principle. It is based not on mechanisms of orderly transmission but on the "mobile, polymorphous and contingent techniques of power" that engender "a continual extension of areas and forms of control" and are manifest "through numerous and subtle relays"—the main vector of which "is the body" (1990: 106–107). The new family is based not on a marriage of order and succession symbolized by the law of exogamy, but on a more plastic and unstable system, driven by an amplification of sex—a "sexing-up" of the nuclear family unit, which "since the eighteenth century . . . has become an obligatory locus of affects, feelings, love" comprising "an economy of pleasure" (108).[17] This is how, according to Foucault, the "traditional technology of the flesh" in the form of Christian pastoral guidance, and the impetus to express penitence through confession, evolves into the "new technology of sex" that is both produced and disciplined by medicine, pedagogy, psychiatry, demography, and the state. This is how "sex became a matter that required the social body as a whole, and virtually all of its individuals, to place themselves under surveillance" (116). It is how the "Anglican pastoral" was replaced by nineteenth-century medicine in the form of "the campaigns apropos of the birthrate [that] took the place of the control of conjugal relations," and similarly how "the question of death and everlasting punishment" became "the problem of life and illness" (117). In the same way that Marx describes the birth of factories by referencing Darwin's comparison of tools to organs, Foucault describes the birth of a new apparatus of sex in this same era as "flesh . . . brought down to the level of the organism"—now a biological force to be managed, and one, as we shall see, that is soon brought down even further.

Sex after IVF

As the history and contemporary evolution of IVF reveal, "sex" in the form of reproductive biology continues to be subject to new forms of proliferation, regulation, and management, which also introduce new forms of biopolitics, as well as identities, norms, and markets. This "disciplining of reproduction," to use Adele Clarke's (1998) phrase, has, if anything, achieved new prominence in the early twenty-first century as an economic priority directly correlated to a redefinition of human health in the context of a more explicit calculation of the value of life and sex as both reproductive and regenerative. In his analysis of the emergence of the human sciences in the late nineteenth century, Foucault argues that a new epistemological space that took "Man" as its object was in part facilitated by the emergence of new biological definitions of life, sex, and population. Arguably the extension of this process is evident today in the effort to realign biotechnology with "the human" and its biological future—a process in which new definitions of these same concepts are once again both means and indices of social change.

What is noticeably different in the contemporary era, however, is the relocation of this nationally governed managerial effort to manage life "down" to the level of sexual substance itself. It is as if the effort to produce and discipline sex via the sexed body described by Foucault for the nineteenth century has "descended" and been refocused at the level of reproductive substance itself, now of course the object of a level of surveillance, management, and handling that is unprecedented in human history. Correspondingly, and as Marx would have predicted, an extension of the state apparatus now administers, polices, and disciplines the detailed biology of gametes and embryos, as in the Human Fertilisation and Embryology Act. Today it is not only the sexed bodies of couples that are at issue in the effort to manage fertility, nor even their individual (or joint) sexual practices or identities. Indeed, this level of management is precisely what IVF technology renders irrelevant. "Sex" in the sense of either sexual practice or sexual identity is not so much regulated through the legislation governing hES research as are the "sexual" substances themselves, such as sperm and eggs. Remarkably today, and just as Foucault described the production of new sexual identities in the past, bodily substances that did not previously have a "sexual" role, such as skin cells, can now be made sexual through forms of experimental technology that render them viably reproductive: their germinal power technologically induced through new regimes of enhancing their potency, as in the induced pluripotent stem cell. Here is "sexing up" on a whole different scale—indeed precisely the kind of scale that would have interested Marx.

We should also note Foucault's concern about the population—that other object of the technologies of sex he describes. This concept too, like Marx's models of labor and value, is significantly altered in the context of biotechnology. If Darwin's theory of evolution provided the logic Foucault argues was required to establish the autonomous principles of "life itself" necessary to enable the birth of modern biology, with its account of speciation as a process of selection across the population, Foucault's embedding of the "anatomical" human in a Darwinian concept of population that becomes newly manageable can be seen to have acquired a very different set of implications today in the context of biotechnology. The analogy of "the breeder's hand" so important to Darwin's account of biological plasticity has been considerably extended in the form of animal populations bred and manipulated as models of what this plasticity can be made to do—that is, how it can be differently managed or disciplined. These model populations are now the screens on which the effort to track biological substances, pathways, and mechanisms can be shown or revealed. Thus, the meaning of "the population" has been amplified by becoming interspecific (across species), at the same time the human populations that matter have been disaggregated and reconstituted as cellular. Moreover, neither the interspecies comparisons nor the banked populations of human biomaterials belong to the same "natural system" as Darwin's speciating finches, or long-necked giraffes. The new biological kinships forged between these populations, like their handmade genealogies, are technological in origin. As the Human Genome Project clearly demonstrated, understandings of the human are increasingly embedded in a nested system of comparative animal model populations that provide the syntax for understanding biological inscription, like so many Russian dolls (worm, fish, frog, mouse, sheep, human). Biomaterials, such as viruses and peptides, provide the handles for manipulating living connections, while reproduction provides the engine of growth. In order to read the principles of biological development in the reproductive substance itself (e.g., genes), it has been necessary to produce the additional hardware or infrastructure in the form of mouse houses, nematode worm colonies, zebra fish tanks, and now also stem cell dish models, comprising sufficiently large populations of living entities to reveal life's hidden codes. This is a very different kind of tool kit for both producing and managing life than crop rotation or pigeon breeding.

This is of course also the new biological tool kit that, by luck as well as effort, delivers the IVF technique, which is a product of changing methods in experimental mammalian developmental biology, and the birth of new model systems, as we shall see in chapter 3. Ironically, it was in part a concern about population growth and the need for more effective contraception that motivated much of the technological innovation leading to successful mammalian IVF. IVF is a technology of sex completely unlike that described by Foucault, much as his hugely original and innovative methodology is highly pertinent to its historical and anthropological characterization. Nonetheless, his "gene-alogical" model of history can allow us to see how a technology devised in the context of limiting the population engendered changes in how the concept of population is deployed. Indeed, this shift can now be seen as crucial to the complete reversal of the situation that gave rise to Foucault's conception of sex as a "technology" to begin with: today it is not technologies of sex that discipline reproduction, but reproductive technologies that discipline sex.

The question of how reproductive technologies such as IVF both imitate and transform technologies of sex thus introduces a new meaning of this phrase (as Foucault might have predicted they would). This is why it is nec-essary to combine a feminist account of technologies of sex and gender with an analysis of how biology has become increasingly technologized—a com-bination I suggest is manifest in both the rise of IVF technology and its new biological relations with other technological innovations, such as stem cells. As we shall see in subsequent chapters, many of the important methodologi-cal tools for such an investigation can be found in the extensive, but largely neglected, feminist literature on new reproductive technologies, and in the feminist analysis of sex and gender as technologies, as well as the anthropo-logical study of kinship (to which I turn in more detail shortly). However, for now it may be useful to explore these themes through a somewhat more con-crete form of exemplification.

The Embryo Workshop

In order to approach the evolution of IVF as a technology of sex more con-cretely, it is useful to visit another workshop, this one in present-day Lon-don, where a new kind of human-tool-machine relation is being forged in the effort to discipline reproductive substance. In the United Kingdom, where the research for this book was based, and where both human IVF and stem cell culture were initially developed, the strong government effort to pro-mote human stem cell derivation is evident in a new generation of bespoke public facilities that have been commissioned and built over the past decade adjacent to IVF units. The new labs embody the goal of enhancing U.K. stem cell derivation, banking, and standardization, with a view to establishing new sources of living human cellular products, as well as conducting basic re-search using human embryonic cells as research models. They manifest a na-tional scientific ambition that is also economic and informed by a perceived social consensus to harness technological innovation in the interests of im-proving the quality of human life. They are thus also part of a broad sociologi-

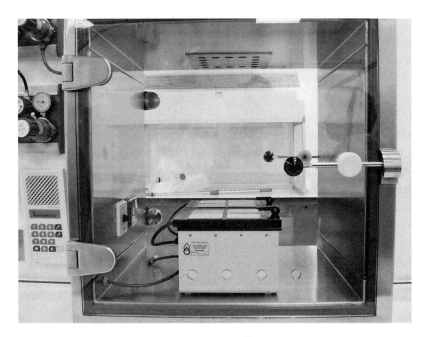

FIGURE 1.3. Looking through the hole in the wall from the IVF surgery into the clean room stem cell laboratory. Photo by the author.

cal process conjoining the management of reproductive substance to the body politic in the name of "future health and wealth deliverables."

I first visited the largest and most state of the art of these new laboratories at Guy's Hospital in London in the autumn of 2008 during its final postconstruction phase before opening the following spring. Professor Peter Braude, a consultant obstetrician, geneticist, and head of the lab, led the tour. The timing was ideal because the lab was just beginning the process of decontamination, so we could see everything and wander around freely without wearing bunny suits and masks. Peter's is the largest of seven new U.K. labs that have been constructed with government funding across the U.K. to bring IVF and hES derivation physically closer together, so that any spare or clinically useless embryos can go straight into a quality controlled clean-room laboratory if a couple decides to donate them to research (which approximately 70 percent of those asked in the U.K. will be likely to do). The new labs are thus designed to join together a so-called dirty surgical room, where eggs are aspirated from women patients undergoing IVF, with a clean laboratory that complies with the highest quality standards of sterility. The two rooms are separated by a hatch, or hole in the wall (figure 1.3). The eggs aspirated from women IVF patients go through the hatch to be fertilized, and, if they grow and develop normally, one of them returns through the door for embryo transfer. Other fertilized eggs or embryos can be frozen for future use, donated to other couples for treatment, donated to research, or disposed of, depending on what the patients decide to do with them.

The new labs are thus seen to offer a path forward—in the current idiom of scientific innovation they represent the cutting edge of biomedical translation. They are where what is referred to as frontier applications and are being developed for what are imagined as the horizon industries of cellular replacement therapies. What the FDA denominates as "the critical path" is the path to successful translation, and thus not only a successful passage "from bench to bedside" but "from bench to market." The new U.K. stem cell labs manifest this ambition as a goal-oriented, purpose-built architecture designed to facilitate a more efficient interface between IVF clinics and stem cell science. At the IVF–stem cell interface a new form of passaging human gametes and embryos is made possible, not only from one dish to another, or even from one room to the next, but from a specific clinical context (a patient having treatment in a surgery) to a new biological order of things (quality-controlled facilities that can be process-validated for the safe handling of human cells). This form of propagating human cells represents the latest evolution of the IVF platform—broadly speaking, it enables IVF to become a source of embryo supply for a much wider range of (nonreproductive) applications.

Following the major shift in scientific understandings of cellular potential emerging out of stem cell research in the 1980s—namely that even ordinary cells can be reprogrammed to become newly embryonic, or "totipotent," the IVF–stem cell interface has become an increasingly important "contact zone" and thus a place where human and technological genealogies are being both reimagined and refashioned (as we would expect from a frontier). The view from the IVF–stem cell interface thus overlooks a new form of coevolution between human reproductive substance, scientific knowledge, laboratory craftwork, and technological innovation aimed at improving control over biological mechanisms, systems, and pathways. Although novel, the transfer of eggs and embryos through the hole in the wall of the clean room is only the latest extension to a chain of embryo transfers that define the origins not only of IVF and stem cell research, but experimental embryology and the study of biological development—especially in the twentieth century, especially in mammals, and especially in the British Isles.[18]

These egg and embryo movements, or transfers, have been a staple technique of reproductive and developmental biology since the late nineteenth century, and their practical applications in livestock breeding have had enormous consequences for world agriculture as well as zoological conservation (especially in combination with cryopreservation, see Friese 2013). Indeed, one of the simplest means of tracking the history of IVF is by tracing the extension of these transfers from animals into humans—or indeed by considering IVF itself as a critical path of embryological knowledge transfer. In other words, IVF was the translational bridge that enabled the technique of embryo transfer to make its "human turn"—initially as a means of redressing the burden of human reproductive and developmental deficits, later for stem cell research, and now for regenerative medicine.

The embryo transfer of "IVF and ET," which is used to describe the surgical transfer of an embryo into an IVF patient's uterus, belongs to a long lineage of related, or ancestral, embryo transfers extending back at least a century.[19] Today, human embryo transfer also belongs to an expanding global diaspora of reproductive trafficking, or tourism, as well as to global networks of international scientific exchange, commercial transactions for research eggs and embryos, and stem cell banking.[20] This global movement of embryos is part of a contemporary dialectic of biotranslation through which new cellular models generate new applications, and vice versa. In vitro fertilization and embryo transfer epitomize this process, having an equally robust importance on both sides of the pure and applied domains of the biological sciences. As I argued in my previous work on cloning, embryo exchanges continue to cement clinical-scientific collaborations in the busily expanding bioscientific present, just as they have done historically by facilitating mutually beneficial veterinary-scientific and agro-scientific partnerships (such as those uniting Britain and Australia in livestock breeding; Franklin 2007a, 2007b). These kinships of scientific technique form a crucial part of the process of embryo transfer in the sense not only that reproductive material is being passed around and shared, but because they are motivated by an ethos of translation—of working up these substances to make them newly (re)productive, that is, translational.[21] At work propelling embryos through the doors of the new labs at the IVF–stem cell interface, then, are historically well-established goals of maximizing efficiency through cooperation, promoting economic growth, exchanging scientific knowledge and materials, and generating technological progress as well as "paybacks" to the general public (who funds much of the research). The new labs express the intention to rationalize the thousands of transfers of research embryos all over the United Kingdom, to standardize and validate derivation procedures, to increase biosecurity and ethical oversight, and eventually to remunerate the British population by delivering into U.K. GDP a larger share of the bioeconomic pie.

For the bioeconomy to become productive, it is necessary for new sources of capital stock to become more streamlined in order that they can be scaled up, banked, and used for manufacturing new therapeutic products on a commercially viable scale. Put simply, the significant appeal of human embryonic cell lines is their importance as the best source of capital stock available, and thus the most likely to repay capital investment. As the King's College team based at Guy's Hospital describes "the best stem cell model for capital investment in stem cell therapy," "pluripotent stem cells . . . can be produced in theoretically limitless quantities, and [are] therefore capable of providing more cells than from any other source, regardless of differentiation efficacy and stabilization. Thus, they are the cell type likely to yield the most from invested capital" (Stephenson et al. 2010: s678). Necessary to the realization of this yield are a number of "banking" issues including: "legislation to allow use of human embryos for stem cell research," "consensus for reporting the quality and type of embryos suitable for stem cell derivation," and "a regulatory route map to facilitate clinical application" (s678). These obstacles "have largely been overcome, especially in the UK" due to the collaboration of a large number of government agencies, again largely financed by the public sector. It is in this way that I have argued the U.K. is creating the equivalent of Greenwich Mean Time for stem cell banking, much as it has historically also set the standards for the global financial sector — in which it continues to occupy a distinctly privileged location because of global time that it streamlined as the first globally prominent capitalist industrial economy.

A Fertile Environment

The critical path of embryo transfers and passages can be traced as a genealogy of tooling up mammalian embryos for over a century (discussed in chapter 3), along which these living technologies evolved from the early investigations of heredity pursued by the early embryo pioneer Walter Heape in 1890 to the mass standardization of hES cultivation and banking in the early twenty-first century. Employed in diverse model systems, across a variety of species, for both basic research and a wide range of actual and projected applications, and benefiting from an ever more sophisticated range of techniques, the coupling of IVF and embryo research now serves as a core component within what a report from the U.K. Department of Health (2011: 45) describes as "a fertile environment for the development and adoption of innovation and scientific advances." The moral and legal justifications for government protection of this sector (which it both funds and promotes in the U.K.) have been driven by essentially pragmatic goals over the course of the past century, while also becoming increasingly economically prominent. Initially these goals were focused on the alleviation of infertility and genetic disease, but today they have greatly expanded—to the point of becoming a new paradigm for the future of health care and national economic growth. Having invested more than 200 million pounds ($300 million) in the stem cell research and regenerative medicine pathway since 2003, the U.K. government describes this sector as having "the potential to provide a step change reduction in health care costs" (Department of Health 2011: 45) as well as generating new sectors of employment and new markets. The development of living cell technologies is hopefully imagined as "a driver for the UK economy and future healthcare" and as an antidote to the "patent cliff" faced by a pharmaceutical industry increasingly disillusioned with the blockbuster model (Department of Health 2011).

As in the nineteenth century, which saw an equally significant government investment in industrial manufacturing and infrastructure, for similar political and economic reasons, these pragmatic goals have been the subject of considerable public debate, often occasioning new public funding initiatives, new regulatory bodies, and new acts of Parliament. The proposal that human embryos should become tools lay at the heart of the protracted legislative debate in the U.K. that lasted for twelve years after the birth of Louise Brown (a debate, it is worth remembering, that was less about clinical IVF than experimental embryology). Although this debate involved considerable deliberation over the need to protect the rights of embryos, the HFE Act ultimately protected a collective human right to human embryos and specifically to their use as tools in the effort to alleviate human suffering.

As the Cabinet Minister for Women, the Right Honourable (Labour) MP from Barking Jo Richardson, argued in the British House of Commons in December 1988, as part of the debate over the first Human Fertilisation and Embryology Act: "It is of course true that the fundamental principles of human IVF were established with the use of animal models, but different animal species—including the human—differ from each other in biochemical and developmental details. That means that however much enormously useful information can be provided by animal models there will ultimately be a point in the research when the human system must be directly examined. That is why it is necessary that we ensure that there is an opportunity for the research to continue" (December 16, 1988, HC c. 1268). Based on more than half a century of experimentation with fertilized mammalian embryos in vitro, the eventual clinical success of IVF confirmed, as Ruth Edwards described at the outset of this chapter, that human ova could be removed from the body, cultured in media, fertilized in vitro, and transferred to the uterus to produce viable offspring. This not only confirmed a transferability of principles from other animal models to humans, but a functional isomorphism between in vivo and in vitro conception. Put simply, IVF proved the viability of a substitution of an in vitro model for the "real thing," and parliamentary decree confirmed the inestimable value of this new tool for human progress.[22]

A Cybrid Manifesto

In order to observe how this logic of IVF has evolved in the U.K. over the past thirty years, and indeed how the management of reproduction, or sex, has descended to the level of substance, it is useful to revisit the most recent round of British embryo debates, many of which were centered on the question of deliberately creating new embryonic tools in the form of so-called cybrid, or human-animal admixed embryos, for basic scientific research into the ground state of cellular renewal.

In the autumn of 2008, not long after I had visited the stem cell lab described above, I attended one of the major demonstrations outside the Houses of Parliament in support of, and against, the new Human Fertilisation and Embryology Act at a key point during its complex legislative passage into law (figures 1.4 and 1.5). It was a beautiful sunny day and it was a short bike ride from my office at the LSE down the Embankment to Old Palace Yard in Westminster, where I arrived just after 1 PM. In the announcement of the May 12, 2008, pro-embryo research demonstration, Show Your Support, organized by the office of (Liberal) MP Evan Harris (the leader of the pro-cybrid lobby), it was suggested, "In recent months there has been intensive lobbying of MPS, particularly from groups who are opposed to embryo research to continue in the UK, including embryonic stem cell science and the animal-human hybrid work. MPS may not have heard quite so clearly from those who strongly support the proposals in the Bill, and know that it is vitally important that the legislation is not watered down." It went on: "A YouGov poll in August 2005 showed that 77% of people accept embryo research for life-threatening diseases. But for far too long, the most prominent shows of feeling on this issue have come from those who wish to impede carefully regulated embryo re-

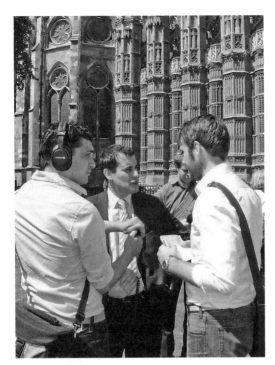

FIGURE 1.4. (left) Liberal MP Evan Harris with reporters at Old Palace Yard opposite the Houses of Parliament for the May 12, 2008, Show Your Support demonstration, organized by his office, to promote the legalization of cybrid embryo tools. Photo by the author.

FIGURE 1.5. (below) Patient groups and families affected by genetic disease attended the Show Your Support demonstration in order to protect scientific research using human admixed embryos to improve stem cell techniques. Photo by the author.

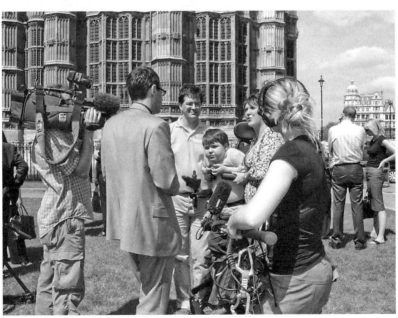

search and important and ethical clinical interventions like preimplantation genetic diagnosis." The announcement concluded that on May 12, 2008, just before the start of the bill's second reading in the House of Commons, "hundreds of patient groups would join with scientists, doctors and other supporters to represent the breadth and depth of support for the Bill, and in particular to confirm support for the government proposal that embryo research should continue in the UK, and should include animal-human hybrid work as well as embryonic stem cell science."

In fact, that day fewer than a dozen patients and representatives of patient groups were available to comment to the assembled media—most of whom had left by the time I arrived. The only scientists present were some members of the Guy's Hospital stem cell lab, who joined the small demonstration but appeared to have nothing to do. The fear that the pro-embryo research lobby would be swamped by a pro-life rally scheduled the same afternoon just before the start of the second reading at 2 PM proved groundless, as it too was poorly attended and lackluster, the weather perhaps too glorious to support a mood of indignation.

Riding back to my office to watch the debate on the bill live on Parliament TV, I reflected on what a different political climate had prevailed in the late spring of 1990, when the first Human Fertilisation and Embryology Bill was at a similar stage. At that time, not so long after a Private Member's Bill by Conservative MP Enoch Powell had attempted to ban embryo research entirely, the question of how Parliament would vote on the amendment to allow embryo research was far from certain. The pro-life lobby was much larger and better organized. In a dramatic show of opposition to abortion, its supporters had showered the chambers of Parliament with postcards showing aborted fetuses.

The reduced size and fervor of the demonstrations for and against embryo research concerning revisions to the Human Fertilisation and Embryology Act during its second passage through Parliament were not the only measure of the difference between 1990 and 2008. Looking back, we can see that although some forms of reproductive technology, such as cloning, human-animal hybrids, and stem cells, still engender controversy, the logic of IVF has been sedimented into a naturalized trajectory of intervention in the name of improvement, in which technological manipulation of human embryos is not only widely accepted as a viable alternative to natural reproduction but is seen as a necessary path to the continued improvement of human health. As Danny Boyle's opening ceremony for the Olympics confirmed, innovative health technologies have become celebrated features of British national identity and linked to its industrial past through the symbolic idioms of rebirth, creativity, and regeneration. A long legacy of increasing public support for increasingly radical forms of human embryo research, combined with explicit cross-party government support for ongoing innovation in this field, has embedded a logic that is now seemingly part of the British national imaginary, and is celebrated as a source of national pride. If severe, debilitating, and destructive diseases can be alleviated through embryo research, the reasons to object to these techniques appear increasingly less persuasive or even credible — especially in the wake of the rapid expansion of IVF, which was developed using precisely such methods. Over time, the connection between IVF and fertility — or even conception — has been superseded (as it was preceded) by a more general isomorphism between improvements to human life and the ability to culture human embryos in glass. This is the biological relation IVF substantializes as both a model system and an ethical consensus, and therefore not only as a translational path but as a public duty. This is the logic of remaking life that appears increasingly to have become a sign of a vital, caring, and creative Britain. The code for conduct that inheres in this logic unites a belief in the value of scientific research with a duty to work up reproductive substance in the name of shared benefits for the body politic as a whole.

Five million miracle babies later, the basic principle of retooling human embryos has come to appear not only obvious but even patriotic. The British (non)debate over the use of cybrid embryos in 2008 indexes a striking cultural shift over the intervening thirty years, during which a new understanding of human reproductive substance as technology gained so much force it can now inspire a public demonstration outside Parliament to promote human-cow embryo cybrids. This cultural shift is directly related to the success and popularity of IVF — a technique that has rendered biology newly relative in the process of making new biological relatives, and which, over time, has made both of these relatives more regular. Three decades post-IVF, human embryo technology has become a normative and nationalized project — and not only in the U.K. The lack of contemporary public opposition to stem cell research in the U.K. increasingly characterizes the dominant worldwide pattern (albeit one to which the U.S. is a significant exception).[23]

Another significant indicator of this normalization effect is the increasing public intolerance of religious denunciations of both IVF and stem cell research. During the high-profile U.K. debate in 2008 concerning human-animal hybrids, or cybrids, the Catholic right-to-life position was relegated to the extreme fringe of public debate. Cardinal Keith O'Brien's strident 2008 Easter sermon condemning the revised Human Fertilisation and Embryology Act was widely perceived to damage the reputation of Catholicism. His characterization of embryo research as "a monstrous attack on human rights, human dignity and human life" appeared tone-deaf, if not hysterical, to the wider society as well as to many of his fellow Catholics.

"It is difficult to imagine," O'Brien claimed, "a single piece of legislation which, more comprehensively, attacks the sanctity and dignity of human life than this particular Bill":

> What I am speaking of is the process whereby scientists create an embryo containing a mixture of animal and human genetic material. If I were preaching this homily in France, Germany, Italy, Canada, or Australia I would be commending the government for rightly banning such grotesque procedures. However here in Great Britain I am forced to condemn our government for not only permitting but encouraging such hideous practices. . . . This Bill represents a monstrous attack on human rights, human dignity and human life. . . . One might say that in our country we are about to have a public government endorsement of experiments of Frankenstein proportion. May God indeed help us to be Missionary at this present time and to hand on the saving message of Jesus Christ in a world which does not seem prepared to receive it. (O'Brien 2008)

O'Brien's attempt to provoke a sense of national shame in relation to human embryo research was as poorly judged and badly timed as Danny Boyle's display of a giant national health baby was perfectly aligned with public sentiment four years later. The response to O'Brien's sermon was particularly vehement from within the Christian community, whose members did not appreciate his interpretation of "the saving message of Jesus Christ" or his references to "public government endorsement of experiments of Frankenstein proportion." Among those challenging O'Brien's view was the prominent geneticist and Anglican priest Mary Seller, whose commentary on cybrids published in the *Tablet* cited the teachings of Jesus Christ as a motivation not only to heal the sick but to marvel at the splendor of God's creation:

> God certainly intends healing of the sick. Jesus always healed when he encountered a person in need: he never passed one by. Indeed he often flouted authority to do so: he healed on the Sabbath, he touched untouchables, and vociferous criticism did not stop him. Furthermore, he gave power and authority to his disciples to go out on the highways and byways to do likewise. If today we are able to heal anyone through our

new scientific endeavors, it is an expression of our discipleship, and can also be construed as another way in which we legitimately "play God." (Seller 2008)

Seller's pragmatic interpretation of Christ's teaching closely follows the mainstream U.K. position of support for science based on a sense of moral duty to explore new avenues for the relief of human suffering. In her view, God's intentions are consistent with instrumental intervention, including scientific experimentation, and the use of biology as a technology—indeed the use of human embryos as life-saving tools. She evokes a tradition of active, mobile evangelism—flouting the state's authority to take to the road, "the highways and byways," with tools to heal the sick. Scientific experimentation, in this view, is no less than a form of discipleship.

In their press release prepared to accompany the debate in Parliament on human-animal hybrid embryos, the Genetic Interest Group (GIG), the largest U.K. organization representing those affected by genetic disease, took a similar view—describing the human in vitro embryo as "a vital tool to advance the progress of research into the potential of embryonic stem cells" and thus as "a potentially vital avenue for research which could greatly increase our understanding of serious medical conditions such as Parkinson's, motor neurone disease, Alzheimer's disease and cystic fibrosis" (GIG 2008). In this endorsement sit side by side the two halves of biological relativity—whereby a very curious tool in the form of an admixed embryo comes to be seen as both a right and a duty. Such a statement strongly reinforces the initial U.K. government position set in place during the 1980s—that embryo research should be protected by law in the effort to provide relief from human suffering—while also confirming, as did the passage of the new pro-cybrid bill unamended, that this position has stood the test of time. As the (lack of) debate over the human admixed embryo revealed, support for the logic of pursuing embryo research has significantly strengthened over time, to the extent that the value of the in vitro human embryo culture system as both a tool and a way has come to occupy the moral high ground. Indeed, the pursuit of this path has become a public obligation. The logic of shared substance indigenous to the context of IVF and embryo research, now part of a high-profile national economic strategy, and linked to the future health and well-being of the nation's sixty million inhabitants, has moved beyond becoming obvious, commonsensical, or regular. This logic is increasingly articulated as a code for conduct mandating more and better future uses of embryos as tools as a national way of life and a scientific duty to future generations.

Conclusion

Although initially controversial, IVF has become an increasingly widely accepted and familiar technique, and can now be seen more clearly to belong
to a cultural legacy it helped to inaugurate and normalize, namely the retooling of human reproductive substance. To the extent that IVF substantializes
a new reproductive model, through which reproductive substance is "taken
in hand," this has also taken place in a highly visible and explicit manner, not
only through the successful worldwide marketing of IVF services, but in the
form of wider public investment in the logic of IVF. The logic of the retooled
human embryo is now established not only as a new norm in both public and
private life, but as a duty to the future—an obligation to pursue the "vital
path" for science, based on the development of a vital tool in the form of the
in vitro human embryo. Indeed, as the biofuturist Stewart Brand suggests, IVF
is the "big example" confirming a new paradigm of biology as technology. In
the context of human embryo research, this suggests that shared reproductive
substance now codes for conduct in the form of signifying a duty to pursue the
alleviation of human suffering. Indeed, this is what stem cells increasingly signify as technologies: they hold out the promise of relief from disease, repair
of injury, cheaper health applications, and new diagnostic models and thus a
distinctive new form of shared reproductive substance.

Home to the development of both IVF and hES derivation, the U.K. case
illustrates how closely linked these two technologies have been in the past,
and how powerful their coupling is imagined to be in the future. I have suggested too that the history of the Industrial Revolution that took place in the
northwest of England in the eighteenth and nineteenth centuries provides a
useful lens on the trajectory of events linking human IVF to the translation of
reproductive substance into new tools and applications. This would be a more
superficial analogy if it were not for some of the strikingly relevant analyses
developed by Marx and Engels from their front-row seats overlooking the dramatic mechanical spectacle of rapid industrialization in the mid-nineteenth
century. Their caution that this process should not be understood as merely
technical, but as the dialectical rolling forward of a more complex apparatus,
which they described as historical materialism, remains highly relevant. The
questions concerning the evolution of machines, the role of scale, the relation of humans to tools, and the substantialization of political economy in the
"exact mechanisms" of manufacturing apparatus yield, for all of the reasons
I have tried to outline in this chapter, an important set of concepts to understand bioindustrialization today.

It is for similar reasons, I have suggested, that we can return to Foucault's model of sex as a technology to ask what further insights it can yield in the contemporary context of biology as a technology, or more specifically, sex after IVF. I suggest not only that his method of analyzing history genealogically adds important dimensions to understanding the histories of IVF, embryo transfer, and embryo research, but that his model of technologies of sex can be productively reworked in this context as well. While Marx and Engels prioritize the division of labor as a crucial apparatus in the emergence of the Industrial Revolution, they pay little attention to the production of sex as a value, or its organization as a means of disciplining bodies. Similarly, Foucault's emphasis on sex as a force that is never merely biological but rather can be activated, amplified, and managed not only has implications for the sexual division of labor, but for reproductive substance itself—especially now that it is not the sexed body or identity, but the exact mechanisms of biological sex, reproduction, generativity, potentiality, and so on, that are the subject of "biopower," to use his phrase. Yet he too overlooked some of the most compelling questions his own analysis raises about the relationship of the sexual division of labor to biopower; the complex relationships between the reproductive sciences, gender, and kinship; the exact mechanisms of producing fertility; or the disciplining of reproductive substance in the context of embryology.

It is in the effort to theorize the condition of being after IVF in its double sense—historically and stylistically—that two workshops are visited in this chapter, one from the nineteenth century and one from the twenty-first. As we shall see in more detail in the next chapter, the self-acting power of the machine-tool, and its relation to both the human hand and its objects, remain useful places to examine the logic of biology as technology. Since this book is largely concerned with IVF as a technology, and as a technological platform, the importance of appreciating its technical aspects—its exact mechanisms—is emphasized throughout this book.

However, both the content and the form of *Biological Relatives* are designed also to emphasize the inseparability of even the most practical aspects of IVF from the wider context of its social logic, manifest as its relation to the body politic and the health of the population, and specifically the production of fertility through technology. In vitro fertilization came into being as a logical plan before it was substantialized as a reproductive model, a working experimental system, or a clinical application. In the final section of this chapter I have argued that Stewart Brand's claim that IVF is the big example of how this logic has become more familiar and regular is illustrated by the recent British debate about a new kind of human embryonic tool. What I argue is evident from the perspective of the U.K., and which I suggest is indeed now a global pattern, is a growing acceptance of the logic of biology as a technology— a logic I argue IVF has done more than any other technology to introduce. In vitro fertilization, to use Heidegger's terminology, has reenframed reproductive substance as a tool.

This enframing is also manifest in the widespread endorsement of hES research as a vital avenue of medical progress, and thus the successor "hope technology" to IVF. Part of my argument, then, is simply to suggest that we may have underestimated the importance of IVF as a technology that has changed not only understandings of the biological, but understandings of evolution, inheritance, and genealogy. In describing IVF this way, I do not intend to suggest it has independent agency, but that its widespread public endorsement and celebration represent a growing degree of consensus about the desirability and legitimacy of mechanizing human biology (as well as the biology of other systems, from cloned livestock to photovoltaic bacteria). In vitro fertilization is in this sense precisely a path or vital avenue, as claimed by the British patient group GIG in their press release supporting a new form of embryonic tool. I have suggested too that in describing the admixed human embryo as a vital tool, the logic of IVF is manifest as a new code for conduct based on a new model of shared reproductive substance.

If so, this also reveals a more curious legacy of IVF—that it has refashioned the relationship between substance and code for conduct not only by making the substance the object of conduct, but by making conduct (e.g., scientific research) *the origin of substance* (e.g., replacement parts, artificial gametes, cultured hES lines, biobanking, etc.). This is also where we might understand the power of IVF as a technology of "genealogical translation," because being after IVF has changed what genealogical and biological are, can do, and mean. In turn, such a hypothesis repositions both the meaning of kinship and its importance to technology more prominently as a dominant sphere of public life. Not only the curious new kinships established through the dissemination of shared reproductive substance, but the biological relation to technology itself established through IVF and embryo research now emerge as "facts of life." The coming into being of this new form of kinship, defying as it does many of the basic tenets of social science, such as the indivisibility of the human subject, the separation of public and private life, or the naturalness of reproduction, requires a theoretical retooling commensurate to a shift that has arguably already occurred, but not yet been fully comprehended.

In turning to the work of both Donna Haraway and Shulamith Firestone in chapter 2, I continue many of the themes raised so far, but explore them in more detail in relation to the actual work of making stem cells in the lab. For this purpose, I also draw more deeply on the insights into labor and tools provided by Marx in his analysis of an earlier period of industrialization. Thus, whereas this chapter has attempted to provide an overview of being after IVF in many of its widest senses, the next chapter looks more narrowly at the hand-tool-embryo relation. Here, where a kind of kinship of biological relations is more ready to hand, is also where we can begin to see through the IVF looking glass, thus shifting our perspective, while keeping many of the same, familiar objects and questions in view.

TWO Living Tools

One of the most powerful analyses of the emergence of contemporary bio-technologies can be found in the work of Donna Haraway, whose theory of cyborg politics and highly influential accounts of human-animal-tool relations reshaped the agendas of feminist theory and science studies during precisely the same period that IVF technology began to become more everyday.[1] Haraway's powerful model of material semiosis, through which technology is interpreted as both expressive and formative of conceptual equipment, draws on her training as both a biologist and a historian, and was first forged in the context of embryology. The question of the relationship of technology to human futures, or more specifically human political futures, that is the major focus of Marx's analysis of historical materialism is also the subject of Donna Haraway's now-iconic late twentieth-century essay "A Manifesto for Cyborgs," published almost exactly a century after Marx's death, in 1985. Haraway's signature method of materialist figuration owes as much to Marxist models as do her politics. But while Haraway's focus on technology, politics, labor, capital, and the human condition shares much in common with the tenets of nineteenth-century historical materialism, her close engagement with information technology, cybernetics, genetic engineering, nuclear physics, and molecular biology places her firmly in the world of twenty-first-century technoscience, as well as transmillennial feminist thought. She is thus the author of a new "biotechnology politics" based on "partial identities" and "ironic communication" that "refuse anti-science metaphysics" and are dedicated to "the skillful task of reconstructing the boundaries of everyday life" (Haraway 1983: 13).

As Haraway noted of the embryological debates described in her 1976 book on the metaphors of organicism that competed to organize twentieth-century developmental biology, the scientific models that inform experimental biology inevitably also model social life. As she observed in *Crystals, Fabrics, and Fields* (following both Thomas Kuhn and Mary Hesse), science cannot function without analogies, and these are inevitably also constitutive orientations:

> The traditional mechanist sees similarities between the organism and actual machines such as the steam engine, hydraulic pump, or a system of levers and pulleys. The neomechanist builds a similarity set from codes, the molecular basis of genes, language, computers, and the organism. . . . The organicist tends to see similarities in the structure of molecular populations, the cell, the whole organisms, and the ecosystem. . . . Concrete analogies are drawn from models, gestalt phenomena, fields, liquid crystals, and also computers. These lists suggest that persons holding one of the three perspectives would be inclined to work on different experimental problems and to interpret the results in a different language. (Haraway 1976: 205)

The scene Haraway describes here, of the enframement of experimental problems, is what has since come to be known as "science in action" (Latour 1987), "laboratory life" (Latour and Woolgar 1979), or "sorting things out" (Bowker and Star 1999). Here too is Haraway's first cyborg figure — the cyborg embryo, not yet denominated as such, but as surely a product of "worlds ambiguously natural and crafted" (1991: 149), "couplings between organism and machine" (150) and a "condensed image of both imagination and material reality, the two joined centres structuring any possibility of historical transformation" (150) as the chip, fetus, gene, seed, database, bomb, race, brain, and ecosystem of her later work (1985, 1991, 1997).

Three and a half decades later, Haraway's cyborg analysis speaks even more cogently to the embryo-strewn world of the twenty-first century. The anxious attention so often directed at "the" embryo, as in the perennial debate over "the moral status of the human embryo," forgets that human embryos are now a vast and diverse global biological population, imaged, imagined, and archived in media as diverse as liquid nitrogen, mouse feeder cells, DVDs, virtual libraries, websites, T-shirts, logos, Hollywood cinema, and brand names. Never very precise, the term "embryo" is ever more of a basket category, now describing everything from a conceptus, a zygote, an "admixed human hybrid cell," or a blastocyst to a reconstructed cell, a fertilized egg, or an embryoid body. We cannot map the complicated social, political, scientific, medical, or ethical lives of human embryos, with all of their increasingly prominent civic and legal entanglements, without the kind of material semiology, or grammar, of the biological that Haraway, uniquely, provides.

As in many other chapters in the history of biological control, the idiom of improvement—and specifically of merging nature with progress—is central to the increasingly prominent role the extracorporeal embryo has played in the reengineering of the facts of life. The cyborg embryo, itself the offspring of a union between reproductive failure and scientific hope, has become, like natural conception before it, something that is seen to be in need of careful management in order to be properly domesticated (Franklin 1995, 1997; Thompson 2005; Throsby 2004). Couples who pursue the assisted conception route can, in a complicated act of affinity with scientific progress and potential communities of future beneficiaries, now also donate their surplus embryos to research to make colonies of immortalized, regenerative, anonymized, and totipotent cells, which will be banked in the aid of an improved human future. This biological reserve, archive, bank, or master stock can be directed to transform into specific types of cell and, in theory, is the seedbed for a previously untapped source of human repair. The improved biology of the future will be more reliable, routinized, and standardized both because technological control of biology is being built into the biological itself, and because other forms of control are being introduced to stabilize and govern the cultivation of these new, rebuilt biologies—such as process validation, good manufacturing practice (GMP), accreditation requirements, and risk assessment strategies.[2] As we shall see in the second part of this chapter, this process now constitutes a specialized form of scientific labor that is in the process of attaining a new scale of application on the verge of becoming industrialized.

In writing of the turn-of-the-century embryo, Haraway demonstrated that we cannot even look at the embryo—objectively, scientifically, in the laboratory, under a microscope—without seeing it through the lens of prefabricated, culturally inherited, constitutive, real, and inescapable frames of reference that incorporate the "external world" into what Evelyn Fox Keller (1996a) describes as "the biological gaze." Nor, as Haraway demonstrated in her work on primatology (1989), is it possible for scientific understandings to escape the interpretive devices, taxonomic conventions, or situated and historically specific conditions enabling us to know anything at all. Today, the evolution of IVF offers similar lessons, not only about how socialized (and socializing) scientific understandings always are, but now also, and ever more visibly, how social values, systems, and aspirations are being engineered and constructed in such a manner that they too become part of what "biological" means.

Technological Kinship

The biologization of human values is as old as horticulture, when human preferences began to be nudged into seedlings, and mutated corn began to be selected for its ears, but the antiquity of bioartifice does not mean that the contemporary transformation of human reproductive substance into technology lacks either specificity or novelty. In showing us a new set of implications of the bioinformatic implosion that enabled the gene to become the master molecule and ultimate coding mechanism, embedded in a "command-control-communication-intelligence" infrastructure that belongs to NASA as much as the National Institutes of Health, Haraway's (1983: 3) work has chronicled a change of kind as well as degree. As we observe the growing population of living human tools, such as reconstructed embryos, in which it is a logic of engineering that guides a project of biological redesign, we are also observing a shift away from "the translation of the world into a problem of coding" (Haraway 1991: 165) and toward a translation of the problem of coding into one of synthesis (a key point throughout all of Haraway's work, and one that could be described as thoroughly embryological). According to this logic, which is also the logic of IVF, "any objects or persons can be reasonably thought of in terms of disassembly and reassembly," and there are consequently "no 'natural' architectures that constrain system design" (1991: 162). The interplay of these two principles, of assembly and disassembly, could be described as the core modeling ethos guiding the effort to take reproductive substance in hand.

Although absent from the final draft of Haraway's most famous article, published in *Socialist Review* in 1985, the logic of IVF played a prominent role in an earlier version of "A Manifesto for Cyborgs" submitted to *Das Argument*, the influential German Marxist journal, in 1983 for a forthcoming volume titled "Orwell 1984." It was in an earlier incarnation of her now-classic manifesto, to which the analysis of both IVF and prenatal screening were central, that the unnatural futures promised by the collapse of the nostalgic nature-culture dualism were first celebrated as part of an "ironic dream."[3] Like other feminists in the 1980s, Haraway was highly skeptical about the various "forms of reproductive technology linked to *in vitro* fertilization (IVF)" and their links to the evolving "infra-structure of genetic engineering" (1983: 6). She is acutely conscious of the capacity for the introduction of new reproductive technologies such as IVF to reinforce existing forms of inequality. However, she is equally skeptical about the political viability of outdated organicist appeals to a pretechnologized nature or body, arguing that these are "kinky mystical illusions" and "illusory" (7). "I think it is not now possible to live in a 'natural' world, and that our most powerful social movements will not grow from such appeals. . . . For better or worse, our form of social existence has permanently displaced the dualisms of nature and science, natural and artificial. . . . It is not clear who makes and who is made in the relation between human and machine" (8, 12). Far from denigrating human-machine coupling, Haraway embraced the possibilities it offered of an alternative hybrid, mosaic, chimeric politics: "I maintain that in so far as we know ourselves in both formal discourse (e.g., biology) and in daily practice, we find ourselves to be cyborgs, hybrids, mosaics, chimeras. . . . There is no fundamental, ontological separation in our formal knowledge of machine and organism, of technical and organic" (12).

Arguing for a political reembrace of the creative connections uniting mind, body, and tool, Haraway argues that biotechnology offers a newly intimate figuration of the machine as us ("it is not clear who makes and is made in the relation between human and machine," 1983: 12), accompanied by a newly potent understanding of ourselves and our own biology as tools: "One consequence is that our sense of connection to our tools is heightened" (12), she claimed.

This new technological, machinic, or "cyborg" consciousness might be particularly important for women, Haraway suggested, given that "up till now . . . female embodiment seemed to be given, organic, necessary; and female embodiment seemed to mean skill in mothering and its metaphoric extensions. Only by being out of place could we take intense pleasure in machines, and then with excuses that this was organic activity after all, appropriate to females. Cyborgs might consider more seriously the partial, fluid, sometimes aspect of sex and sexual embodiment. Gender might not be global identity after all" (1983: 12). This reference to gender not being a global identity refers to both its conventional biologism and its traditional binarism — both implicit in gender's relationship to sex, with its global presumption of the two sexes, and the necessity of their complementary polarity for sexual reproduction. But what if genetic engineering is, as in Haraway's ironic dream, not only a new sex, but a more radical, more pleasurable, and politically improved sex that could change the very meaning of sexual reproduction? And what if genetic engineering is inherently "a technology for the production of meanings, as well as for the production of bodies" (Haraway 1983: 6) and one in which "our sense of connection to our tools is heightened" (12)? If so, Haraway claims, "intense pleasure in skill, machine skill, ceases to be a sin, but [becomes] an aspect of embodiment. The machine is not an it to be animated, worshipped, and dominated. The machine is us, our processes, an aspect of our embodiment" (12). Consequently, Haraway argues, a refashioned feminist politics must imagine a new kinship with technology, and indeed celebrate this new "ironic" model of kinship as the ground for a different version of sisterhood, to which a conventional gender politics is no longer central. Linking the politics of gender, kinship, and race directly to those of science and technology, Haraway calls for a refashioned socialist feminist politics that will "tak[e] responsibility for the social relations of science and technology [and refuse] an anti-science metaphysics, a demonology of technology, [by] embracing the skillful task of reconstructing the boundaries of daily life, in partial connection with others, in ironic communication with all of our parts. . . . Cyborg imagery can suggest a way out of the maze of dualisms in which we have explained our tools to ourselves. This is a different dream of a common language" (1983: 13).

In such arguments for a new politics of gender, kinship, and race via science and technology, Haraway is much closer to Shulamith Firestone than to any of the feminist writers addressing assisted reproductive technologies and IVF in the 1980s (whose work is discussed in chapter 5). Like Firestone, Haraway advocates not only the embrace of transgressive technological pleasure and connection, but a transcendence of the binding naturalisms inevitably associated with "global" (fixed, binary, permeating) models of sex and gender. For Haraway, as for many feminist science fiction writers, there is a revolutionary purpose to be achieved through tools, machines, instruments, and biology, and indeed through their union—they are not the enemy but the path to "a different dream of a common language" and to a radical rescripting of technologies of gender and kinship—indeed to "the material power to draw our own lines in the world" (1983: 7). We would be better off if we reimagined ourselves through these transgressive idioms to begin with, rather than resisting them, she suggests, adding that we need to make better personal and political use of our lively, and often queer, equipment. This sexual politics not only is more pleasurable than purity, wholeness, or back-to-nature nostalgia, but it has a better sense of humor: it is ironic, parodic, impertinent, playful, noncompliant, and unpredictable.

Feminist Biofuturism

For Firestone, who similarly proposed a controversial technological embrace in the 1970s, the importance of technology to assist women to gain control over reproduction, and thus to challenge the fixed biological model of binary sex, was the self-evident starting point of modern, twentieth-century feminism. Since the origin of the sex distinction, in her view, was "biology itself—procreation," its elimination required technological control of the means of reproduction in order for the tyranny of biology over women to be ended.

> Just as to assure elimination of economic classes requires the revolt of the underclass (the proletariat) and . . . their seizure of the means of production, so to assure the elimination of sexual classes requires the revolt of the underclass (women) and the control of reproduction. [This will require] not only the full restoration to women of ownership of their own bodies but also their (temporary) seizure of control of human fertility—the new population biology as well as all the social institutions of childbearing and childrearing. And just as the end goal of the socialist revolution was not only the elimination of the economic class privilege but of the economic class distinction itself, so the end goal of feminist revolution must be, unlike that of the first feminist movement, not only the elimination of male privilege but of the sex distinction itself. (Firestone 1972: 11)

The "new population biology" invoked by Firestone in this passage, and elsewhere in her highly influential 1970 manifesto, refers to the new sciences of reproductive endocrinology, reproductive physiology, and reproductive biology that all emerged during the first half of the twentieth century, and gained momentum in the postwar period, fueling hopes for many applications related to both agriculture and medicine. To Firestone, the pace of developments in the life sciences, and in particular understandings of the reproductive process, was both breathtaking and full of promise. For her, like many of the British "biofuturists" of the pre- and interwar periods, the promise of reengineering reproductive substance was at one with the broadly confident empiricist goal of deciphering the secrets of the universe. The triumph of Cartesian mechanism was at hand, offering a "full mastery of the reproductive process" no feminist worth her Ringer salts could fail to celebrate.

> Now, in 1970, we are experiencing a major scientific breakthrough. The new physics, relativity, and the astro-physical theories of contemporary science had already been realized by the first part of this century. Now, in the latter part, we are arriving, with the help of the electron microscope and other new tools, at similar achievements in biology, biochemistry, and all the life sciences. Important discoveries are made yearly . . . of the magnitude of DNA . . . or the origins of life. Full mastery of the reproductive process is in sight, and there has been significant

advance in understanding the basic life and death process. The nature of aging and growth, sleep and hibernation, the chemical functioning of the brain and the development of consciousness and memory are all beginning to be understood in their entirety. This acceleration promises to continue for another century, or however long it takes to understand the goal of Empiricism: total understanding of the laws of nature. (Firestone 1972: 180)

At the same time that Firestone advocated a much greater feminist engagement with technological progress as a means of overcoming female subordination, she was equally concerned by the rampant sexism within the sciences and made it perfectly clear that a technological revolution would be impossible without a cultural one to match. As Firestone writes in *The Dialectic of Sex*,

> The absence of women at all levels of scientific disciplines is so commonplace as to lead many (otherwise intelligent) people to attribute it to some deficiency (logic?) in women themselves. Or to women's own predilections for the emotional and the subjective over the practical and the rational. But the question cannot be so easily dismissed. It is true that women in science are in foreign territory—but how has this situation evolved? Why are there disciplines or branches of inquiry that demand only a "male" mind? . . . When and why was the female excluded from this type of mind? (1972: 154)

Although inspired by figures such as Gregory Pincus, and motivated by a Marxist-based scientific humanism similar to that of Waddington, J. D. S. Haldane, the Huxleys, Naomi Mitchison, and H. G. Wells, Firestone was, like them, all too conscious that although technology could play a role in social change, the relationship was dialectical: only in a radically changed society could new definitions of technology be born. In contrast to the oft-repeated characterization of Firestone as having put too much faith in the capacity of new reproductive technologies to liberate women, her assessment of their potential precisely anticipated that they would reinforce existing inequalities if their use were not accompanied by a radical redefinition of gender, sex, kinship, parenthood, and the family. As she presciently warned, "in the hands of our current society and under the direction of current scientists (few of whom are female or even feminist), any attempt to use technology to 'free' anybody is suspect" (1972: 206).

Indeed, on the topic of the "revolutionary" consequences of new reproductive technologies, Firestone is most accurately prescient in her prediction that they were instead much more likely to reinforce the status quo. Technology alone, however radical its possibilities, would not itself eliminate patriarchal family structures, the sexual division of labor, or the institution of marriage. And as long as these technologies of sex remained in force, embryology was likely to follow suit. Wrongly often characterized as naive, Firestone's arguments about technology (like those of her bellwethers Marx and Engels) are as focused on its propensity to fail as its potentially transformative capacities.[4]

Firestone was equally conscious of the complicated place of the female reproductive body in relation to masculinist science. It was as unlikely in her view that scientific research would become more feminized as it was that scientific research agendas would prioritize female concerns. As she noted of the history of birth control (a topic that concerned her far more than the distant prospect of cybernetic reproduction), "the kinds of research [for which] money [is] allocated . . . are only incidentally in the interests of women when at all" (1972: 197–198).

Haraway is similarly cautious about the possibility of radical scientific or technological change occurring without a corresponding transformation of social values, which is why, like Firestone, Haraway's politics explicitly foreground and prioritize a more potent and explicit feminist engagement with science and technology:

> Active feminist reconstruction of science and technology requires immersion in forms of knowledge and practice not now friendly to most women, feminist or not. But we are present and active in constructing the social relations of science and technology, like it or not. By the late 20th century, there is no choice in this matter. Our politics and livelihoods are significantly determined by science-based social orders— whether we are a clerical worker at the Lawrence Livermore weapons laboratories, an engineer on the MX project, a witch in Santa Rita jail for blockading a weapons lab, or a grocery clerk using automated inventory and check out systems. Our problem is to be less serviceable and more determining of the structure of objects of knowledge and of forms of scientific social practice. (1983: 10–11)

Haraway was initially trained as a biologist, and has often referred to the biology lab as the origin of both her love of biology and her inability to conceive of any life form as purely natural:

Politically and historically, I could never take the organism as something simply there. . . . I was extremely interested in the way the organism is an object of knowledge as a system of the production and partition of energy, or as a system of division of labor with executive functions. This is the history of the ecosystem as an object that could only have come into being in the context of resource managements, the tracking of energies through trophic layers, the tagging apparatuses made possible by the Savannah River Nuclear facilities, and the emergence of war-time inter-disciplinarities in cybernetics, nuclear chemistry and systems theories. (2006: 136)

Haraway's early penchant for unnatural histories, in other words, was politically and intellectually materialist: it stemmed from her inability to perceive ecosystems or organisms as separate from the laboratory context, or the worldly context of the lab, in which they were identified through specific means of intervention and denomination. To think otherwise proved impossible: "It was never really possible for me to inhabit biology without a kind of *impossible consciousness* of the radical historicity of these objects of knowledge. . . . For me it was always about the materialities of instrumentation of organisms and laboratories" (2006: 136, emphasis added).

Importantly for Haraway, these materialities are never "things in themselves," but always constituted through relationships—what she calls "constitutive relationalities." Everything in the lab comes into being in this way—as Latour (1987) also shows so consistently in his work.[5] These constitutive relationalities demonstrate the inextricability of the human—as a population, as individuals, or as a species—from other companion realms, including the nonhuman, the nonliving, and the machinic or synthetic domain of what Haraway calls "the built world." In this way too, technologies themselves are always already socialized—they are crucially, unmistakably, and dialectically agentic nonhuman "actants" in the lab and its hybrid onto-epistemic bench life composed of Bunsen burners, petri dishes, and the proprietary culture medium that serves as soil for the cultivation of new, increasingly quasi-human, bioproducts.

Culture Media

A good sense of the integration of living entities, including living human entities, with their tools and machines in the lab can be derived from almost any visit to one. Also notable to a novice lab visitor is the enormously disciplined choreography governing not only the use of space, equipment, and materials, but the intense attention to technique. Here, at a remove from the manifesto, and more closely in touch with the laboratory manual, a different kind of biofuture is being forged, in the context of a more quotidian kind of affinity. At the same time, the lab is a very sociable place. The most ordinary thing about these otherwise very unfamiliar settings is the banter among the staff, who, especially if they are in a clean room, inhabit each other's space like the long-term, cloistered crew of a submarine. Like artisans, they know their equipment intimately, their workshop like an extended pair of hands. Far from being excluded, in many of the stem cell labs in the United Kingdom and elsewhere in which new embryonic tools and lines are being cultivated, women scientists and lab technicians often predominate in what is a noticeably feminized arena of highly specialized bioexpertise. The culture of embryo culture in the stem cell lab is by definition highly routinized and regimented, its discipline second nature to its inhabitants. Paradoxically, it is highly sterilized, while also being dedicated to the cultivation of cellular fertility—both in terms of handling eggs and embryos that will potentially be used for treatment, and in coaxing those that have been donated to research into successful colonies of healthy stem cells. In the following extract from my field notes, I describe my first visit to the fully functioning stem cell lab at Guy's Hospital, where I was introduced to the culture of embryo culture by observing some of the basic procedures that are undertaken on a daily basis.

Field Notes, Guy's Stem Cell Lab, March 12, 2010
I arrive at the lab with my camera and am escorted in by Emma, a postdoctoral researcher, through several air locks, discarding my "street" clothes in the first one, acquiring a new sterile lab suit in the second one, and finally stepping into my new shoes. Everyone is wearing blue bunny suits, hats, masks, gloves, and sterile plastic clogs. They sterilize my camera with a special spray. It's very hot and hard to hear because of all the noisy hoods sucking in air. We go from the main (clinical) area into the smaller derivation space, known as Research Lab One, where the filtered air is even purer.

Vicky is about to show me how she amplifies the feeder cells they are using to grow the human stem cell lines they have successfully derived from embryos donated by patients in the adjacent clinic. The wells containing the feeders are kept in the incubator and Vicky is just about to get some out when another lab technician arrives at the door to the lab directly behind her. "Helen is coming in," warns Emma. (Helen enters very carefully, holding a dish of cells.) Incongruously, the incubator looks like a small refrigerator. Helen opens the door very gently and deposits her dish in one of the six heated compartments, each with its own mini-door, and swaps it for another, which she removes with the same very slow, deliberate, and concentrated comportment with which one would handle a hot bowl of soup (which it sort of is). She closes the door with one hand, holding the dish protectively with the other, and exits backwards through the lab door to cultivate her carefully guarded colony.

The six compartments in the incubator each have a separate line in them to avoid cross-contamination. The feeder plates for each line are also kept in their respective sterile quarantines. Vicky stops talking as she removes two feeder plates and a small vial of media from the incubator, moving so cautiously it looks like she is in slow motion. On the front of the incubator are magnets made of square colored photographs of embryos attaching paper notices to the top rim of the hood, beneath which Vicky seats herself, while gently setting down her plates and vial. She settles herself on the stool in front of the hood. Its glass front reaches down almost to the bench top, leaving only a few inches for her hands to go through into protected airspace. The binocular scope of the manipulation bed protrudes through the glass—separating but connecting her to what lies beneath the hood. Vicky drops her vial of fresh nutrient media into a red holder, which already holds another empty vial for the used media, and positions the dish of feeder cells in the bed of the microscope. The metal base of the hood—the bench—is heated to match the incubator temperature, as is the culture media in the vial, so that the cells do not experience a change in temperature (which they do not like). At the front of the bench is a vent, drawing air down through the hood, which has a higher air pressure inside, to minimize the risk of contamination.

Each dish contains four wells of feeder cells. The cells are stuck to the bottom of the well, and the media is on top. As the cell lines grow, they need to be passaged, namely cut into pieces and transferred to new wells with more room and new media. This is how cells are amplified—through the extremely laborious and time-consuming process of passaging them, also referred to as propagation.

Vicky opens a yellow box of fresh pipette tips and snaps one on by stabbing it with the end of her pipette. She is now going to remove the used media to discard it—one well at a time. With the pipette clamped in her right fist, she unscrews the top of the empty vial using her thumb and index finger. She then repositions her right hand to begin removing the used culture media, holding the pipette like an ice pick, her thumb on top to operate it, while with her left hand she holds the dish. Tipping the dish forward to pool the liquid media at the front of the tiny chamber, she takes three delicate sips of used media, dumping each one in the waste vial. She then removes the tip, discards it, and opens the vial of new media to begin the process of replenishing the feeder cells with fresh, carefully heated, and meticulously standardized nutrients.

"Do you have a favorite type of pipette?"

"Um, the P1000 is very handy," she says, laughing. "But we've run out of them at the moment."

"What do you like about those?"

Speaking slowly as she concentrates on transferring new media into the well, using a new tip, and holding the media-filled vial close to the dish with her left hand, she explains, "They're just easier because you can fit up to 1 ml in them, so you have a lot more range to work with."

"Oh, right, the other ones have less, so you keep having to go back and forth with them."

"Right, exactly," she says, changing tips again, and beginning the process of removing the used media from the second well, working left to right, while tipping the dish forward with her left hand.

"So each time you switch media you throw out the tip?"

"Yes, to avoid contamination, just general contamination, I use two pipette tips per well."

"It's quite handy they stick to the bottom of the well, so you don't have to worry about inhaling them."

Vicky is now working slightly faster and is on to the third well, emptying it, and then adding two big dollops of new media. Her manual dexterity is impressive: fast, confident, precise, and practiced. But the work is obviously laborious and fiddly.

"So how long have those cells been in there?"

"They have been on these plates just since yesterday. So they were plated just yesterday afternoon. They were just growing in a big flask, and then we plate them out."

"So how long will it take you to harvest these cells?"

"It takes about four–five days to get them confluent enough to make enough dishes that we need so I've got about twenty dishes out of four days' growth of a T75 flask."

"So this is a constant activity."

"Yeah, every week."

"Growing the food for your lines."

"Yeah, keeping them happy."

Keeping Them Happy

Even this very brief glimpse of daily work in a stem cell lab gives a clear sense of the inextricabilities described by Haraway—the radical sense of context that makes it impossible for her to imagine organisms as "simply there," only inhabiting their own pure, singular, and unadulterated ontology. The complex bench sociality involving living, human, nonliving, nonhuman, and machinic "companion" entities has as its animate metronome the ticking metabolisms of the bespoke colonies of human cells that are being carefully tended in this state-of-the-art propagation lab—or human hothouse. The lab is dedicated to making cell lines that can model human diseases, while also establishing a viable procedural infrastructure, standardized techniques, and quality control criteria for this production process. It is like a giant human petri dish. The viability of these interlinked projects both emerges from and relies upon a continuous evolution of technique maintained through effort, discipline, and diligence. This advanced lab, in a state of permanent symbiotic innovation and evolution, is thus both the offspring and the matrix of accumulated high-specification culture techniques, while its daily life remains largely focused on repetitive, routine, and uniquely skilled manual labor.

At one level the lab is designed to cater to the needs of cells—with its incubators, heated benches, specially prepared nutrient media, graded air, and specialized equipment. But the propagation of cells that might be used for clinical purposes also requires the cells to be subjected to procedures they "don't like," such as being moved about, exposed to light, cut up and replated, and potentially contaminated. What Haraway calls the "constitutive relationalities" of the lab are thus not only disciplined, standardized, and highly controlled (this is a world-class, bespoke laboratory incorporating state-of-the-art equipment and there is a comparatively large, very highly trained staff working here with donated human material), but these relationships can also be, by turns, intense, intimate, unpredictable, personal, boring, or exciting. Also, they frequently fail: lines go off or die, equipment gets contaminated, and computer backup systems crash. The choreography of the lab is highly specialized, rigorous, and demanding—precisely because it is dealing with the familiar trio of known knowns, known unknowns, and unknown unknowns. Every single thing that is moved into or out of the lab has to be specially selected, prepared, cleaned, and logged, using equipment that is also precisely designed, built, decontaminated, documented, and coordinated. Everything in a GMP lab has to be quality controlled (maintained to strict standards) and "process validated" (i.e., performed to a documented and reproducible protocol that is part of the lab's accreditation, and thus of the lab products' scientific, clinical, and commercial viability). At the end of the day, biological control in a GMP lab is quality control: quality-controlled biology is the name of the game in tissue engineering and regenerative medicine. The engineering model that drives this workplace requires maximum predictability and control. Even the plastics have to be low emission.

Such quality control requires constant attention to the maintenance of the highest compliance standards, in terms of not only the sterile dress code and tight protocols that must be followed by lab personnel, but also the embryologists' comportment in the lab. The adherence to a strict discipline of movement is very evident to anyone observing routine procedures in a stem cell lab, where even ordinary movements such as opening a door require intense concentration. Awkward new habits have to become ingrained through constant repetition and practice (such as performing delicate tasks wearing gloves, communicating over the noise of hoods, and breathing through face masks). This constantly evolving choreography is one in which human activity is being tightly coordinated with that of cells, machines, and tools, which all have well-established roles in the daily life of the lab's elaborate ecosystem. This is the culture of cell culture described so beautifully by Hannah Landecker (2007) in her account of "how cells became technologies." It is the legacy of what Philip Pauly (1987) describes as the "engineering ideal in biology," or Adele Clarke (1998) calls the "disciplining" of reproduction. The cells, the cultivation of which is the lab's main function, are both instruments and products: the feeder plates are the carefully prepared soil on which the human embryonic cell lines will be propagated. The clean human stem cells, which are the viable offspring of highly evolved techniques, themselves become tools when they are employed to model rare human genetic diseases such as Huntington's or Tay-Sachs. The complex quotidian labor of lab technicians, with their stylized, repetitive, slowed-down, tooled-up, bespoke systems and cycles, connecting humans, cells, and machines, is both thoroughly technoscientific and thoroughly human. Even the tools are human in this biotechnological ecosystem, where life is being grown to order, just like forced rhubarb in a heated potting shed.

It is noticeable too how even in this ultramodern lab, full of noisy respiring machinery, there is also a profound sense of craft—indeed traditional manual craftsmanship, in the sense Richard Sennett (2008) discusses in his monograph widening our awareness of the still-pervasive artisanal culture of craftwork even in the high-tech industries where it is imagined to have disappeared. The art of propagating cell cultures evokes a sense of both traditional and communitarian pride in work that depends for its success on being undertaken to the very highest standards by a team, and thus, to a certain extent, and in spite of the rampant commercialism of high or late capitalism, for itself. A sense of satisfaction in what the practiced "green" hands of a skilled propagator can do (with or without a P1000) is constantly evident in the stem cell lab, where, as we shall see below, live toolmaking over the forge is still routine. Such handmade tools are crucial to the ultraprecise work of lab technicians, whose care for the cells, and skilled manipulation of them, is ideally manifest as successful growth—as in horticulture.

Field Notes, Guy's Stem Cell Lab, March 12, 2010
Emma next shows me how to passage a cell line, initially by placing it in the bed of the bench microscope, which is attached to a video screen. Pointing to the sea of blue on the screen, she explains her procedure, pointing out the feeder cells, the colonies of stem cells, the dead cells that are coming off the established colonies, and the method she will use to cut these up with a handmade microtool to establish new colonies in new plates.

"So every day we come in to inspect our cell lines, to see if they need any care or attention. We come in and check them daily. On the screen you can see the feeders all the way around the edge here. And then the colonies of stem cells growing on top of those feeder cells. The feeders are these long, thin cells, all around the outside, and then you can just about see there the defined edge of a colony. That's one colony, and that's another there (she points to lumpy, round islands of stem cells). One here, and one there. So the dark bits that you can see are cells that are beginning to die, and they curl up, lift off, and go into suspension. And that happens when the colonies get big enough to be cut up and moved onto fresh feeders. So I'm about to passage these, and what I will do is use a glass pipette, and I will score through the colonies like that (she traces a cross-hatch pattern with her index finger on the screen), and then each of those separate sections gets put into a fresh dish to regrow again, exponentially, to give me, hopefully, six colonies out of each one."

"So how old is this line?"

"This line? This line was derived in about June last year. So it's only eight months old."

"And how come there are four colonies?"

"We replate, so, once I chop this one up into maybe six, I'll move all of those into another well, so all six of those will grow and give me another colony."

"So, did this start out as six pieces and now it is four pieces? Or there were only four pieces to begin with?"

She scans the well for other colonies. "I think in this one there were only four. So it was probably a smaller colony that we didn't cut up quite so much."

"I see, I see, because they grow at different rates, so . . ."

"Yes."

"I guess that's part of the art—you know how many pieces to cut it into."

"It does take time, yes, to see what they're doing, knowing when they're happy, knowing when there's something wrong, when to cut them, when to leave them, when to add a bit of extra something in the media."

"Is this a happy one?"

"This is a happy one, yes." She pauses, nodding, looking at the screen. "Yep, this one. Because we, ah, try whenever possible," she pauses and turns to look at me, somewhat self-consciously, "not to come in every weekend. So I am cutting this one up today, so it will be happy for a couple of days, so when I come in on Monday, it will be ready to go again."

"So they are happy because they are growing steadily and regularly."

"And the morphology is very good."

"Right."

"So I am just going to pop these in again, while I get ready to passage them."

She picks up the two dishes and puts them very carefully back into the incubator.

"So they are probably not happy if they get moved around too much?"

"When you have just passaged them, they really are very delicate, but once they're attached to the plate like that, they're not so sensitive. But because we have got so many lines growing, and people are passaging on different days, it's best practice just to always be very careful. Like even just shutting the door very carefully (she makes a very slow, gentle movement with her arm, as if shutting the door in slow motion), so you don't disturb anything that's growing."

"So you always have to be very gentle."

"Yes, always assume there is something in there that needs extra attention."

"Well you are obviously very good at it, because you get a lot of lines."

Emma's knowledge of her lines, and their needs, is crucial both in order to grow high-quality cells, and to give her some control over her own time. She and her team check their cells daily in order to see "if they need any care or attention." But she also needs the cells to be especially "happy" over the weekend so she can have some time off herself. She knows when they are happy, or not, both by their appearance and through her own experience over many years of cultivating cells under tightly controlled conditions. Consequently she is also aware of how much she doesn't know about their needs, and for both of these reasons much of her work is performed as an extreme discipline of care: "it's best practice just to always be very careful," and to assume that some of the cells might need "extra attention." It takes time to develop this sort of relationship with the cells—to come to know and understand their likes and dislikes. As in any relationship, it is important to know when they need a bit of attention and when they need to be left alone (and especially how to treat them right if you are going to abandon them for the weekend).

Emma's relationship to the cells is heavily mediated by machinery, including the incubator, the bench, and the microscope. Her ability to culture her lines successfully depends on all of these, and in particular the video screen that is attached to the microscope. Although sophisticated—indeed, state of the art—the machinery is also crude: she can see the outlines of the cells, and enough to cut up the colony into pieces to replate it, but she cannot see any of the crucial metabolic processes that would tell her if the cell is truly happy.

In a sense, Emma can know her machines better than her cells: she can diagnose and repair a broken incubator more easily than a contaminated cell line, or one that simply fails to thrive. Similarly, she can know her lab team well enough to diagnose changes in their routine that might be necessary, and these can be communicated, implemented, rationalized, debated, changed, or written down as instructions. The relationalities of the clean lab are all about this kind of intense coordination between humans, their machines, and their work objects—indeed it is the fusion of these three that creates what Landecker describes as "technologies of living substance" (2007: 1).

Lively Relations

For Haraway, as for Marx, it is the situated character of the "constitutive relationalities" out of which new entities, such as human stem cell lines, make "the human" a necessarily historical category, but by its very hybridity also establishes new forms of "kinship" connecting humans, organisms, tools, "and much else." As Haraway claims: "'Human' requires an extraordinary congeries of partners. Humans, wherever you track them, are products of situated relationalities with organisms, tools, much else. We are quite a crowd, at all of our temporalities and materialities. . . . How many species are in the genus Homo now? Lots. And there are several genera for our close and ancestral parallel kin as well" (2006: 146). Haraway's emphasis on the hybrid historicity of the human acknowledges both novelty and continuity. Recollecting the sense of the liveliness of tools, tool use, and technique that pervades the writing of both Marx and Haraway, we might note this is a crucial feature of how they both theorize technology—and thus be reminded that this is why the evolution of technique reveals deep historical continuities despite the fact that it is often changing radically. In the same way that relationality is described by both Haraway and Marx as the smallest unit of analysis in the study of human sociality, so too this could be said of technological devices, which are always part of larger systems—the vital linchpins, cogs, crankshafts, axles, or pumps always already interrelated through a kinship with their wider machinic environment. In terms of the "exact mechanisms" by which the stem cell lab functions, what is notable is the tight integration between them—uniting human gestures and tools, tools and cells, machines and equipment, and the calibrating of the timing and sequence of their functions.

The manual labor of the lab workers is also reminiscent of the synergy between the human body and the machine described earlier by Marx. This proximity is one of the original contexts of posthuman anxiety, as it also is for transhuman or cybernetic optimism. For Marx, the situation was unquestionably human — no less than heroic, even — but also almost superhuman in its symbiotic vigor.[6] Indeed, it is the liveliness and vitality of the lab environment that recalls the way in which Marx conceived of technology both as a kind of organism and as alive, which in turn comprise core elements of his (very early) theorization of the human as a technology. "He opposes himself to Nature as one of her own forces, setting in motion arms and leg, head and hands, the natural forces of his body, in order to appropriate Nature's productions in a form adapted to his own wants. By thus acting on the external world and changing it, he at the same time changes his own nature" (MECW, Vol. 35, *Capital*, Vol. 1, Book 1, C 7, section 1).

According to the technological dialectic at the heart of Marxist theory, humans are allied with their environment through tools; the environment is revitalized through human activity; and both are substantially reshaped as both nature and human nature are remade and instrumentalized. (There could hardly be a better description of a stem cell lab.) In the Marxist model of labor, humans are part of the force of nature, but in turn humanize nature, by adapting it to their own wants, thus also changing themselves (add instruments, raw substances, and machines and you have the basic ecosystem of historical materialism). Had Marx, instead of Foucault, coined the phrase "life itself," it would have described the fusion of human and tool, rather than of human and animal (indeed, this is arguably what he did, according to Bernard Stiegler [1998]). In contrast to the anthropocentrism of some of his depictions of the human-machine relation, there are hints in other passages of the greater emphasis on the agency of objects too, as has been emphasized within some branches of science studies (such as the work of Latour). As noted in the introduction to this volume, Marx describes the earth as both an organ and a tool house annexed to his own organs:

> Thus Nature becomes one of the organs of his activity, one that he annexes to his own bodily organs, adding stature to himself in spite of the Bible. As the earth is his original larder, so too it is his original tool house. It supplies him, for instance, with stones for throwing, grinding, pressing, cutting, etc. The earth itself is an instrument of labour,

but when used as such in agriculture implies a whole series of other instruments and a comparatively high development of labour. No sooner does labour undergo the least development, than it requires specially prepared instruments. Thus in the oldest caves we find stone implements and weapons. In the earliest period of human history domesticated animals, i.e., animals which have been bred for the purpose, and have undergone modifications by means of labour, play the chief part as instruments of labour along with specially prepared stones, wood, bones, and shells. (MECW, Vol. 35, *Capital*, Vol. 1, Book 1, C 7, section 1)

Contrary to Scripture, according to Marx, the earth is a paradise for homo faber—the earth "his original larder" and itself "an instrument of labor." Yet his description also moves beyond the notion of nature as mere supply, in particular in his reference to the increasingly complex "development" of labor's relationships to its instruments and objects. In a distinctly anatomical idiom, which acquires new implications in the context of regenerative medicine and stem cell science, Marx describes mechanical tools as the "bones and muscles" of production, and more primitive tools, such as baskets and jars, as its "vascular system"—thus imagining the productive economy as the outcome of increasing development and specialization of organs. "Among the instruments of labour, those of a mechanical nature, which, taken as a whole, we may call the bone and muscles of production, offer much more decided characteristics of a given epoch of production, than those which, like pipes, tubs, baskets, jars, etc., serve only to hold the materials for labour, which latter class, we may in a general way, call the vascular system of production. The latter first begins to play an important part in the chemical industries" (MECW, Vol. 35, *Capital*, Vol. 1, Book 1, C 7, section 1).

Widening his evolutionary vision to include the "conductors of activity" necessary for the labor process to function, Marx describes the earth not only as a larder but as an instrument—a prosthetic technology functioning as a "*locus standi* to the laborer and a field of employment for his activity": in sum, less a "standing reserve" in the Heideggerian sense than a live earth stock ready to be quickened into productive purpose by the laborer's activity.[7]

In a wider sense we may include among the instruments of labour, in addition to those things that are used for directly transferring labour to its subject, and which therefore, in one way or another, serve as conductors of activity, all such objects as are necessary for carrying on the labour-process. These do not enter directly into the process, but without them it is either impossible for it to take place at all, or possible only to a partial extent. Once more we find the earth to be a universal instrument of this sort, for it furnishes a *locus standi* to the labourer and a field of employment for his activity. Among instruments that are the result of previous labour and also belong to this class, we find workshops, canals, roads, and so forth. (MECW, Vol. 35, *Capital*, Vol. 1, Book 1, C 7, section 1)

In a particularly notable passage referring to "labor's organism," Marx describes the extraction of use value out of brute nature as regeneration, and imagines the living laborer rousing the rusted machine from its "death-sleep" through his "fire." This aspect of labor—its role in activating both machines and materials—describes not only the outcome of the labor process, but its "elementary constituents." It is out of these connections—between labor, technology, its energy, and its objects, that "things" are "made alive" by "labor's organism":

> A machine which does not serve the purposes of labour is useless. In addition it falls prey to the destructive influence of natural forces. Iron rusts and wood rots. Yarn with which we neither weave nor knit, is cotton wasted. Living labour must seize upon these things and rouse them from their death-sleep, change them from mere possible use-values into real and effective ones. Bathed in the fire of labour, appropriated as part and parcel of labour's organism, and, as it were, made alive for the performance of their functions in the process, they are in truth consumed, but consumed with a purpose, as elementary constituents of new use-values, of new products, ever ready as means of subsistence for individual consumption, or as means of production for some new labour-process. (MECW, Vol. 35, *Capital*, Vol. 1, Book 1, C 7, section 1)

At the heart of this complex set of analogies, in which machines are depicted as prey to the destructive, passive, entropic waste imposed by nature, against which living labor is depicted as rousing and seizing the machine to make it live again, is a vivid reproductive imagery, in which it is the coupling together of things with labor that produces a new kind of life. This feature of Marx's depiction of labor's connection to its objects is most explicitly captured in the semimythic, quasi-procreative image of the blacksmith at his forge. As Marx puts it succinctly: "The blacksmith forges and the product is a forging" (echoing Engels's [1962: 81] similar claim that the human hand is not only an organ of labor but a product of it). In Marx's archetypal, neoclassical, and pre-Christian image of the forge, "labor's organism" is depicted not only as the offspring of a historical materialist system, but of a natural historical, or even biological one (not unlike Darwin's) in which machines, instruments, materials, and tools are "made alive" again through use (as he notes later in Volume 1 of *Capital*, "labor-power in use is labor itself," Marx [1990]: 283). "In the labour-process, therefore, man's activity, with the help of the instruments of labour, effects an alteration, designed from the commencement, in the material worked upon. The process disappears in the product, the latter is a use-value. . . . Labour has incorporated itself with its subject: the former is materialised, the latter transformed. That which in the labourer appeared as movement, now appears in the product as a fixed quality without motion. The blacksmith forges and the product is a forging" (MECW, Vol. 35, *Capital*, Vol. 1, Book 1, C 7, section 1). The power to give life through movement is analogized to the blacksmith's ability to forge new tools in this figurative comparison representing the laborer's ability—indeed imperative—to "take in hand," to mind, to shepherd the idle, wasted natural potential that is equated with death.[8] In this version of labor as reanimation there is a continuum between anthropocentrism (function, efficiency), instrumentality (tools), nature (resources), and generativity (animation, development). As Marx makes clear, the action (force, cause) is dialectical—humans are reshaped by the reshaping they do, ditto the machines, the material, and the environment. And this process is also situated, or concretized: each tool is made as part of a larger system and as the outcome of a specific history, the traces of which it bears, and which hold it in place, giving it its biology, or genome, as it were.

Marx's model of the living labor that quickens nature's elementary resources into useful animate existence is historically cumulative, and, like Darwin's model of natural history, tools, bodies, and materials are molded and adapted through live action. Concrete technological forms, like species, evolve in this process of gradual transformation through the filter of labor:

> Though a use-value, in the form of a product, issues from the labour-process, yet other use-values, products of previous labour, enter into it as means of production. The same-use-value is both the product of a previous process, and a means of production in a later process. Products are therefore not only results, but also essential conditions of labour.
>
> With the exception of the extractive industries, in which the material for labour is provided immediately by Nature, such as mining, hunting, fishing, and agriculture (so far as the latter is confined to breaking up virgin soil), all branches of industry manipulate raw material, [including] objects already filtered through labour, [or] already products of labour. Such is seed in agriculture. Animals and plants, which we

are accustomed to consider as products of Nature, are in their present form, not only products of, say last year's labour, but the result of *a gradual transformation*, continued through many generations. (MECW, Vol. 35, *Capital*, Vol. 1, Book 1, C 7, section 1, emphasis added)

In this passage, both the materials and the instruments of "living labor" are depicted as evolving "through many generations" so as to acquire their present form. This sense of the traces of the human hand can likewise be seen in the Darwinian model of natural selection, which was derived less from his account of either sexual selection or competition than from selective breeding—or what he called the influence of "the breeder's hand." Likewise, it is the propagator's hand in the stem cell lab that is refashioning natural organisms as tools, in what is an increasingly hybrid technological matrix. Against the image of the "invisible hand" of economic competition proposed by Adam Smith, Marx offers the forge at work making forgings, the blacksmith's hand at work leaving traces, echoed today by the handmade cells fueling the microscopic productive economies of bioindustrialization.

Field Notes, Guy's Stem Cell Lab, March 10, 2010
While the colonies waiting to be passaged sit in the incubator, Emma prepares her tools. She is standing in front of an eleventh-floor window overlooking south London in her clean room uniform: dark blue body suit, white-gloved hands, light blue head cap and mask, blue lab shoes. Several boxes of pipette tips and a small forest of vials in stands adorn the shelves beside her, while a cluster of electric appliances and a pile of spiral-bound notebooks sit on the countertop below. Emma removes a small glass alcohol burner from the shelf and casually ignites it with a plastic cigarette lighter. "So there are various ways to passage the cells," she begins, explaining that: "Passaging means lifting them up off their current feeder layer and placing them onto a fresh one. I prefer to use a glass pipette. Other people will use some other tool, some tips, or needles; there are various methods that have been developed in different labs." As she speaks she inserts a thin glass tube into the flame and begins heating it until it is soft enough to pull into an even thinner strand.

"Do you like to make your own pipettes?"

"I prefer it because your end is really, really fine" (she inspects the end of her newly made pipette and delicately props it into a plastic stand alongside three others). "And when you have pulled about 400 and you're quick at it (she caps the flame, extinguishing it, and replaces the burner on the shelf) you can get a whole range of tips—some with very sharp corners on them, some that are slightly fatter or some that are slightly thinner, so that I can use the one that's most appropriate for the cells I am cutting." She picks up the pipette stand carefully with both hands and turns around to face the hood.

"So is it a little old fashioned to make them that way? Is that considered what you might call a traditional way to do it?"

"I think it's fairly common, and I think probably for me, coming from embryology, [it's normal] that you make your own pipettes. The problem we have with all of the methods people use at the moment is none of them qualify for GMP. Because it has to be a medical product, and if you can't record [exactly what] it [is] (she gestures to the pipettes) it's no longer a medical product. So we are going to have to find a different way of doing this, for GMP."

"If you pulled one yourself that you quite liked, could you then give it to a company and they could manufacture one just like it?"

"We have done that actually, um, there was someone who worked with a company to make tips like the biopsy and the ICSI pipettes, [which] are made by a company now. We don't make our own, but it is the same idea. If we can make them in a standardized way, we could overcome the problem of their not being a product. The problem is that not enough people are buying them. So they cost about six pounds each. And I've got four there, to do one plate, and you multiply that by the number of plates you're going to use (she starts shaking her head) and it's just going to get astronomical. But the idea is spot on. That's what we are trying to do. So it is in a packet, and sterilized."[9]

"Because to process validate it for GMP you have to document its origin."

"What has happened to it, where does it come from."

"So I am just going to get that dish again."

She walks to the incubator and carefully removes the dish of stem cells from the top right-hand corner compartment, and a feeder dish from the bottom left, closing the doors to each compartment, and the unit, with almost glacial slowness.

"So I have the dish with the stem cells, and the dish with the feeder. And everything stays within the heated area of the surface so that they stay warm. And we have the phenyl red indicator in the media so that we can see if they have been out too long. Because if it goes really, really pink we know it is time to put them back in. It means that they are becoming too alkaline because you are losing the CO_2. So it's coming back out. Because they are in 6 percent in the incubator. So they lose their CO_2 after a while."

She focuses the microscope on the dish, which is illuminated from below by a light built into the bench — a well beneath a well. Turning away from the microscope view piece, she carefully inspects her pipettes, examining them with her naked eye, and putting two back before settling on a third — a bit like a snooker player selecting a cue.

"So I just pick the one I like the look of most to start with."

She is stabilizing the dish with her left index finger and thumb, while holding the chosen pipette in her right hand like a pencil. She could be about to sign her name on the stem cell colony.

"And I go in and score them into pieces that I think are the right size. And then because the pipettes are in the shape of a hook, I can use the bottom of the hook to gently lift them off the feeders."

"Right. So you can score and hook with the same tool?"

"Yep, that's why I like using them."

"So do they stick to the feeders?"

"If they are beautifully undifferentiated and good-quality colonies, then they generally come off very easily. If they've started to differentiate then because the cells — if they start making contact with each other, and start making contact with feeders, and the intracellular matrix becomes quite strong, then they become very sticky."

"So you can almost also begin — not to characterize them exactly, but to learn about them by the feel of how much they stick?"

"Yes, for me it is definitely a fifty-fifty combination between how do they look and how do they feel. And then I know if they are good quality or not, and then I know what to do with them."

"So it is partly what you can see and it's partly what you just get a sense of by manipulating them."

"Yes, and then the ones that are, generally, the ones that come away really nicely and [are] good quality I put in a well together. The ones that aren't so nice go in a well together, so that you know where your perfect ones are."

"So you are kind of sorting them as you go along."

"Yes. So then if you get some with not such good growth in one of your wells you know that it's because you didn't start off with particularly brilliant cells. So the ones I've just cut I'm going to transfer into a fresh feeder plate. So we label the plate with the ID of the cell line, and the date, and the passage number. And these were passage 6, so they are now passage 7. That gets labeled first. And then we just use a yellow tip. And suck up the pieces one by one."

"And move six pieces to each well?"

"Yes, we will put them all in here together. And then I would repeat that for all of the colonies that are ready in that batch. Then they go back in the incubator. And we leave them untouched for about forty-eight hours. So they have plenty of time to stick, spread out, be happy. And then we check them, and we feed them and keep our records in our lab books."

"So they won't be hugely happy right now. But they might get quite happy over the weekend?"

"Yes. Yes."

"And by Monday they should be very cheerful."

"Yes, by Monday they should."

"Great, and then you can start again!"

"It is continuous!"

In the same way the organism was reenvisaged as a lab at the origins of synthetic chemistry (and the cell as a technology at the dawn of tissue culture), so too in stem cell labs today are some of the oldest manufacturing processes, such as the forging of tools, still in use in the context of contemporary bioscience. The primordial arts of forged tool manufacture aid the propagator's hand in what has become a vast project of recultivating human cellular efficiency—a key sector of today's bioeconomy. This neoagricultural technology of assisted generation is not one in which either tools or materials exist independently of their histories or immediate, and more distant, contexts of use.

The hand-forged hook pipettes evoke the early agricultural tools so crucial to Marx's definition of capital as stock, and of capitalism as the linkage of inanimate stocks of techniques, machines, devices, and tools to the live stocks

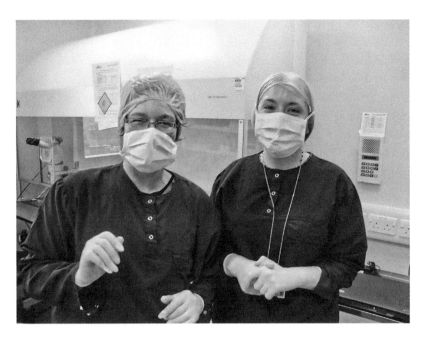

FIGURE 2.1. The author with Emma in the lab. Photo by the author.

of selectively bred crops (cotton, corn) and domesticated animals (cattle). The lifeblood of this system was human labor and the accumulated technical expertise needed for manufacture. Its vasculature was the infrastructure of roads, buildings, canals, storehouses, and transport vehicles. This is exactly what is happening in the bioindustrial revolution today, in which new automated machinery plays a crucial role alongside delicate, bespoke, handmade surgical tools for micromanipulation and cellular reconstruction. The crucial shift that will next take place will be successful financialization of this sector, and thus commercialization. DHL and FedEx will be as crucial to the regenerative medicine market as proprietary culture media and P1000 pipettes. Already the hospital infrastructure for replacement parts markets is being established in the form of new telerobotic virtual surgeries that can operate on a global scale. This too will be part of the crucial step change in scale needed to fully industrialize human biological products, just as it was for cotton and wool in the 1800s.

Fueling this scale-up in the ability to rebuild human beings will not be any one particular sector or component or entrepreneur or technique, but their integration. The quasi-organismic quality of successful industrial systems, which become increasingly systemic as they develop in scale and degree of internal organization, is not a new phenomenon—as Marx's eyewitness accounts of an earlier period of intense industrialization attest. Neither are the outcomes of such dramatic changes in mode of production unprecedented—indeed they are by now cliché.

The main difference in the stem cell lab is that "labor's organism" is being forged through a new fusion of the human and human reproductive substance as equipment. Not only are living human laborers making live human tools out of living human colonies of cells, but this project, and myriad like it all over the world, is being undertaken in the name of the most humanitarian of purposes—to provide improved health for future generations. In Marx's terms, this task is also being undertaken for the purpose of "labor itself"—still a very relevant model, since cells in general, and human cells in particular, are increasingly being recruited for their untapped labor power. Indeed, the new lab is exclusively dedicated to their preservation, in order that they be more efficiently harnessed into service for an ever-widening range of purposes.

These purposes include the effort to establish new markets, as chapter 1 demonstrated, by emphasizing government support for this new industry—as yet not a major, or even significant, source of new commodities. It will remain to be seen how effectively the development of new human tools purpose built to improve human health or new human stem cell labs designed to convert human reproductive substance into marketable products can be converted into a successful integration of public health objectives supported by private sector markets. For now, in the absence of a market in human stem cell products, the empirical question that is arguably part of the effort to chart the emerging political economy of biocapital is simply the relationship between tool, labor, and stock.

This is where both Marx and Haraway's perspectives are especially helpful in identifying the kinds of questions we might ask of the new living human tools being manufactured in laboratories worldwide. In particular, what is helpful to understand about these newly technologized substances is their complex biological relations, manifest as both specific modes of reproduction and renaturalization as technologies of kinship. In order to parse the complex moral, economic, and political questions that will attend to the mass marketing of human stem cell products, and other tissue and cell commodities, it is arguably important to recognize how much this economy depends upon a retooling of kinship and reproduction, as well as of cells and substances.

"The Best Tool You Can Get"

As Haraway notes in her account of new genetic technologies, one of the most important tools at work in the conversion of living substance into either a commodity or tool is the scientific model. "Models," she argues, are powerful conversion devices, "instruments built to be engaged, inhabited, lived" (Haraway 1997: 135). It is a similarly central premise of this book that the logic of IVF is powerful not only because IVF provides a working model of a reproductive mechanism, or because this model is itself productive of new offspring—and thus a means of reproduction, as well as a depiction of it. In vitro fertilization is a powerful model in the synthetic sense, in that it is not only a bridge between theory and practice, between in vivo and in vitro, between imagining and touching. It is a model that has become a platform—a globally disseminated platform with a life of its own, now serving science, medicine, industry, the media, government, and even the entertainment industry. Through this model a kinship is established also to the most intimate features of family life—indeed the basis of family life itself, in the form of producing biological offspring.

Yet while the modeling role of IVF is already, for all of these reasons, a singularly compelling example of Haraway's claim that "fundamentally, models are more interesting in technoscience than metaphors" (1997: 135), there is still more to its significance in the realms of bioscience, where the connections between IVF and modeling appear to grow ever more complex. More than a model either "of" or "for," in Clifford Geertz's (1966: 56) terms, IVF is a source model, or stem, for new generations of models and modeling. It is an example of what Haraway (1997: 135) describes as one of the "lively matrices" of technoscience. At the IVF–stem cell interface are new connections of shared reproductive substance to both tools and the ethical protocols that govern their use to intervene in genetic diseases. The new dish technologies being manufactured in labs connected to IVF clinics rely not only upon new biological connections to tools as offspring, but new technological definitions of being human. At the same time, tools are differently humanized through this process. As we trace the provenance of a human dish model of disease, we thus follow an increasingly familiar path of engineered human reproductive substance—brought into being, as before, through a union of reproductive hope, future promise, and scientific innovation. To make what the scientific director of the Guy's Stem Cell Lab describes (below) as "the best tool you can get" to develop cures for genetic disease, a dish model of that condition derived directly from an affected human embryo is beyond compare.

Making Natural Human Mutation Models for Science and Industry
Dr. Dusko Ilic, senior lecturer in stem cell science in the Guy's Stem Cell Lab, explains to me why human embryonic stem cell models of disease ("dish models") are "the best tool you can get."

SF: So maybe if you could just give me an idea of what the advantages of a dish model would be, say compared to an animal model?

DI: So if you are talking about different monogenic diseases, they can be modeled the best with human embryonic stem cells or induced pluripotent cells. These cells can be differentiated into different cell types such as neurons, muscle cells, or whatever is the cell type that carries the most pathology. With these cells we can then model disease in vitro, in the laboratory. The advantage of this system when compared with animal models is working in the human system avoids species-specific differences. Although animal models are invaluable and irreplaceable for studying disease in a whole-body context, they provide a limited representation of human pathophysiology. In addition, stem cells are an ideal tool to reduce the number of animals, complexity, and costs associated with animal experiments in drug development and toxicology.

SF: So if you were looking at a particular mutation, would it be an advantage that the mutation was, as it were, a natural mutation as opposed to say a knock-in mutation in a mouse?

DI: It would from one point. I mean, there is no difference whether mutation occurs naturally or it is generated in the lab. As I mentioned, animals cannot replicate everything that is going [on] in the humans and obviously the best way that you can do lab work is with a human source of cells. It is still technically challenging to make specific mutations in human embryonic stem cells. This is easy to do in mouse, because mouse embryonic stem cells are more prone to homologous recombination, et cetera. You can do knock-in technologies or knock out genes. In human cells it is almost impossible and has a very, very, very [much] lower efficacy, so that is why we are aiming to get natural mutations.

SF: Right, right, right. So that is why you would be using PGD [pre-implantation genetic diagnosis] embryos.

DI: Absolutely. Absolutely. So those embryos, and cells from those embryos, they can be used. They are clinically unsuitable, and they are not used. And so the other option would be just discarding them. Like this they can be converted into very, very useful tools to address mechanisms of disease and also be a very good model for potential drug discovery. If you get a new drug, develop a new drug, you want to see how harmful or how beneficial the drug is, for this particular disease. Currently tests are done in animal cell lines, which are not the same as humans, as I mentioned before, or in human lines that are transformed that carry various mutations and that are more closer to malignant cells than to normal. Thus, the data may not be as clear and strong as one would wish. Therefore, cell lines derived from PGD embryos are actually the best tool that you can get.

At work in this description of why harnessing natural mutations is far preferable to using animal cells or microbiology models are both a highly technical and a commonsense logic—just as in the case of IVF, which relies on a similar combination of obvious mimesis and alteration. Not surprisingly, models of genetic disease made from embryos donated by couples undergoing PGD, in order to avoid commencing a pregnancy with an embryo affected by serious genetic disease, are superior to those using either nonhuman animal cells or subcellular protocols. It is precisely this logic that compels many PGD patients to donate these embryos to research scientists working on means to treat serious genetic diseases that are often fatal. Most of Emma's lines are thus derived from the context of PGD—a technique that was developed via IVF, but also a therapeutic procedure that was crucial in the social legitimation of IVF in the U.K. (its potential use for the alleviation of genetic disease as well as of infertility strengthening the case for the legalization of human embryo research in the 1980s; see Franklin and Roberts [2006]).

People working in the lab are very conscious of the combined reasons why the human reproductive substance they are using is "special": it is scientifically unique ("the best") and also personally unique (it comes from a couple having treatment). At the heart of the merging of the world of IVF (its history, its logic, its technical pedigree, and its evolution as a research platform) with stem cell research, in a future-oriented lab built like a giant human petri dish, to hothouse new mechanisms for human repair, is thus a new kind of kinship linking reproductive substance to regenerative medicine—a biological kinship through which this substance is shared, cultured, and reproduced technologically. The dish model of disease that results—the human model that is better because it is naturally human, the model that is "the best tool you can get"—is not just a model of molecular pathways, or a model of human disease. It is a model, and even a proof, of a promissory future, in which the tool kit of human biology is put to work more efficiently and economically. It is thus not only a model tool, but a conception model of the visionary promise of human repair forged in human cells (Franklin 2013). If it is thus also a new model of technology as kinship, and of kinship as technology, it might also be a useful looking glass into the question of what it means to be "after IVF" in all of the senses of this term.

Conclusion

From all of the perspectives rehearsed in the past two chapters, we can see how the logic of IVF is at once that of technology and yet also transformative of how we understand this important term sociologically and historically, as well as philosophically. Echoing many of the arguments within science and technology studies, IVF emerges as a case study in both biosociality and bio-power, while also extending some of the more established meanings of these terms. Similarly, "reproductive technology" is widened to include more than fertility treatment, to encompass a process that can be instructively observed both close up and from the distance of as far away as Marx's understandings of the human-tool-substance relationships that informed his account of the emergence of industrial manufacturing technologies. As Haraway's description of technoscience as a world dependent upon, and emergent through, the formation of newly hybridized historical kinships of biological connections and living tools suggests, the social relationships that comprise the smallest unit of analysis are never separate from the workings of the technological systems that may appear to have an independent, reified existence as forces in the world.

If, as I have attempted to show in this chapter, the IVF–stem cell interface reveals not only how new technologies of reproductive substance emerge out of established norms, but also how the logics of these norms evolve and change. A more specific question is how the traffic through the hole in the wall can yield some insight into what kind of making of what kind of life is occurring as this novel gateway delivers new biological technologies. How does the life of the lab relate to the life being cultured inside it—what originary technics animate the reproduction of living tools? How are these received and translated, and what are they pointed toward? In the following chapters, some of the exact mechanisms by which we might begin to approach these

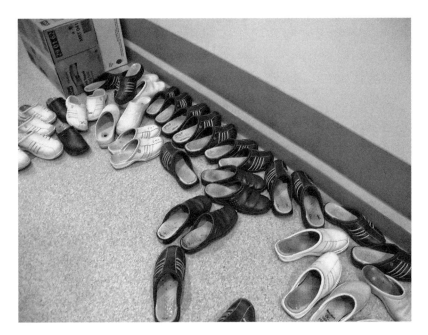

FIGURE 2.2. All members of the lab have their own clean shoes that are left in the changing area when they leave the lab. Photo by the author.

questions of technological life are explored with a view to foregrounding a richer intersection between them. It is from these perspectives that the promise of both Haraway's and Firestone's technological politics can be more fully realized, particularly in terms of their attention to the intersections of sex, gender, kinship, reproduction, and science. It is in the space of the widened biological relations these entail that we can better understand and characterize the condition of being after IVF.

THREE Embryo Pioneers

On November 17, 1944, U.S. president Franklin Delano Roosevelt commissioned a report from the Office of Scientific Research and Development intended to "make known to the world as soon as possible the contributions which have been made during our war effort to scientific knowledge." His intentions were both reparative and translational. As one of his last acts in office, the author of the New Deal sought to turn swords into plowshares by bringing the science of war into the service of peace, "with particular reference to the war of science against disease" and an emphasis on "what the government can do now and in the future to aid research" (Roosevelt 1944). The resulting report, "Science—the Endless Frontier," authored by Vannevar Bush, head of the Office of Scientific Research and Development, was published in Washington in 1945, shortly after Roosevelt's death and just before news of the atomic bomb was released to the American public.[1] An "instant smash hit," as one of Bush's colleagues is reported to have remarked on the day following its release (Kevles 1977: 23), the report's contents would not only guide science policy in the United States throughout the twentieth century and beyond, but would define an enduring worldwide ethos—and lasting idiom—for the scientific pursuit of the unknown in the name of the public good.[2]

Roosevelt's letter introduced the now-famous frontier analogy that would guide his final mission on behalf of science. Evoking the spirit of national repair that infused many of his speeches during the Depression era, he imagined the progress of science as a new American frontier. The letter ended with a call for a new kind of pioneering on the "frontiers of the mind": "New frontiers of the mind are before us, and if they are pioneered with the same vision, boldness, and drive with which we have waged this war we can create a fuller and more fruitful employment and a fuller and more fruitful life" (Roosevelt 1944). Bush began his ensuing report with reference to the defining historic role of the U.S. government of protecting access to new frontiers, claiming it was an "American tradition" that "has made the United States great": "It has been basic United States policy that Government should foster the opening of new frontiers. It opened the seas to clipper ships and furnished land for pioneers. It is in keeping with the American tradition—one that has made the United States great—that new frontiers shall be made accessible for development by all American citizens" (Bush 1945).

Bush was an engineer from New England, educated at MIT, and deeply involved in the scientific contributions to U.S. military efforts during both world wars. He later became the first director of the National Science Foundation in 1950, on which organization's website his famous report remains prominently accessible more than half a century later. The American frontier analogy he was bequeathed by Roosevelt to guide his task of redefining the postwar role of American science would quickly become one of the most frequently employed idioms to describe the pursuit of scientific knowledge and discovery, as well as the translation of science into useful applications, now defined by the National Science Foundation as the "critical path."[3] Today the frontier analogy is ubiquitous in descriptions of scientific exploration, and is virtually synonymous with scientific discovery. It is the dominant trope of many countries' science policy discourse, and much academic scholarship on science as well as media coverage, corporate mission statements, and product advertising. Everything from stem cells to nanotechnology is today described as a new frontier—indeed it might be even argued the concept of the frontier has been reborn in these contexts (see figure 3.1).[4]

The Reproductive Frontier

Reproductive biomedicine is a good example of a twentieth-century science that came of age on the postwar scientific frontier mapped out by Bush. Indeed, given its agricultural origins and often pragmatic aims, reproductive biology could be a poster science for the frontier ethos on which Bush's report is based. Control of reproduction, or what Philip Pauly calls "culturing nature," was a prominent American frontier concern because of its importance to both horticulture and husbandry during the transition from settlement to industrialization.[5] To a large extent it was an experimental science that began on the farm in the form of agricultural improvement—or what Deborah Fitzgerald (1990) calls "the business of breeding." Both plant and animal reproduction were dominant concerns at newly formed, postsettlement Midwestern U.S. colleges such as the University of Illinois—founded in

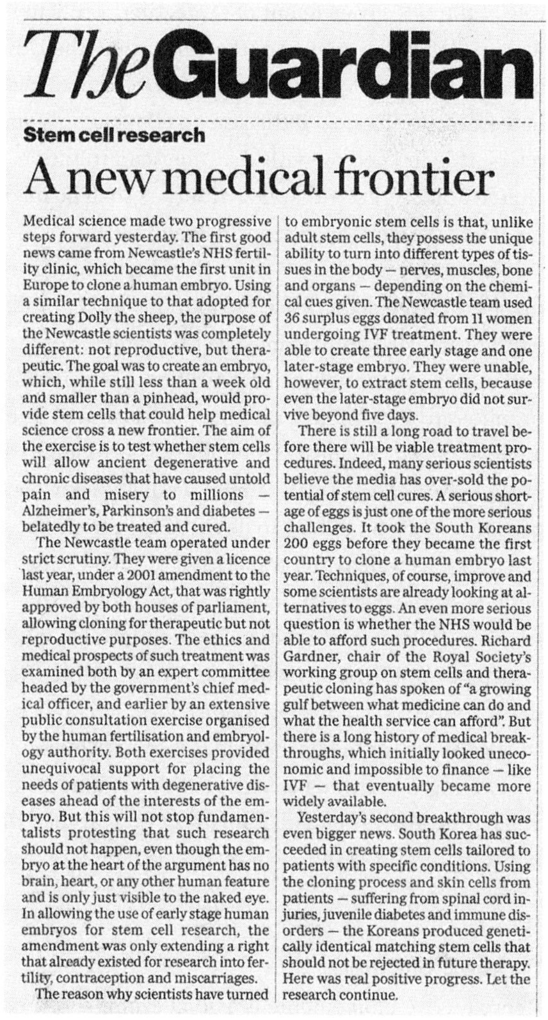

FIGURE 3.1. In this editorial from May 20, 2005, the *Guardian* emphasizes both the desirability and the legality of pioneering human embryonic stem cell research involving the cloning of human embryos using the "Dolly technique." As the editorial points out, the goal of this initiative was primarily technical—and there remains a "long road to travel before there will be viable treatment procedures." Copyright Guardian News and Media Ltd., 2005 (www.guardian.co.uk).

The figure reproduces a Guardian newspaper editorial:

The Guardian

Stem cell research

A new medical frontier

Medical science made two progressive steps forward yesterday. The first good news came from Newcastle's NHS fertility clinic, which became the first unit in Europe to clone a human embryo. Using a similar technique to that adopted for creating Dolly the sheep, the purpose of the Newcastle scientists was completely different: not reproductive, but therapeutic. The goal was to create an embryo, which, while still less than a week old and smaller than a pinhead, would provide stem cells that could help medical science cross a new frontier. The aim of the exercise is to test whether stem cells will allow ancient degenerative and chronic diseases that have caused untold pain and misery to millions — Alzheimer's, Parkinson's and diabetes — belatedly to be treated and cured.

The Newcastle team operated under strict scrutiny. They were given a licence last year, under a 2001 amendment to the Human Embryology Act, that was rightly approved by both houses of parliament, allowing cloning for therapeutic but not reproductive purposes. The ethics and medical prospects of such treatment was examined both by an expert committee headed by the government's chief medical officer, and earlier by an extensive public consultation exercise organised by the human fertilisation and embryology authority. Both exercises provided unequivocal support for placing the needs of patients with degenerative diseases ahead of the interests of the embryo. But this will not stop fundamentalists protesting that such research should not happen, even though the embryo at the heart of the argument has no brain, heart, or any other human feature and is only just visible to the naked eye. In allowing the use of early stage human embryos for stem cell research, the amendment was only extending a right that already existed for research into fertility, contraception and miscarriages.

The reason why scientists have turned to embryonic stem cells is that, unlike adult stem cells, they possess the unique ability to turn into different types of tissues in the body — nerves, muscles, bone and organs — depending on the chemical cues given. The Newcastle team used 36 surplus eggs donated from 11 women undergoing IVF treatment. They were able to create three early stage and one later-stage embryo. They were unable, however, to extract stem cells, because even the later-stage embryo did not survive beyond five days.

There is still a long road to travel before there will be viable treatment procedures. Indeed, many serious scientists believe the media has over-sold the potential of stem cell cures. A serious shortage of eggs is just one of the more serious challenges. It took the South Koreans 200 eggs before they became the first country to clone a human embryo last year. Techniques, of course, improve and some scientists are already looking at alternatives to eggs. An even more serious question is whether the NHS would be able to afford such procedures. Richard Gardner, chair of the Royal Society's working group on stem cells and therapeutic cloning has spoken of "a growing gulf between what medicine can do and what the health service can afford". But there is a long history of medical breakthroughs, which initially looked uneconomic and impossible to finance — like IVF — that eventually became more widely available.

Yesterday's second breakthrough was even bigger news. South Korea has succeeded in creating stem cells tailored to patients with specific conditions. Using the cloning process and skin cells from patients — suffering from spinal cord injuries, juvenile diabetes and immune disorders — the Koreans produced genetically identical matching stem cells that should not be rejected in future therapy. Here was real positive progress. Let the research continue.

1867 and originally named Illinois Industrial University. The founding of the Society for the Study of Reproduction at the University of Illinois at Urbana-Champaign in 1967 reflects the field's significant and ongoing links to the land grant universities established to provide education in the settlement areas, with their prominent emphasis on agricultural improvement, the veterinary sciences, and medicine—as well as industry.[6] Postwar reproductive bioscience, as both Adele Clarke (1998) and Evelyn Fox Keller (2002) have shown, was part of the shift to biology that characterized the second half of the twentieth century, with its emphasis on the logics of life rather than the physics of death—thus in some ways confirming exactly the transfer Roosevelt envisaged from the sciences of war into a war on disease. The development of IVF, like the earlier introduction of artificial insemination into livestock breeding, recapitulates many of the definitive features of technological innovation that characterize postwar reproductive biology and its translation into more widespread commercial and industrial applications.[7]

However, and as this chapter charts, the evolution of IVF was also — perhaps more like an actual frontier — often haphazard and fortuitous (as is the business of breeding). Among other reasons for its meandering path, its history can be read as the evolution of technique through hands-on exploratory experimentalism, as much as the advance of basic scientific understanding or clearly specified practical goals.[8] Not a few of the major techniques used in reproductive biomedicine were discovered by accident, such as intracytoplasmic sperm injection and the ability to freeze mammalian gametes (Gordon 2003). It is, as noted earlier, one of the most prominent historical ironies of IVF that much of the research leading to its eventual transfer "into man" was originally intended to restrict, not promote, fertility. As we shall see in this chapter, several of the most prominent figures associated with the development of human IVF, including Robert Edwards, were funded by philanthropic institutions such as the Ford Foundation in order to improve the efficacy of contraception. The "developments in embryology" referred to by Shulamith Firestone (1972) in chapter 2, for example, were aimed at population control — a topic that she, like many political activists and social commentators in the 1960s and 1970s, considered to be the single most important issue facing the human race.

Although the frontier idiom as it is used to describe scientific progress is associated with the steady march of knowledge "forward," other definitions of the frontier, like many frontier histories, emphasize the opposite — namely the frontier as a site of confusion, hybridity, destruction, and conflict. Both meanings of the frontier have relevance to the history of disciplining reproduction. In attempting to depict the early history of IVF in this chapter, I have emphasized both the search for knowledge that would offer a critical path to applications, and the haphazard quality of research in the area of human reproduction — arguing this was preceded by a similar pattern within experimental embryology. Generally lacking a unified hypothesis or theory, the history of embryology was characterized by Joseph Needham in the 1930s as largely "ad hoc" (1935: 17). In part this is because embryology, like most experimental sciences, is highly tool dependent. Episodes from the history of experimental embryology are thus presented in this chapter not only because they illustrate the technologization of reproductive substance that precedes clinical IVF, but because they confirm the importance of what Clarke and Fujimura (1992) describe as "the right tools for the job."[9] Even Wilhelm Roux's work on "developmental mechanics"—often cited as the origin of experimental embryology—is more often celebrated for the innovative experimental technique he introduced than his often inconclusive scientific results.[10] This emphasis on the importance of technical skill, and the invention of new tools, is very striking in the history of the reproductive frontier, and is defined by Needham (1935: 17) as the core "limiting factor" in the advance of embryology.[11]

Of course the interdependence of knowledge and technique characterizes all sciences, and it is not uncommon for technological discoveries encountered either by accident or by sheer luck to redirect scientific inquiry down new paths—paths that emerge in the wake of technological advances that make them both possible and passable, only acquiring a direction in retrospect. Interestingly, some of these new paths appear because technologies are passed around, being put to new uses that expand their remit, and thus acquiring value, like capital, through circulation. A chief means of technological passaging or transfer in embryology is the movement of technique across species—through interspecific technology transfer. For example, in the long-unsuccessful effort to fertilize a human egg in vitro, Robert Edwards eventually borrowed the culture media one of his graduate students (Barry Bavister) had developed for hamsters. Following its success with human ova, Edwards described this medium as a "magic fluid" that had helped not only to pave the way to human IVF but to topple scientific orthodoxy: "Once again orthodox scientific opinion had been proven wrong" (Edwards and Steptoe 1980: 82). Here, as is typical of the history of embryology, and of IVF, is the sequence whereby a cherished hypothesis falls in the wake of a successful, application-led, technical breakthrough.[12] In vitro fertilization is not unusual in having a rather fumbling as well as an eventually distinguished scientific ancestry. This is what arguably makes it interesting from the point of view of understanding both science and reproduction as frontiers that are shaped by open-ended exploration largely based on the use of handmade and hand-held tools.

This chapter thus addresses "the question concerning technology" in relation to IVF by using the frontier idiom to explore what is meant by technological pioneering, manifest as the technical exploration of reproductive mechanisms. While offering a background of technique to IVF and embryo transfer, this chapter also focuses on what the terms "frontier" and "technology" mean in relation to each other, and what happens to this relationship when it is reproductive interiority that is being charted, mechanized, and domesticated. How do we understand the concept, for example, of embryo pioneering? What does it mean for reproduction to be "made available for development" in order to produce a more "fruitful way of life"? What work does the frontier analogy do in the context of experimental embryology, and what kinds of contact, conversion, and contingency does an analysis of this analogic idiom reveal?

Like Marx, Joseph Needham argued that "the Carlylean tendency to regard the history of science as a succession of inexplicable geniuses arbitrarily bestowing knowledge upon mankind has now generally been given up as quite mythological. A scientific worker is necessarily a child of his time and the inheritor of the thought of many generations" (1935: 1). More recent science studies scholars, such as Joan Fujimura, similarly argue that the "problem path" of any particular experiment evolves through "situated interactions," emphasizing, like Needham (1935: 7–8), that experimental embryologists' problems coevolved with their instruments (Fujimura 1996: 156; and see also the work of Suchman 1987, 1995, 2007). Technology, in these models, cannot be separated from conceptual equipment, historical conditions, cultures of the workplace, or the wider social milieu. Scientific apprehension is based on a prosthetic imagination: experimental practice relies on inherited cultures of technique, and the maintenance of the traditional artisanal skills needed to reproduce vital equipment and devices. Inevitably, technological "probing" or "reaching" also implies a gap between the immediate conditions of work and a future yet to be shaped. As the British social anthropologist Alfred Gell pointed out in his essay on technology in 1988, "technology is coterminous with the various networks of social relationships that allow for the transmission of technical knowledge, and provide the necessary conditions for cooperation between individuals in technical activities" and these conditions, he adds, by definition involve "a certain degree of circuitousness." He continues: "Techniques form a bridge, sometimes only a simple one, sometimes a very complicated one, between a set of 'given' elements . . . and a goal-state that is to be realised making use of these givens" (Gell 1988: 6). In other words, "technical means are roundabout means of securing some desired result" and "tools . . . are an important category of elements which 'intervene' between a goal and its realization" (6). In chapter 4 I return to Gell's analysis of technology in the context of what he describes as "Technology of Reproduction," namely kinship — "a set of technical strategies for managing our reproductive destiny via an elaborate sequence of purposes" (7). For the purposes of addressing IVF as a technology in this chapter, however, it is his discussion of technology's connection to magic and free play that concern us first.

Following both Malinowski and Lévi-Strauss, Gell defines magic as a form of free play: "Magic consists of a symbolic 'commentary' on technical strategies," he suggests, comparing it to the spontaneous imaginative play of children's pretend games. This type of play is characterized by its imaginative projection ("Look, I am an airplane!") that reaches "beyond the frontiers of the merely real" (Gell 1988: 8). Play, in this sense, is a prosthetic—a reaching, probing, exploratory exercise—to engage with what is beyond its actual conditions. Like magic, it "sets an ideal standard, not to be approached in reality, towards which practical technical action can nonetheless be oriented." Gell continues:

> Technology develops through a process of innovation, usually one which involves the re-combination and re-deployment of a set of existing elements or procedures toward the attainment of new objectives. Play also demonstrates innovativeness—in fact, it does so continuously, whereas innovation in technology is a slower and more difficult process. Innovation in technology does not usually arise as the result of the application of systematic thought to the task of supplying some obvious technical "need," since there is no reason for members of any societies to feel "needs" in addition to the ones they already know how to fulfil. Technology, however, does change, and with changes in technology, new needs come into existence. The source of this mutability, and the tendency toward ever-increasing elaboration in technology must, I think, be attributed, not to material necessity, but to the cognitive role of "magical" ideas in providing the orienting framework within which technological activity takes place. (Gell 1988: 8)

One way to understand the frontier idiom, according to Gell's description, is as a form of magical thinking, which sets an orientation to the task of exploration beyond the reach of existing elements or procedures "toward the attainment of new objectives." This orientation is what directs the frontier exploration toward a reconciliation of mental and material equipment. Notably, as an orienting framework, the frontier is by definition temporary: eventually, frontiers become something else. An important feature of the frontier is that it is, like the horizon, a temporary line, establishing a relationship rather than a place—indeed its definition has less to do with an actual place than an imagined space. Above all the frontier describes a set of possibilities: like Gell's imaginative play, it is a magical idea. Unlike the reach of Gell's imaginative play, however, the frontier can be used to reimagine both the future and the past—thus functioning as a kind of conversion device, in both time and space. The frontier idiom is most specific or real when it is imagined in the past, invoking an actual historical scene that serves as an originating ground of present-day conditions. This has been especially true of the frontier narratives of the New World, such as in the United States and Australia, where the frontier idiom has been accompanied by a distinctive national ethos. Here, the frontier idiom is at its narrowest and least imaginative—functioning as a defensive panacea or apologetic myth.[13] At the other end of the spectrum is the translation of the lost frontier that is behind into a future-oriented idiom—such as that of endless scientific progress that lies ahead. In this context, the frontier that is still ahead is recharged with the promise of unexplored territory offering an open-ended prospect onto a promising unknown, the core symbol of which is discovery.

The translation of a historic frontier narrative into a future-oriented invitation is one reason why, despite its parochial and ideological American origins, the endless frontier analogy is today equally British and European in its widespread use as an aspirational discourse of scientific innovation. Indeed, the frontier analogy is among the paramount examples of idioms that have traveled back to Europe from the colonial context.[14] The same can be said of the "manifest destiny" ethos that the frontier idiom expresses—the moral imperative to defend technological progress in aid of human betterment, also a colonial Americanism.[15] Like the Californian vines expatriated to restock their *terroir d'origine* on the Continent in the wake of phylloxera, the American frontier analogy has gone inconspicuously native, even (and perhaps especially) in Europe.

The colonial connotations of the frontier idiom are, of course, not entirely absent from its current usage as an idiom for scientific progress. The image of "walking hopefully into the scientific foothills" is one that still carries with it the sense of duty and conquest that is as recognizably British or European as American, especially when it is used to describe medical or scientific exploration of the unknown. We need only listen to Sir Ian Lloyd in the British House of Commons in the spring of 1990, as Parliament debated the future of embryo research, at a turning point in the passage of legislation that has since made the United Kingdom a leading center of innovation in the life sciences, to be reminded of how seamlessly a moral sense of necessity, responsibility, obligation, exploration, and progress can be woven together by using the frontier idiom to evoke a sense of both destiny and duty. Describing the technologization of reproductive substance as a map, Lloyd argues its completion signifies no less than the successful passage into a new phase of human civilization:

The discovery of DNA, the very blueprint of life, is certainly awe-inspiring, and when the full map of the human genome is known . . . we shall have passed through a phase of human civilization as significant as, if not more significant than, that which distinguished the age of Galileo from that of Copernicus, or that of Einstein from that of Newton. . . . We have crossed a boundary of unprecedented importance. . . . There is no going back. . . . We are walking hopefully into the scientific foothills of a gigantic mountain range. Hitherto, man has had no option but to come to terms with a serious burden of human impairment, but now he can look ahead, perhaps a long way, to its eventual elimination. . . . For us to forswear the assistance which science can provide in modifying that code to the advantage of the human race would be an indefensible abdication of responsibility. It would cross the portcullis of this place with a most sinister and destructive bar. (Sir Ian Lloyd, HC, 23.4.90, cols. 96–98)

Significantly, the image of "walking hopefully into the scientific foothills of a gigantic mountain range" evokes the quintessentially American frontier landscape with figure (in Europe a frontier is a border between two nation-states).[16] It invokes the equally American manifest destiny model of future progress to be gained through the risks and potential costs necessary to chart the unknown. Importantly, it is not only the process of discovery that is being evoked here, but its reward in the form of scientific and technological progress: in this case the "awe-inspiring" full map of genetic interiority that will inaugurate a significant new phase of civilization. The progressive, linear conception of history evoked in the image of looking ahead, "perhaps a long way," conflates the time and space of progress into the single figure of a forward-marching pioneer, who in turn invokes the custodial, protective duty of Parliament. It is on behalf of both the lone explorer and the lives of future generations that Parliament must perform its forward-looking duties. Indeed, there is no going back.

As this chapter argues, there are many reasons why the history of IVF is imagined through the frontier idiom, particularly in its American form, in which the frontier is a crucible of rebirth. This was the meaning of the frontier that was pivotal to Frederick Jackson Turner's influential hypothesis establishing the American frontier as the soil out of which a new kind of man was reborn—a man with his back to Europe, a new outlook, and a distinctive intellect (essentially that of an enterprising engineer). In the contemporary period, as we shall see, it might be argued that the frontiers of reproduction and regeneration have become yet again a different kind of crucible, indeed a literal set of containers for rebirth—the test tubes, petri dishes, and new labs in which the future of humanity is being regenerated and remade, in order to enact a duty, once again, of cultivation in the name of human progress. It is here too that we see in the idiom of the frontier the clear outlines of a model of technology as kinship, providing both the ethos and the map of civilized regeneration manifest as the cultivation of human reproductive substance.

Cultivating Technique

As well as providing an instrumental means, a cognitive orientation, and a kind of prosthetic reach, technology is a form of material culture—a legacy of technique as substance, inheritance, or stock. Just as the tools by which the soil is cultivated in any particular field or region of settlement are inseparable from its more general mode of reproduction, so any form of cultivation can be characterized, in part, by its technological culture—the specific form of its technological arts, tools, and devices. The history of embryology is not dissimilar to agriculture in having evolved as a tool culture as well as a conceptual one: its technical characteristics and its craft have developed inconsistently, and variously, but cumulatively and interactively across diverse fields of innovation and experimentation—not unlike viticulture, milling, or weaving. Although technological evolution is never purely technical, there is nonetheless a genealogy of technique that can be followed, in the form of a substantialized legacy of skill and knowledge—and one that is passed around as well as passed down. Such genealogies of technique can be seen in the development of experimental embryology as it is employed variously to investigate reproduction, heredity, animal and plant breeding, development, determination, growth, and myriad other topics on its way to generating the possibility of IVF "in man." As noted earlier, this evolution is not simply linear but circulatory—we might even think of experimental embryology as an accumulation of techniques that evolve through circulation, as they are passaged through a range of contexts, becoming interwoven with a diverse set of fundamental and practical problems in the process. This is also how we might approach the sociology of technology: in the same way that Lévi-Strauss (1969: 479) borrows Maurice Leenhardt's image of "the action of the needle for sewing roofs, which, weaving in and out, leads backwards and forwards the same liana, holding the straw together," so do the tungsten steel needles and Spemann pi-

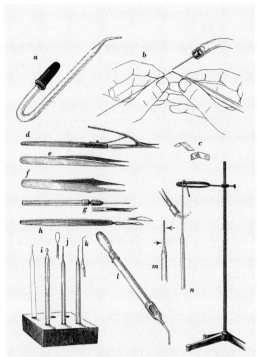

FIG. 1.—Instruments for operating on embryos. *a*, micropipette; *b*, preparation of glass needle on the microburner; *c*, glass bridges; *d*, iridectomy scissors; *e*, *f*, watchmaker forceps; *g*, fine steel knife, prepared by sharpening of sewing needle; *h*, Knapp iris needle; *i*, glass rod with ball tip; *j*, hair loop; *k*, glass needle; *l*, Spemann micropipette; *m*, *n*, preparation of capillary pipette (see text).

FIGURE 3.2. Embryological tools including a Spemann micropipette. From Keen A. Rafferty Jr., *Methods in Experimental Embryology of the Mouse*, p. 3. Copyright 1970 by The Johns Hopkins University Press. Reprinted with permission of The Johns Hopkins University Press.

pettes of the embryologists (figure 3.2) substantialize a technological kinship, or tool genealogy, uniting nineteenth-century science with techniques that are still in use today, and agricultural applications with those of clinical medicine. The historical examples presented to illustrate this interwoven fabric, or texture, of technique in this chapter are thus not meant to imply that there is, in the conventional progressive sense, a linear process of embryo research culminating in the triumph of the miracle baby. Rather, in a more anthropological style of episodic or indicative description, and with Gell's sense of play in mind, the techniques of embryology can be observed, like the famous circulating connubium, as transferable, interspecific relations that together substantialize a kind of technological kinship.[17]

In an attempt to explore these kinships of embryological technique as a background to contemporary IVF and embryo research, the following descriptions are intended to provide neither a Darwinian narrative for technology nor a progressive chronology of innovation driven by necessity and utility. The effort instead is to put under closer inspection the development of specific cultures of embryological technique, such as those discussed in chapter 2, in the depiction of how to passage a stem cell line, and to mine these examples for resources that are pertinent to the question of what it means to be after IVF.[18] This chapter thus also emphasizes that despite its association with contemporary biomedical novelty, many of the basic techniques involved in IVF can be traced back to the nineteenth century and beyond. In terms of their development over time, what we can observe in the history of IVF is a pattern of technological transfer that circulates through diverse model organisms and animal models, creating a distinctive animal-tool interface in this interspecific field by interconnecting reproductivity across widely disparate sites of intervention. It is on the basis of this accumulated experimental and technical knowledge — of what works in one model system, and the extent to which it can be transferred (by analogy, model, or tool) to another — that much of the work leading to human clinical IVF was founded. This "inter" work principally involved the removal of mammalian ova, their culture in vitro, in vitro fertilization of the egg, and transfer of the resultant embryo either to a recipient uterus or to another glass container.

The process we can thus observe is one of building up an interspecific system of reproductive workings that combine technology with substance in the name of both exploration and control. As a work object, reproductivity thus acquires a new meaning and scale as a biotechnical entity that is at once both sub- and suprahuman, while technology in this system becomes a shared substance that can no longer be seen as separate from reproductive matter. One of the reasons it is in some ways surprising that IVF was not applied to humans much earlier is because of the intensity of research in the field of embryology in the first part of the twentieth century, followed by an equally striking concentration on early mammalian development in the postwar period. But human reproduction per se was not the primary goal of much research leading up to human IVF. At issue was the constitution of a much larger system of biotechnical reproductivity — and not so much a mode of reproduction as a model of it. It is in the context of this more general effort to model reproductivity that the unity of biology and technique are substantialized as its workings or mechanics.[19]

The late nineteenth and early twentieth century are renowned as a dense period of embryological investigation, conventionally associated with the technological and conceptual shifts that give rise to experimental embryology as an emergent modern scientific field (later giving way, as Haraway [1976] chronicles, to the organicism and cybernetic feedback loops of the systems analogy that still predominate in biology today). It is during this period that the tool kit of embryology underwent one of the most important changes that would later enable the development of a huge variety of practical reproductive applications, as well as fundamental research experiments, namely the process through which the embryo is transformed from an object of study into a means of intervention. Rather than being simply passive unexplored anatomical terrain, which could be mapped and charted in the manner of a newly discovered geographic region, the interior of the embryo comes to be seen during the late nineteenth century more in terms of an organized mechanical system—subject to dis- and reassembly, with parts that can be extracted and transferred into other embryos.[20] In other words, this is the point at which parts of embryos themselves become tools, a new species of investigative apparatus: they are no longer simply worked on or even worked up but become recombinant working models of themselves.

The shift away from mere description is conventionally associated in the history of embryology with the *Entwicklungsmechanik*, or "mechanics of development," of the German zoologist Wilhelm Roux, or the Swedish anatomist Wilhelm His—both of whom were inventive technicists as well as theorists. The shift was codified by turn-of-the-century biologists such as Oxford's J. W. Jenkinson, who began his 1909 textbook *Experimental Embryology* with an account of "a new branch of biological science," concerned with "the origin of form," which the author dates back to a specific experiment: "It is with the origin of form that [experimental embryology concerns itself], and in particular with its origin in the individual. The endeavour to discover by experiment the causes of this process—as distinct from the mere description of the process itself—is a comparatively new branch of biological science, for Experimental Embryology, or, as some prefer to call it, the Mechanics of Development . . . really dates from Roux's production of a half-embryo from a half-blastomere, and the consequent formation of the 'Mosaik-Theorie' of self-differentiation" (Jenkinson 1909: iii).

In contrast to the "mere description" of embryos via dissection, or classification of embryological processes via observation, experimental embryology is distinguished by its emphasis on direct interference with the internal mechanics of the embryo using manual or chemical intervention, such as investigation through fusion, stress, constriction, grafting, or recombination.[21] Experimental embryology is also characterized by the attention paid by its practitioners to deviant, monstrous, and pathological formations—an interest that early on is envisaged as a means of exploring not only part-whole relations but the extent and character of innate organic plasticity. It emerged in the period during which Darwin's, Weismann's, and later Mendel's models of inheritance were being debated in relation to morphogenesis—the acquisition of form—with an emphasis on experimental means of identifying causal mechanisms and thus the workings of heredity. Much of the experimental work in experimental embryology was thus also highly conceptually—indeed to many philosophically—motivated, while at the same time becoming more boldly instrumental in disrupting natural trajectories and inventing, or forcing, new recombinant ones. New microsurgical tools and techniques were developed as part of an expanding culture of wrench-in-the-works experimentalism based on the transfer of substances between whole organisms in order to study the parts of organisms, or to create new mosaic organisms that were deliberately designed to be different from what would emerge normally. This newly interventionist embryology enabled mechanical parts of embryos to become tools of investigation to understand, or probe, the causal dynamics of morphogenesis, reproduction, regeneration, development, and heredity.[22] Experimental progress could be made either by putting cells together or taking them apart—a constructivist ethos that was designed to elicit and explore the forces that controlled embryonic organization, growth, and the acquisition of form. Naturally existing forms and substances were increasingly viewed as biological mechanisms that could be imitated, inverted, reassembled, reverse engineered, or otherwise manipulated, while new things that had never existed could be created and observed in vitro in order to isolate individual controlling variables, units, or factors through the artifice of experimentation.

The ethos of experimental embryology, then, was not so much one of understanding how form followed function, or vice versa, as of manipulating both, often by transposing them—thereby converting the resulting organism into a double window onto development: the object of study (e.g., a fertilized egg) in its controlled environment (the experimental system) was one window, whereas what went on inside the entity (e.g., the mechanics of embryogenesis) became another. In the same way the in vitro dish renders entities that would be invisible in vivo amenable to observation and manipulation, so too do such entities themselves become in vitro containers for experimentation (its "vasculature," as Marx might have said).[23] Thus, Wilhelm Roux, a student of Haeckel, conducted experiments with amphibian embryos by recombining their parts to make new wholes (mosaics), while Hans Driesch, his contemporary, separated two sea urchin cells to demonstrate they could produce two independent organisms—manually splitting a whole entity to reveal its innate properties of regeneration.[24] The once-flat world of embryological observation had erupted: it was now a tooled-up experimental vivarium. As well as a looking-glass world, in which the workings of morphology were subject to remechanization, this is equally a push-me-pull-you experimental field of entities built through collision in order to model the invisible, otherwise imperceptible forces at work in the processes of reproduction, regeneration, and development.

Embryo Pioneers

As late nineteenth-century embryologists increasingly sought to tackle questions of organization, morphogenesis, differentiation, and recapitulation, embryological experiments became more technically ambitious and more prolonged over time — eventually leading to the in vitro dish window of tissue culture in the early twentieth century. As well as being tedious and time consuming, such experiments were in other respects also similar to highly skilled manual crafts — based on precise, repetitive techniques and prolonged exposure to specialist tools and familiar research materials. Like that of jewelers, embryologists' labor required excellent eyesight, dexterity, practice, and tenacity. As in other mechanical workshops, embryological artisans required tools to make tools, as well as accumulated knowledge about how to use them, often acquired through lengthy apprenticeships through which such knowledge was passed on to a new generation of experimentalists. A wide variety of optical techniques were used to visualize embryos, and new instruments were constantly being developed to manipulate them, as well as containers and solutions in which to keep them (figures 3.3 and 3.4). Chemical forms of preservation, marking, labeling, and interference were used, as well as handheld microtools. Equipment derived from watchmaking and eye surgery was adapted to embryological experimentation, and remade by hand. Staining, dyeing, and tattooing techniques were used, as well as wax modeling and sectioning. Passed on, remastered, and handed down again, these genealogies of artifice composed the technological infrastructure of increasingly adept manual control of reproduction.

These accumulated techniques can be interpreted in more Marxist terms as means of getting a better handle on reproductive substance, achieved through mechanical evolution. The constant redesign of specialist tools in the embryology lab is in this sense no different from any other artisanal setting, where practical and spontaneous innovations are constantly being made

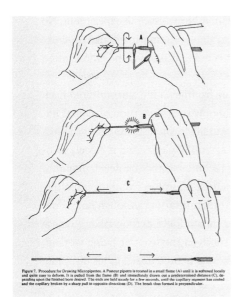

Figure 7. Procedure for Drawing Micropipettes. A Pasteur pipette is rotated in a small flame (A) until it is softened locally and quite easy to deform. It is pulled from the flame (B) and immediately drawn out a predetermined distance (C), depending upon the finished bore desired. The ends are held steady for a few seconds, until the capillary segment has cooled and the capillary broken by a sharp pull in opposite directions (D). The break thus formed is perpendicular.

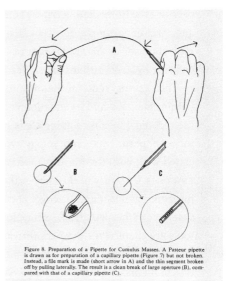

Figure 8. Preparation of a Pipette for Cumulus Masses. A Pasteur pipette is drawn as for preparation of a capillary pipette (Figure 7) but not broken. Instead, a file mark is made (short arrow in A) and the thin segment broken off by pulling laterally. The result is a clean break of large aperture (B), compared with that of a capillary pipette (C).

FIGURES 3.3 AND 3.4. Techniques for the hand-forging of microtools, such as those described in chapter 2, are passed down over time through lineages of technique for handling cells, as is here illustrated in the preparation of different types of "Pasteur" pipette. From Keen A. Rafferty Jr., *Methods in Experimental Embryology of the Mouse*, pp. 16 and 17. Copyright 1970 by The Johns Hopkins University Press. Reprinted with permission of The Johns Hopkins University Press.

with a view to securing more purchase on the object being worked. Similarly, we can also approach these techniques, and their relations to their objects, as frontiers insofar as they constitute a zone of encounter characterized by contact and conversion—themselves also generative processes. From this perspective, we can appreciate why the idiom of the frontier—of open-ended exploration, unknown territory, and unexpected encounters—usefully emphasizes the fruitfulness of indeterminacy, particularly in the context of experimental science. From the point of view of the artisan, technician, or experimentalist, in other words, the frontier is never "toward"—for it is precisely the indeterminate nature of experimental outcomes that gives them value to the scientist. If, in other words, the idiom of science as a frontier as used in the British Parliament to describe "walking hopefully" into "a gigantic mountain range" conveys the helicopter view of science that is external to it, the experimentalist's much more constrained outlook can only barely perceive the immediate territory at hand, in other words, the experiment. No airy, Archimedean panoptic is available to the lone experimentalist—whose tools themselves are always part of what is being explored, and who is often working by habit rather than sight.

This internal sense of the frontier—the frontier as it is encountered from within science—and its equation with not only the exploration of objects but the technical means of doing so, is substantially evident throughout the history of experimental embryology, where scientific pioneering is closely associated with both the mastery of existing techniques and the development of new ones. Contrary to the view of the scientist as explorer walking hopefully into unknown lands, to discover and chart their interior (although not inconsistent with this depiction), is the pioneer embryologist as toolmaker—whose tools are themselves the path forward—or even the frontier being worked. Hence, for example, the biologist and historian Scott Gilbert, in his introduction to *A Conceptual History of Embryology*, writes that developmental biology is the offspring not only of "embryology's concepts, organisms and sense of wonder" but of the "new set of tools with a resolving power far greater than what was available a generation ago." Deploying a developmental analogy for the science itself (and echoing the reproductive double entendre of his book's title), Gilbert describes the increase in "resolving power" available to a new generation of experimentalists as the result of a combination of new model organisms, new tools, and new molecular methods: "Frogs, chicks and sea urchins (along with nematodes, flies and leeches) are now being dissected with monoclonal antibodies, antisense mRNAs, and confocal microscopes. We are presently seeing a return to those old embryological enigmas that were abandoned for lack of such specific tools. The morphogenesis of the discipline continues. . . . Glory, indeed, to the science of embryology" (Gilbert 1991: ix).

The sense of the tool itself as a frontier is similarly captured by the use of the adjective "pioneering" to describe the development of tools and techniques in science—hence, for example, the description of Patrick Steptoe as the "laparoscopy pioneer" on his Wikipedia page. Thus also the frequent references to technical advances that open up new research opportunities and pathways forward in understanding. The pioneer awards common to scientific societies, health organizations, and academia are commonly associated with the development of new technology.

The annual Pioneer Award of the International Embryo Transfer Society (IETS), established in 1982, provides a useful picture of the range of embryological techniques that have been seen to pave the way to new research advances in this field, as the frontiers of knowledge yield to new working methods. Specifically chosen for their technical contributions to science, the current list of thirty Pioneer Award winners includes many of the most eminent figures in modern reproductive and developmental biology (table 3.1). As can be noted from this list of the IETS embryo Pioneer Award winners from the 1980s and 1990s, advances on the reproductive frontier were often achieved in the form of both technological innovation and technology transfer. Although celebrated for the paths they individually opened up to other researchers, the general pattern of advance can equally be characterized as one of technological exchange — of sharing and comparing techniques to explore different biological mechanisms, at different stages of development, under varied conditions, and across a wide range of different animal species or models.

Also notable from this list is the striking number of Pioneer awardees who were centrally involved in the development of human IVF. Indeed, in its award to Robert Edwards in 1993, the society noted that it is "no accident that human IVF clinics are well populated by scientists and technicians who began their work with members of [the IETS]" (IETS 1993). As Edwards himself has noted, the road to IVF was not only long and bumpy, but also often haphazard and even directionless. As noted in chapter 1, Edwards did not initially set out to achieve human IVF, just as Chang did not originally intend to pursue IVF in rabbits. Indeed few of the scientists listed in table 3.1 had a clear path ahead of them as they moved forward, often instead being redirected as technical obstacles were overcome, opening new instrumental possibilities, and — equally haphazardly — new and unexpected avenues of inquiry.

Of the many questions that can be asked about the depiction of science and technology as frontiers, then, is how many there are. Taking the frontier to comprise a set of relationships, for example, we might consider at least three primary frontiers: between tool and object, object and knowledge, and knowledge and tool. Pioneering can occur in any one of these contexts, opening a way for others to follow or a new avenue of inquiry. A breakthrough can similarly transform any one of these frontiers, or more than one of them, in the way that the discovery of a viable culture medium for an embryo can enable it to be grown in vitro, cultured, transferred, frozen, or stored. What is made visible in the context of embryo pioneering, in other words, is the necessity for constant circulation of technique across a series of frontiers. More important, it is the inextricability of tools and objects that make of re-

TABLE 3.1. Selected embryo Pioneer Award winners 1983–1999 whose work contributed to the successful development of human IVF.

AWARD WINNER	CONTRIBUTION	YEAR AWARDED
Min Chueh Chang, Worcester Foundation for Experimental Biology	First successful IVF in mammals (rabbits, 1959) using capacitated sperm; codeveloper with Pincus of the contraceptive pill.	1983
Lionel Rowson, ARC Unit of Reproductive Physiology, Cambridge University	Use of rabbit incubator for long-distance transport of sheep embryos; development of media for bovine eggs.	1985
Christopher Polge, ARC Unit of Reproductive Physiology, Cambridge University	First successful cryopreservation of sperm and embryos; founder of the science of cryobiology.	1987
Anne McLaren and Donald Michie, Institute of Animal Genetics, University of Edinburgh	Refinement of embryo transfer methods to explore uterine effect on genetic development (epigenesis).	1988
John Biggers, Harvard University	Contributions to embryo culture, first mammals born using cultured embryos (with A. McLaren).	1990
Andrei Tarkwoski, Warsaw University	Development of micromanipulation techniques; transfer of half-blastomeres; production of mammalian chimeras.	1991

productivity a complex work object in which tools themselves become working model systems.

Hair Loop

Hans Spemann's experiments, conducted in close cooperation with his doctoral student Hilde Mangold, are often used to illustrate the importance of an evolving conceptual and technical experimental approach during the period

AWARD WINNER	CONTRIBUTION	YEAR AWARDED
Ralph Brinster, University of Pennsylvania	Development of embryo culture systems; transfer of stem cells into blastocysts; transgenic embryos.	1992
Robert Edwards, Physiological Laboratory, Cambridge University	First IVF of human ova (1969); development of human IVF and preimplantation genetic diagnosis.	1993
Neil Moore, Department of Animal Husbandry, University of Sydney	Live offspring from frozen sheep, goat, and cattle embryos; zona drilling and microinjection of sperm to assist IVF.	1994
C. R. "Bunny" Austin, Physiological Laboratory, Cambridge University	Codiscoverer (with Chang, but independently) of sperm capacitation; confirmation of the mammalian acrosome reaction.	1995
Wes Whitten, University of Sydney and Australian National University	Contributions to embryo culture media; twins by blastomere splitting; contributions to reproductive endocrinology.	1996
R. M. Moor, ARC Unit of Reproductive Physiology and the Babraham Institute, of Cambridge University	Improvement of superovulation, in vivo follicular signaling, oocyte reprogramming and maturation, maternal messaging.	1999

Source: Compiled from the records of the International Embryo Transfer Society.

when embryology began to focus more intensely on causal mechanisms, such as induction factors—that is, how particular organizational steps were triggered by either internal or external stimuli guiding overall development of the early embryo. In 1906 Spemann developed a glass needle for surgery that has since proven a versatile and indispensable tool that is still in use. He also invented a microburner for pulling the glass tubes such as the capillary pipettes used for microtransfers in vitro. In a modification of his earlier constriction methods, Spemann famously designed a hair loop by threading both ends of a single human hair into a specially fashioned capillary tube and fixing them in place with wax. Mounted on a handle, this microtool could be used to move, flip, or roll eggs and embryos during experimental procedures, thus itself coming to play a developmental role in the biological workings of his model system.

Spemann also developed round molds to impress wax holders for eggs and glass microapparatus to facilitate grafting. These handmade microtools and associated techniques, including an early form of nuclear transfer, facilitated the exploration of individual differentiation for which Spemann was awarded the Nobel Prize in 1935, recognizing his efforts to experimentally chart the organizer effect by grafting part of one embryo onto another. Spemann's experiments are in many ways the archetypal example of the importance of transplantation and transfer to experimental embryology and developmental biology, and the corresponding epistemic shift described by Jenkinson from anatomical description to experimental interference that marks the emergence of a field that relies more fully on techniques that today would be described in terms of bioengineering. Since the logic of this shift remains fundamentally embedded in modern reproductive biology, it is worth revisiting one of these now-celebrated classical embryological experiments that took place in Germany in the first half of the twentieth century.[25] Importantly, Spemann's grafting experiments involved the fusion not only of different parts of embryos, but of tools with reproductive substance.

The manual mastery of fine tools necessary for microsurgery, and the ingenuity involved in devising new experimental techniques, are often emphasized in textbook reproductions of Spemann's famous constriction experiment (a predecessor to his grafting work), undertaken in three stages and published in 1904. "Developmental Physiological Studies on the Triton Egg" begins with a technical description of the methods and materials used in a series of experiments designed to bisect fertilized amphibian eggs at the early blastocyst (two-cell) stage using fine hair loops (in Spemann's case using strands of hair from the head of his infant daughter Margrette; figure 3.5).[26] The aim of the experiments was to characterize the relationship between the differentiation of structures (in particular the axial organs) by manipulating the interaction of their component parts. In order to understand how a radially symmetric egg acquires axial polarity and bilateral symmetry (and also switches from one to the next), Spemann devised a series of interventions into the earliest stages of development using constriction to explore axis formation by manipulating it.

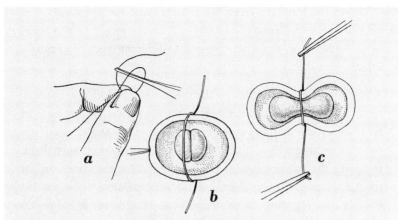

FIG. 20.—Constriction of urodele egg in 2-cell stage. *a* = preparation of the hair loop; *b* = orienting the egg in the loop; *c* = constricting.

FIGURE 3.5. Illustration of the hair loop methods used by Spemann to produce "dividuals" using a ligature made of his infant daughter's hair. Illustration taken from Viktor Hamburger, *A Manual of Experimental Embryology*, rev. ed. (Chicago: University of Chicago Press, 1962), p. 81. Reprinted with permission of the University of Chicago Press.

Largely by perfecting techniques that had been less successfully employed by previous experimentalists, Spemann showed that by constricting newt (salamander) embryos at different stages of development with his hair loops, he could create wholly separate organisms, partially separated organisms, and a variety of asymmetrical organisms. In his hand-tied embryo experiments, Spemann observed that both the timing and the plane of constriction (median or sagittal) played a role in determining which kinds of developmental modifications could be induced by his precise micromanipulations. By so doing he elaborated one of the basic principles of experimental embryology described earlier by Jenkinson, namely that reproductive substance could be mechanically manipulated not only with tools, but as a tool. For Spemann, the constricted newt egg was a probe, a device, and a crucial piece of equipment. More than a model in the sense of being a static replica, the tied egg system functioned over time to enable — indeed to produce — visual data that yielded insights into the causal bases of morphological plasticity. Growth became a means to test the limits of form.

In his detailed reconstruction and analysis of Spemann's experiments, the biologist and historian Victor Hamburger (who was Spemann's student at the University of Freiburg) describes his findings as "a graded series of anterior duplications" that corresponded to different types of manual constriction:

> A medium deep constriction in the median plane gives two heads; if the constriction is somewhat deeper, there may also be two pairs of fore limbs and a merging of the two parts in one posterior trunk and tail with a single pair of hind limbs. If the constriction is very slight, then only the anterior head is duplicated. . . . On the other hand, if the constriction cuts very deep, and only a narrow bridge connects the two blastomeres, then the two embryos are fused only at the region of the anus. [A] complete separation of the two blastomeres results in identical twins. . . . Whereas constrictions in the early gastrula still produced anterior duplications, the capacity for regulation decreased with the progression of gastrulation, and constrictions in the early neural plate stage resulted merely in an indentation without duplication. Since regulation implies that embryonic parts can give rise to structures different from those they would form in normal development, the loss of regulation capacity at the end of gastrulation means that the axial organs become irreversibly determined during gastrulation. (Hamburger 1988: 17)

In this description are evident the two planes of force being explored in relation to one another through the coupling of the tool and organism to reveal form through growth. The interpretation of results relies upon a contrast between the inside and the outside of the model system. On the one hand, the developing embryo is subjected to a range of carefully controlled surgical forces, such as constriction, the results of which are observed over measured periods of time through visual inspection. On the other, this handmade model system is designed to explore the inaccessible, invisible, or hidden mechanisms of development or organization, described by Hamburger as regulation or regulation capacity—the factors or variables that are presumed to exist within the embryonic structures but cannot be observed. Like hand shadows projected against a wall, the precise manual micromanipulations are designed to reveal the workings of internal, invisible forces (factors) that cannot be observed directly but can be made to appear as biological form by reworking them. The retooled organism thus models, in sum, not only the outcome of these invisible factors but a new kind of biological control that employs the mechanics of reproductive substance as both its means and proof, and in which the tool itself plays a developmental role.

While much commentary continues to surround the significance of Spemann's experiments, the simple point for our purposes here concerns the shift they are understood to exemplify to commentators such as Jenkinson (1909)—which is not only a change in the understanding of the role of technology in manipulating an object, or its use as an extension of the microscopic gaze as a kind of probe, but the fusion of tool and object into a live model system. The second important point to notice in the context of understanding how technology comes to be merged with reproductive substance, as in the example discussed in chapter 2 in a contemporary stem cell lab, is the complex technological layering—or archaeology—here made visible, whereby tool, organism, and experimental system perform the work of modeling the fusion of internal organizing forces and externally imposed mechanical technique. It is because it is not the model organism per se, but the fusion of organism and tool into a model system that functions as a live apparatus, in effect, for recording life, that the question of what, exactly, the experiment represents becomes rather complicated. As noted earlier, the artificial generation being modeled here as a working system is always recursive, serving as a model in which the workings of technology and reproductive substance are fused to reveal their combined agency as biology. Yet the biotechnical artifacts that are produced by this method complicate the meaning of "biological" in the very effort to reveal the principles guiding the underlying mechanics of development. What are revealed instead are the results of fusing tools with reproductive substance.

As Nick Hopwood has illustrated in his analysis of the nineteenth-century embryological studies of Wilhelm His, the concept of development was as much a product as a precursor of experimental studies such as those of Spemann—it is in part what he worked to produce. Whereas "development is often taken for granted as what embryologists study," argues Hopwood, it is instead what researchers such as His "labored to produce" (2000: 31). The account of IVF offered in this book shares Hopwood's contention that the mundane practices and routine work of embryology cannot be separated from the material production of ideas that might otherwise appear entirely prior to these labors. Indeed it is a central argument of this chapter that the human application of IVF is as much a product of its history as a working model in the effort to work up reproductivity as of a guiding vision of this end during most of its development. As we shall see, the history of IVF as a technique is both continuous and inconsistent, translational and transient, migratory—but perhaps above all it was "handy," which is equally the appeal of this technique today.

In the same way that Spemann's laborious study of constricted and recombinant embryos coupled technology and biological substance in order to explore the frontiers of organization, so too were concepts of heredity being manually and analytically refashioned during this period using a wide variety of embryological methods. Not all of these were directed at either development or organization. Some were directed to questions of heredity, while others had practical, agricultural applications (or combined the two, as had Mendel). Spemann's grafts and constrictions concerned the origin of form, or morphogenesis, as well as the internal mechanics of these forces, which he investigated both by fusing parts of embryos, and by manually manipulating development, using tools. For other researchers, reproductivity was more explicitly engaged as itself a tool in the process of experimental proof. In turning to this context of more explicit reproductive technologies, we also observe the principle of biological transfer reworked somewhat differently.

Maternal Models

Among the embryo pioneers who are most directly relevant to the history of IVF (much as they might not have expected to have been) is the English embryologist Walter Heape. In his account of Heape's now-celebrated embryo transfer experiments, undertaken between 1890 and 1899, the reproductive biologist and contemporary embryo pioneer John Biggers (1991) emphasizes their relationship not only to the conflict between Darwin's Lamarckian model of pangenesis and the theory of germ line independence propounded by August Weismann, but to the much older debate that epitomized this conflict—namely that concerning "telegony," the effect of prior fertilization upon reproductive outcome, or the ability of offspring to inherit the characteristics of their mother's previous mates. "Many biologists of the time," Biggers writes of Heape's contemporaries, "including Darwin, believed that 'if the male element can act directly on the female form,' it would provide strong evidence for the inheritance of acquired characters" (1991: 179). The theory of telegony, in circulation since antiquity and propounded by Aristotle, remained influential well into the twentieth century. Its most celebrated airing is a famous letter by Lord Morton to the Royal Society in 1821 concerning his prize thoroughbred mare's pairing with a quagga (a now-extinct equine species), causing all of her subsequent offspring (sired by horses) to bear striped coats, stiff hair manes, and thus signs of the "preponderance" of her original mate.

The persistence of traits from a prior coupling, also referred to as "infection of the germ," "fetal inoculation," or "saturation," exercised widespread concern among livestock breeders because of its deleterious consequences for otherwise valuable female stock. However, the controversy over Morton's mare's offspring gained disproportionate significance in the context of late nineteenth-century debates about inheritance because of the extent to which telegony served as a placeholder for much wider disagreements over the precise mechanics of conjoined reproductive substances in vivo (or, in this case, in utero). This question encompassed a broad area of uncertainty, namely how fertilization affected hereditary transmission of traits. Whereas Darwin had earlier advocated a model of heredity based on diffused particles (pangenesis) that allowed for the inheritance of acquired traits (according to which telegony was a plausible theory), Weismann proposed his doctrine of the continuity of the germplasm in 1893, insisting upon the absolute independence of the reproductive cells, as well as their immortality. Weismann used the theory of telegony specifically to denigrate "the doubtful effects of heredity" he claimed his experiments had disproved, arguing that the "throw back" model was, in effect, mythological. Herbert Spencer, whose theory of evolution preceded Darwin's and was much more strongly Lamarckian, was one of many prominent nineteenth-century figures for whom the telegony debate took on great importance, for social as well as scientific reasons, in a debate that has been the subject of both enlightened and entertaining commentary by many historians of biology.

Heape's experiments, like those of Spemann, employed a type of part-whole dis- and reassembly, similarly harnessing transplantation as a method. His scientific goal was to disprove telegony, but he also sought to confirm a new means of investigating it using what is now known as embryo transfer. Unlike Spemann, Heape's part-whole transplantation involved the surgical removal of an intact fertilized egg from a rabbit and its transfer into the uterus of a hare — thus using the uterine environment as his experimental crucible. Like Spemann, Heape relied on the bodies of his experimental offspring as his morphological map or proof to reveal the internal forces he was investigating — thus employing reproduction in a working (animal) model system to reveal heredity forces. He was also instrumentalizing the species boundary between two model organisms as part of the research design for his novel and laborious test cases.

The Heape technique for the recovery of fertilized ova from the fallopian tube was developed at the Morphological Laboratory in Cambridge, where Heape both trained and worked as a demonstrator under Michael Foster and Francis Balfour.[27] To complete his project, Heape combined delicate manual technique with sophisticated animal husbandry in his hometown of Prestwich, near Manchester, where his technically demanding and unprecedented series of embryo transfers were conducted between 1890 and 1899. In a series of papers read to the Royal Society (which funded his work), Heape described the outcome of his experiments as a success, both in terms of producing viable offspring and confirming an absence of uterine effect (no telegony). He concluded his 1897 Royal Society paper on a technical as well as scientific note, suggesting, "It is possible to make use of the uterus of one variety of rabbit as a medium for the growth and complete foetal development of fertilized ova of another variety of rabbit."[28]

Although Biggers emphasizes that Heape did not envisage any practical application of his experimental methods (in the sense of using embryo transfer for livestock breeding, for example), his lasting contribution has in fact been a highly practical technical innovation for the pursuit of experimental science as well as the business of breeding.[29] Heape is today celebrated as a pioneering technician. F. H. A. (Francis Hugh Adam) Marshall, whose 1910 textbook *The Physiology of Reproduction* is considered to mark the emergence of the new discipline of reproductive biology, draws heavily on Heape's work and cites its pivotal importance in linking the study of animal breeding to the experimental study of reproduction—or what he denominated as a new field of science. Marshall, who wrote Heape's obituary in 1930, dedicated his landmark textbook to him in recognition not only of his innovative and technically demanding experiments combining the analysis of reproduction and heredity, but for his substantial contribution to embryological methods.[30] Despite his primary orientation toward a purely scientific question, Heape's work, in a migration that is typical of embryological techniques, has become the foundation for the embryo transfer industry, which is currently the world's largest embryological enterprise—and one of the closest kindred sectors to the global market in IVF (Gordon 2003). Indeed he is today acclaimed as the Patron Saint of embryo transfer and responsible for the twentieth-century "rekindling of interest in artificial insemination and the laying of a scientific foundation to the animal breeding industry with emphasis on its economic importance" (Betteridge 1981: 1). In the making of modern reproductivity, embryo transfer is a foundational technique that, along with the airline industry and cryopreservation methods, facilitates the purposeful and profitable circulation of reproductive substance, passaging it across both time and space to maximize the benefit of prized genetic stock.

Stem Technologies

An important feature of Heape's embryological experiments was not only that they combined an interest in heredity and reproduction, and pioneered a new technological means of transferring reproductive substance, but that they were conducted in mammals. From an embryological point of view, detailed knowledge of the events involved in the earliest stages of reproduction and development is more difficult to obtain in mammals for the simple reason that these events take place inside a living body. Unlike salamanders, frogs, axolotl, chickens, sea urchins, worms, tortoises, fish, or other common model organisms in embryology, the majority of mammals are distinguished by hemotrophic viviparity, or development of the embryo within the mother. Heape did not use specialist culture media, and he was not seeking to remove particular mechanisms, parts, or processes from the interior of live mammalian bodies in order to examine or observe mammalian development or fertilization through an in vitro window.[31] This effort would await a later period and in particular, as is discussed below, the improvement of in vitro culture methods. Heape's contribution had been to introduce a different medium in the form of another animal's reproductive system, and to prove the viability of this system for experimental purposes. His contribution could be described as the generation of a new species of technique — a technique that has acquired a life of its own, so to speak, and is now so widespread and fundamental in its uses as to be considered a stem technology.[32]

The role of stem technologies in the evolution of technique that Heape's contribution exemplified in the form of embryo transfer similarly characterizes the development of IVF techniques, which can be viewed as sharing a technological kinship with each other, in spite of their enormously varied uses. As Barry Bavister notes in his account of the history of IVF, it begins its life as a specific kind of experimental technique: "A potentially useful technique is to recover fertilized eggs or early embryos from the female reproductive tract, and to study their subsequent development *in vitro*" (2002: 182). This technique becomes particularly useful in mammals by enabling the ex vivo modeling of reproductive events. In vitro culture of mammalian eggs, Bavister explains, allows for continuous and close observation of events that would be inaccessible in vivo both by replicating them artificially and by introducing systemic control mechanisms. "Information can be derived much more readily from the study of eggs that are fertilized and then developed *in vitro*. Not only can the process of fertilization be closely observed, but factors contributing to normal and abnormal fertilization and development can be examined. The progress of fertilization or embryogenesis can be frequently, if not continuously, observed and the conditions of culture can be varied to examine their effects on development. Thus a wealth of information is available from studies *in vitro*, given the technical ability to accomplish them" (2002: 182). As Bavister, whose "magic" culture medium enabled the first successful fertilization of a human egg in vitro in 1969, notes in this description, the wealth of information that can be gained from in vitro studies depends primarily on "the technical ability to accomplish them." The technical ability to experimentally manipulate mammalian reproductive substance within the in vitro observation chamber became increasingly various and sophisticated during the twentieth century, confirming the increasing inseparability between reproductivity and tools. In the case of IVF, it cannot simply be said that reproduction is assisted by tools, since the tools are part of the reproductive process—they are how it works. Predictably and, as Marx would probably have said, spontaneously, the experimental use of in vitro model systems for the study of mammalian development became increasingly intimately interrelated (or we might even say crossbred) with another crucial stem technology, namely cell culture methods. Versions of these methods, as noted earlier, were already part of late nineteenth-century embryology in the form of the various solutions that were used to maintain live cellular material in vitro, such as the salt solution developed by Sydney Ringer using the chlorides of sodium, potassium, calcium, and magnesium. Wilhelm Roux had also developed an early cell culture method using a mineral salt bath in a watch glass.

In the early twentieth century the American embryologist Ross Harrison, based at Johns Hopkins University, improved these methods substantially, demonstrating that live tissue fragments could be sustained in culture media for weeks at a time, through what is now known as tissue culture. As Hannah Landecker writes of Harrison's work in her account of how cell culture systems became independent and autonomous "living technologies," he established new methods to observe, control and manipulate living matter in vitro, thus "proving the possibility of observing internal body events without the body itself—observations that had been previously assumed to be impossible" (Landecker 2007: 15). She describes Harrison's contribution to the development of in vitro systems as continuous with the "increasing emphasis on artifice in science" that is the hallmark of "what Philip Pauly has called 'biological modernism'" (16). This means of cultivating life ex vivo in its own media required a working in vitro system combining control of temperature (incubation) and of infection or contamination (asepsis), as well as housing this controlled system in glass apparatus facilitating both manipulation and observation to make a looking-glass world. Like the development of dyeing and staining techniques in an earlier period, the goals of tissue culturists such as Harrison were essentially technological—to devise methods of seeing life develop within a controlled, external, closed, and transparent experimental system.

Prior to the ability to observe mammalian embryos in vitro, the main approach to understanding their early development was derived from the procedures introduced by experimentalists such as Spemann—which were not viable for mammals. As Waddington and Waterman note at the outset of their 1933 article "The Development *in Vitro* of Young Rabbit Embryos": "Very little experimental work has as yet been performed on the early stages of the mammalian embryo. The two main methods of experimental analysis, isolation of the primordia and transplantation of fragments into different situations in the embryo, which have been applied with such success in the Amphibia, both present great technical difficulties when applied to the embryos of warm blooded animals" (1933: 355).

While Waddington and Waterman experimented in the 1930s with explantation of rabbit blastocysts to analyze early mammalian development in vitro, Gregory Pincus, while visiting Cambridge in the same period, took a different approach by revising Heape's methodology of embryo transfer and combining it with in vitro culture methods more similar to those developed by Harrison to study extracorporeal mammalian fertilization. Whereas Heape had devised embryo transfer methods to investigate the relationship between gestation and heredity, by analyzing the effects of maternal environment upon transplanted offspring, his techniques were redeployed by Pincus using IVF as well—thus coupling together three stem techniques to create a powerful experimental platform. Substituting unfertilized mammalian eggs for embryos, Pincus attempted to achieve mammalian fertilization in vitro. Unlike Waddington and Waterman, who, like Harrison, sought to understand processes of "self-differentiation" and morphological development through an early method of cell culture, Pincus sought both to observe and to successfully replicate the entire process of mammalian fertilization, using surgically recovered rabbit eggs that, after what he mistakenly presumed to have been successful IVF, he then transferred to host rabbit does to obtain proof of his success in the form of viable offspring, just as Heape had done.

Pincus's early attempts at IVF in mammals in the 1930s, and his later success in producing "fatherless offspring" via parthenogenic reproduction (dubbed Pincogenesis), provide useful examples of the modern biological study of reproduction as it emerged in the first half of the twentieth century and was transferred into mammalian systems by fusing together an increasing number of stem technologies. The effort to replicate the process of fertilization in glass reflects the continuing emphasis on combining biological substance with technology that had become more common during the last decade of the previous century, now adding the traction gained through experimental embryological studies that employed improved cell culture methods. These models both worked better and could do more work. They also circulated more widely across both species and continents, as well as lines of experimental investigation. From the perspective of the history of technique, a noticeable feature of the evolution of human IVF out of studies such as those conducted on both sides of the Atlantic by Pincus between the wars is their complex imbrication within so many otherwise unrelated experimental trajectories, or what we might call their very mixed, or hybrid, technical parentage.[33] These thick genealogies of IVF, while intriguing in and of themselves, are also helpful in illuminating the instabilities that remain at the heart of human IVF today—for example in terms of what is meant, exactly, by fertilization, epigenesis, potentiality, or, for that matter, biological reproduction at all, once these workings have been increasingly technologized.

It is the technological kinship established through both meticulous training in received technique and the passing around of these experimental methods into different hands that enables experimental innovation to proceed along its continually meandering path—just as Needham described for the ad hoc embryology of an earlier period. What is visible from this point of view are the complex relationships linking ideas or concepts (experimental questions) with technical means (tools, technologies, or technics), and their various milieus—including both those that are inside the experimental system (e.g., culture media) and those that condition the experimentalist within a specific culture of science (e.g., developmental biology). These are what Andrew Pickering describes as "the continual reconfigurations of the material, conceptual and social strata of science that make it impossible to specify the relativity of scientific knowledge to any substantive variable"—a pattern that constitutes the "structure of practice" in science, and which he describes as "path dependency" (1995: 208–209). Thus we return again to the "magical" frontier space of a reaching beyond both the substance and the technology at hand—a practice that arguably takes on additional importance when the frontier is the human conceptus in vitro.

Taking Fertilization in Hand

Gregory Pincus had been a student of W. Z. Crozier, who in turn had been trained by Jacques Loeb, the German American scientist who developed "artificial parthenogenesis" at the Zoological Station in Naples in the 1890s, during the same period Heape was conducting his embryo transfer studies in mammals in Prestwich.[34] Working with the traditional embryological model organism, the sea urchin, Loeb had sought to use experimentation as a more direct means of biological translation—driving biological processes forward to new speeds, as it were, by not only exploring but harnessing the developmental mechanics of eggs and embryos. Loeb pursued a philosophy of biological invention based on forcing biology into new shapes—much as a breeder might attempt to shape or mold an organism to develop to order. In pursuit of his bioartifice, Loeb developed experimental methods (based on botany) enabling him to chemically induce parthenogenetic division in sea urchin eggs by modifying the salt content of their nutritive medium—that is, by controlling internal events via manipulation of the *milieu exterieur* in an early version of what later became known as cell or tissue culture. Unlike Heape, whose interests lay in elucidating the basic principles of heredity as they would have occurred naturally and internally, Loeb's experiment has been described as a more explicit turn toward an engineering ethic in biology that had the production of novel, synthetic, and unnatural biological forms as its goal. As the historian Philip Pauly describes Loeb's interest in the artificial induction of parthenogenesis, it made manifest a new role for science and a new self-image of the scientist as the origin of biological control: a "conscious engineering standpoint" that "considered the main problem of biology to be the production of the new, not the analysis of the existent" (1987: 8). The author of *The Mechanistic Conception of Life* (1912), Loeb sought to exploit the analogy of mechanics from the problem-solving vantage point of a creative engineer: like the successful agricultural biotechnologist he later became, Loeb was less concerned with what biology is than what it could be made to become or do. He considered "successful experimental control [to be] functionally equivalent to scientific explanation" (Loeb, quoted in Pauly 1987: 9). He similarly considered audacious pioneering to be the best way forward on the uncharted biological frontier of the early twentieth century—an analogy he saw as properly American, and through which he believed biology could be rendered more thoroughly technological.

Pincus was a scientist very much in the Loebian tradition, and Pincogenesis exemplified the engineering mentality described by Pauly, which prioritized the isolation and observation of a specific mechanism in order to establish "a constructive or engineering biology in place of a biology that is merely analytical" (Loeb, cited in Pauly 1987: 93). Whereas amphibian model organisms, with their useful capacity for regeneration, were well suited to illustrating the complex developmental mechanics of Roux, His, and Spemann, the ability to manipulate fertilization held out a more pragmatic promise to Loeb, who compared the production of whole, new, manmade biological constructions to the bold and unprecedented tunnels and bridges built by heroic Victorian engineers such as George Stephenson or Isambard Kingdom Brunel (or the steam engines designed by Watt). As Landecker points out in her account of the history of "culturing life," Loeb argued that such experiments held out the promise of "a technology of living substance" (Landecker 2007: 1), the deliberate, creative redesign of which was no more unnatural or monstrous than motorcars or telegraphic communication. In this model, technology did not assist biology so much as produce a new definition of biological control. As Pauly stresses, Loeb was explicit in his goal of creating "new forms whose properties depended solely on scientific action" (Pauly 1987: 51). He was less interested in the character or properties or principles of biological entities and processes in themselves than what could be achieved through manipulating them toward specific ends—a position that, as Pauly observes, "reversed the priorities of analysis and control" (51). As a consequence, argues Pauly, Loeb sought to engineer biological substance beyond its merely natural limits purely in order to see how far it could be reengineered: "Loeb's project was not applied science. It was a refocusing of biological inquiry itself around what Loeb conceived as the activity of the engineer. . . . He considered the distinction between natural and pathological irrelevant. . . . Breaking down the distinction between natural and monstrous would be a necessary preliminary to the development of an engineering biology" (51).

As Hannah Landecker has observed, this definition of biology as engineering emphasizes the importance of the tools and techniques the experimentalist can use to manipulate synthetic living systems, with the express purpose not only of observing their mechanisms or mimicking their functions but of redesigning and remaking new biological systems and tools. It is not only the difference between the natural and the pathological that is irrelevant to such a pursuit. Crucially, it is also the importance of the synthetic or artificial that is emphasized in and of itself as a singular goal. In other words, it is the collapse of a distinction between biology and technology that specifically distinguishes the mode of reproduction this definition of biology as artificial synthesis prioritizes. As a consequence, the differences between what is biological, what is a biological mechanism, what is an experimental apparatus, and what is an experimental tool are deliberately rendered opaque. In a word, biology is relativized. Within an artificial, handmade in vitro system such as Harrison's hanging drop experiment, in which a fragment of tissue is enclosed in a droplet of lymph on a glass cover slip, inverted over a hollowed-out slide, sealed with paraffin, and incubated at the correct temperature to allow the tissue to grow for up to a month, it becomes entirely unclear where the biology ends and the technology begins. Self-evidently the entire setup is simulated: a bespoke synthetic, in vitro propagation of an organic mass that serves as a model biomimetic system. It no longer matters whether this bioartifice is about seeing or making, being or doing, knowing or controlling, or nature or culture — the point of this working model of life is that it is viable and accessible, that it can be observed and manipulated, and thus that it can be reworked. Such a system exemplifies the principle Hannah Landecker describes in her account of how living substance comes to be taken in hand, which is not only that life or biology come to be regarded differently in vitro, but that biology is changed by becoming a component within an artificial system. As she puts it more concisely, "biotechnology changes what it is to be biological" (Landecker 2007: 223). Arguably, as we shall see, what the history of experimental embryology and IVF also demonstrate is the extent to which biology changes what it is to be technological.[35]

Indeed, the process by which biology changes what it is to be technological is exactly what both IVF and embryo transfer model as technologies of reproductive substance. Arguably what is also evident is the extent to which technology is biologized in the form of new living tools — a new species of tools that comprise a distinctive form of technological evolution. From the point of view of the evolution of technique, it is irrelevant that much of this work was experimentally inconclusive, misleading, or failed — because much of it was not result but technique driven to begin with. Its larger object was not only modeling biological mechanisms, or for that matter reworking them, but building a new biology in which tool and substance work together biologically. Gregory Pincus and Robert Edwards were remarkably similar in this respect — both were iconoclastic, antiestablishment, and controversial biological engineers, very much in the Loebian tradition of seeking social progress through controlling life. Pincogenesis, for example, was most successful technologically, establishing the viability of an ex vivo model system to replicate a biological process, despite the fact that it ultimately failed to demonstrate successful IVF. Biologically, in terms of what this term generally refers to at the level of fundamental biological processes, it remains unclear today what, if anything, Pincogenesis revealed about the primal scene it was designed to illuminate. What it confirmed instead was how different species of technique could be successfully crossbred in the effort to manipulate life more skillfully.

Pincogenesis

Ironically, it is precisely the technological success of Pincogenesis that obscured the very process Pincus was trying to observe in a telling example of how technology cannot reveal the workings of biology, because it changes them. In his 1961 reassessment of the literature on mammalian IVF, Austin cites thirty-five articles by twenty-one authors dating back to 1878. In only three of these studies were live offspring obtained, the earliest of which were the experiments by Pincus and Enzmann in rabbits in 1934. As Chang writes in his 1968 appraisal of these three experiments, none could reliably be confirmed to have been successful. "Due to the technical difficulties involved in conducting such studies [of mammalian IVF] and lack of confirmation of [the results of] these experiments by others, together with the unreliability of the criteria of fertilization used by some investigators, the evidence for fertilization of mammalian eggs *in vitro* even at present may still be in doubt, and it becomes to some extent a controversial issue" (Chang 1968: 15).

Ostensibly, part of the confusion concerned the precise mechanisms of fertilization and how they should be characterized, but much of it inevitably concerns the technical means by which this process is documented and analyzed. For example, in the early studies of both in vivo and in vitro fertilization, as Chang points out, "most investigators considered fertilization to mean the penetration of a sperm into the cytoplasm of an egg, but in reality this phase is only the beginning of fertilization" (1968: 15). "*Biologically*," he continues, "fertilization is a physiological process, which starts with the penetration of sperm into the cytoplasm of the egg, and includes the subsequent formation, development and syngamy of the male and female pronuclei until the union of maternal and paternal genetic materials" (1968: 15, emphasis added). Austin, in his 1961 review, further emphasizes that the egg can only be considered to have been fertilized when it has begun to cleave. Pincus, in his early experiments on fertilization in the rabbit (1930) had observed not only cleavage but penetration of the spermatozoon into the vitellus, as well as the existence of two polar bodies, although he did not claim at the time to have achieved fertilization in vitro. Both lack of sufficient knowledge of the definitive criteria for confirming fertilization, and inadequate technological control of the in vitro model system (it is very difficult to determine by sight alone if the spermatozoon has passed fully through the zona pellucida, for example) created uncertainties.

Serial failure, as much as serial success, then, was required to bring biology and technology sufficiently into alignment in order to both identify and achieve all of the necessary steps in the process of *in vitro* fertilization.[36] In his later experiments with Enzmann, Pincus claimed to have successfully obtained live offspring using IVF and embryo transfer in mammals for the first time. However, since they only mixed the eggs and sperm together in vitro for half an hour, and then washed the eggs before transferring them to a surrogate doe, it is likely the offspring were the result of undetected sperm clinging to the eggs' surface, which were then able to capacitate and fertilize the egg in vivo (an early version of what is now known as gamete intrafallopian transfer). Indeed, it would not be until the successful codiscovery, separately by Austin and Chang, of sperm capacitation (the need for mammalian sperm to be exposed to the female reproductive tract for a period of time before they are capable of fertilizing an egg) that successful mammalian IVF could be confirmed by Chang in 1959. Over time, the fertilization of mammalian eggs was only fully characterized and successfully confirmed as a result of a lengthy process of experimental repetition and innovation. Successful IVF in mammals resulted from the intergenerational acquisition of sufficiently elaborate knowledge and technique necessary to model the event in question. In other words, the ability to replicate the union of egg and sperm depended upon the success of a prior union between biology and technology, and this synthetic modeling project was itself an offspring of combined lineages of scientific expertise. The elaborate apparatus required to induce ovulation, surgically remove a ripe egg from the reproductive tract, culture it in vitro, fertilize it in vitro, and transfer it back into the uterus to establish a pregnancy could only be achieved through an increasingly intimate merging of technology and reproductive substance—to the extent that it is not clear which is the more successful coupling involved in IVF, that between the egg and sperm, or between artifice and biology. More to the point, it means that the only biology that can be fully characterized in the context of such modeling is that produced when reproductive substance can be brought into a successful working relationship with experimental techniques. That this forced, harnessed, or cultivated biology is at once more fully characterized and more surprising is the result of the kind of biology it is—namely a biology that only works when it is coupled to the right tools.

In addition to the domestication of semistandardized (well-trained) experimental methods (for animal husbandry, surgical procedures, culture techniques, incubation temperatures, etc.) and agreed-upon criteria for processes such as fertilization, another crucial feature of mammalian in vitro experimentation familiar from other histories of equipment is the effect of accumulated scale. The greater project of characterizing how reproduction works needed to be undertaken on a vast comparative basis, achieved through the circulation of both model organisms and proven techniques through many hands and over many generations, in order to fine-tune the workings they could reveal, or produce, in the laboratories of highly trained experimentalists. Scale is of course particularly important to science in terms of evaluating and reproducing experimental results, and in the identification and elucidation of missing factors—such as egg maturation or sperm capacitation. Gradually, over time, the differing reproductive cycles and mechanisms of various mammalian species have become part of a much larger archive of know-how that has in turn yielded new factors: how conception happened for hamsters, for example, could not be relied upon to establish its precise workings in mice, never mind goats, deer, or dogs. It was only over time, and with the benefit of increasing cross-species (interspecific) comparison (scale) that the early events of mammalian development could be more reliably characterized as a linear series of stages or steps—in order that they could be reliably (technically) reproduced. In their own cyclical way, basic techniques and experiments—including both IVF and embryo transfer—are also scaled up, thus sedimenting into place a stable base of stem, or platform, technologies that is endlessly repeated. These lineages of technique were literally fused with the lineages of model organisms used in embryology (which often became model organisms through the repeated application of particular techniques) thus comprising the inherited technical physiology of developmental biology. It is in the merging of these various tools and models that a new ability to work biology becomes more practiced and reliable—even if it is not at all clear what this functionality reveals in the curiouser and curiouser world of early mammalian development.

Thus, for example, Pincus begins his book *The Eggs of Mammals* (dedicated to Crozier) by typically comparing two very different model organisms through the same technology. "The fundamental control of the cleavage mitoses is alike in rabbit and sea urchin ova" (1936: 98), he notes. One lineage here is his direct academic descent from Loeb via Crozier, while another is a technological inheritance—or kinship of technique—through the reprise of classical experiments, such as artificial parthenogenesis (à la Loeb) and embryo transfer (à la Heape). Despite the fact that Pincus's book is largely descriptive and offers no obvious engineering solutions (and might even appear to be dedicated to the use of in vitro methods in order to return to an earlier era of classical or descriptive embryology characterized by "mere" observation[37]), his Loebism is apparent in his overriding emphasis throughout the 160-page monograph on the means of investigation. "The investigative aspects are what interest and intrigue me," he writes (1936: vii). Here, then, as Hannah Landecker points out, the "cycle of artificial parthenogenesis" is proof of "a genealogy of plasticity [that] structures today's experimental probing of the manifold potentiality of living matter and the practical experimental milieus in which cells are made to live" (2007: 8). However, we might add that this genealogy of plasticity is also one in which technology acts as a kind of shared substance of descent, remaking the science as scientists remake their work objects and technical objectives.[38] This technical evolution, while linear, is thus also cyclical—endlessly recapitulating the alliance between the objects and methods that constitute its lineage—and recombinant, as it recirculates these elements, by passing them around, as it were, through a kind of experimental exogamy. The means of investigation—the constant remixing of known model systems and model organisms with new animal species and genres of technique—are thus as much an object of study, and source of discovery, as the processes they are designed to investigate.[39] This circulatory recycling of technique fused with substance is, indeed, how reproductive biology reproduces itself as a science. The importance of passaging and transfer partially explains why the biological phenomena this branch of science investigates—be they fertilization, cleavage, ovulation, or heredity—are never purely biological, or for that matter never fully "understood." Indeed, as Pincus says himself, his book about the eggs of mammals is as much about techniques as ova. It is "an examination [of] the *experimental investigations of* the growth and development of the mammalian ovum during the various stages of its life history in the ovary and oviducts" (1936: 128, emphasis added) (figures 3.6 and 3.7).[40]

Landecker's emphasis, like that of other historians of twentieth-century biology, on "those practices that exploit and explore the plasticity of living things" (2007: 8) is evident in Pincus's use of IVF and artificial parthenogenesis in combination with techniques of both explantation (tissue culture) and transplantation (embryo transfer) to explore oogenesis across a range of model organisms from different animal species subjected to repassaged

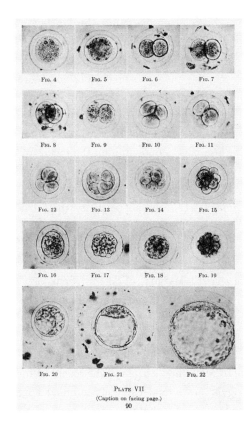

PLATE VII
(Caption on facing page.)
90

FIGURES 3.6 AND 3.7.
Mammalian ova in culture documented by Gregory Pincus in one of the numerous tables of experimental data contained in his *The Eggs of Mammals* (New York: Macmillan, 1936).

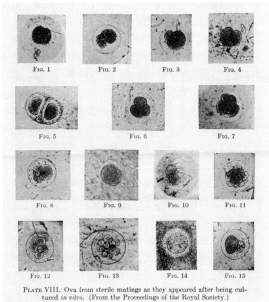

PLATE VIII. Ova from sterile matings as they appeared after being cultured *in vitro*. (From the Proceedings of the Royal Society.)

and recycled species of technique. Pincus, like Robert Edwards, was strongly motivated by a conviction that inadequate attention had been paid to the living mammalian egg due to a technical deficit, or, as he put it, "because no technique was developed for preserving it intact *in vitro*" (1936: 2). Pincus was determined to remedy this technical deficit, and he provides an exhaustive review of existing tools and technologies (including cinematography) alongside those he has invented himself (such as a new form of pipette for removing ova during lapararotomy; 66–67). The outcomes of hundreds of experiments are meticulously recorded through "standard motion picture cameras adapted for microphotography" (66) in Pincus's *Eggs of Mammals* over the course of ten chapters containing twenty-six tables, thirty-three figures, and thirty-six original photographic plates that together document a technological history as well as a physiological one. Throughout his technologically adventurous researches, Pincus was dedicated to an instrumental genealogy of technique: to "the experimental investigation of the growth and development of the mammalian ovum during the various stages of its life history" (1936: 128).[41]

On the one hand, this question for Pincus concerned "the problem of the origin of the definitive ova" (128, also referred to as the origin of the "so called 'primordial' germ cells of the embryo," 6), while on the other it was dedicated to another kind of development entirely, namely of the technical means available to pursue these obscure origins, ranging from the use of ultraviolet light and radiation (X-ray sterilization) to the injection of bespoke hormonal preparations. Both what Pincus classed as the "essentially descriptive" (1936: 5) observation of egg cell morphogenesis and the more explicitly interventionist "experimental investigation of the growth of egg cells" (6) achieved by "varying the conditions . . . and deducing from the derived data the nature of the factors concerned in the production of functional eggs" (6) relied on the constant development of new techniques, including those of visualization and calculation, as well as surgery, tissue culture, and the ability to artificially simulate both chemical and physical events relevant to "the physiological processes occurring in developing eggs" (53). As a record of what the effort to take living mammalian ova "in hand" involves, his portrait of an evolving technological milieu is as thorough as that provided by Marx of Adam Smith's famous pin factory.

The experimental work for *The Eggs of Mammals* had taken place largely in the absence of any detailed understanding of the endocrinology of mammalian reproduction, but nonetheless made significant contributions to this field that would later be applied to the development of the first successful oral contraceptive pill—the achievement for which Pincus is historically most well known. His own interests continued to focus on parthenogenesis, and it was his aim to produce live offspring from unfertilized eggs that had been artificially induced to begin development when he left Cambridge, Massachusetts, for a sabbatical in Cambridge, England, in 1937. He had noted in *The Eggs of Mammals* that although "we have seen that rabbit ova may be fertilized and cultured *in vitro*" it remained unclear "whether such ova may give rise to normal rabbits"—noting that on the basis of his published work with Enzmann (Pincus and Enzmann 1934) the "transplantation of such ova into the oviducts of pseudopregnant rabbit [reveals] that [only] ova fertilized *in vitro* and also normally fertilized ova kept in culture during the cleavage period apparently resumed normal development after transplantation as evidenced by the production of normal young at term" (Pincus 1936: 96). Pincus had concluded on the basis of this work that "it would seem then that parthenogenetic development may be induced *in vivo*" and that "presumably normal embryos might develop if a diploid cleavage nucleus could be induced to form," suggestively adding that he and Enzmann had "in fact, found indications that such a process may occur in activated rabbit eggs" (1936: 111).

These published observations were the source of significant media coverage, including a *New York Times* editorial that compared "Dr. Gregory Pincus of Harvard" to the character of Bokanovsky, the Director of Hatcheries and Conditioning, in Aldous Huxley's *Brave New World*. In 1937 Pincus was the subject of a sensationalist article in *Collier's* magazine unfavorably depicting him as a well-resourced, impatient young scientist with a name "borrowed from a detective novel," with "slender, almost feminine hands" and the grand vision of fatherless offspring: "the mythical land of the Amazons would then come to life. A world where women would be self-sufficient; man's value precisely zero," the article concluded (cited in Speroff 2009: 88). This negative publicity, combined with the advent of the Second World War, the demise of Harvard's Department of Physiology and the Bussey Institution, and "the fact that he was Jewish" (Speroff 2009: 89), led to the termination of Pincus's employment at Harvard while he was in England.

During 1938–1941, while Pincus was involved in a lengthy relocation to what would eventually become the Worcester Foundation for Experimental Biology (where both the first successful mammalian IVF and the birth control pill would later be born), another émigré biologist, Min-Chueh Chang, was earning his PhD in John Hammond's Animal Research Station at Cambridge. Unbeknownst to either of them, and never having met in Cambridge, Pincus and Chang would spend the rest of their working lives dedicated to a lengthy series of experiments on the endless frontier of reproductive science, much of it applied to American medical and agricultural problems, just as FDR had imagined. Indeed, Chang was to arrive at the newly established independent biological research facility in central Massachusetts, an hour outside Boston, almost coincidentally with the publication of Vannevar Bush's influential report in March 1945. Together, Pincus and Chang would contribute to the curious evolution of IVF largely through their work on contraception—exactly the kind of applied project Roosevelt would have applauded, although with an outcome he is likely never to have imagined.

The Birth of IVF

As noted at the outset of this chapter, there are many reasons why the frontier analogy might be considered particularly apt to describe the postwar development of reproductive biology and its translational offspring in the form of human IVF, for it is possible to sketch the outlines of something very much like what FDR appears to have envisaged when we consider the postwar development of reproductive biomedicine and bioscience. However, I have also suggested that the frontier idiom is in some ways more complicated than it seems—at times even paradoxically so. These complications, I suggest, may be apt, since they provide a useful interpretive perspective from which to examine some of the more paradoxical aspects of the development of IVF and experimental embryology, as well as biology and the life sciences more broadly. The mixed idioms of the frontier and pioneering may help us to appreciate that being after IVF is not simply to be in a position to potentially benefit from a successful clinical application that was deliberately achieved at the end of a lengthy process of translational scientific advance. Instead, I have suggested, it may be helpful to distinguish between the frontier as it is encountered going forward and how it is reckoned in hindsight—in the same way we might somewhat skeptically view the technological progress narratives that are likely to appear more goal oriented from the point of looking backward, or from the standpoint of a proven technological success story (the miracle baby). This distinction is similar to that separating the forward-looking anticipation of the frontier as a gigantic landscape of opportunity, and the experience of probing more experimentally with the tools at hand. The difference between these two perspectives allows us to approach the question of the technological frontier less in terms of a specific goal, or aim, and instead, as Gell suggests, through the magic of an imaginative reach, or play, that extends beyond the merely real in an approach to the edges of the known. The resulting, ambivalent and fortuitous, model of scientific development is more consistent with the haphazard evolution of IVF than the this-discovery-led-to-that-landmark-result model of technological development—as if it were a chain reaction, or even inevitable.

The second reason I have employed the frontier idiom as hermeneutic guide in this chapter is to exploit its traction as an analogy for conversion, through which what is beyond the merely real can become the "regular real"—as have airplanes traveling over the North Pole, or babies conceived in a dish (to name but two examples). From this point of view we can appreciate the process by which technology domesticates its objects—by making them workable and tractable, as well as viable and populous, through the sedimentation of relationships of technique that often have the reproduction of technology as their immediate goal. As is explored further in chapter 7, this transfer, or conversion, of the unknown into the known is what the idiom of the frontier delivers, or performs, as a representational device, or metaphor, to naturalize new relationships—such as those between biology and technology as evolving ways of life. By invoking this representational work of conversion and retrospective sedimentation, I want to suggest that the paths established in and through technological inheritance—what we conventionally think of as the advance of technology—is, like the frontier, more complex and multifaceted than it may seem. In vitro fertilization is a good example of this kind of complex evolution, as is the history of embryology, because the conversions and transmutations that occur in these realms (among others) not only stretch but frequently exceed the frames of the models, idioms, or metaphors used to represent them.

Like other technologies, IVF stretches and exceeds the frame of existing understandings—for example, by enabling an unusual transfer "into man" not only of a high-tech reproductive substance (an in vitro fertilized egg) but a living human tool. For in addition to being a biological relative, a much-desired would-be take-home baby, or a precious human embryo, the in vitro fertilized human egg cell is also a technology, in the most conventional sense of the term. But it is clearly also an unusual technology—a fusion of biology and engineering, a mechanization of substance that establishes a new biological relation to and as technology—and one that arguably becomes curiouser and curiouser even as it is more fully characterized in a scientific sense. What are we to make of the miracle baby's complex ancestry on the technological frontiers that made his or her existence biologically possible as the offspring of a vast, interspecific project of reworking reproductivity? What are the implications for either biological or technological evolution of their union in the form of several million human offspring?

Before moving any further with this question, the final section of this chapter briefly completes the tool history of the world's most famous embryo transfer, conducted by Patrick Steptoe in his Oldham obstetrical ward, following the successful fertilization of Mrs. Brown's egg in Robert Edwards's lab next door. It is Chang, working in Pincus's lab, who is now acknowledged to have achieved the first live births following IVF in mammals in 1959 — an accomplishment that was itself the offspring of a long lineage of successful embryo transfer experiments in the rabbit (1891), rat (1933), sheep (1934), goat (1934), mouse (1942), cow (1949), and pig (1951). It would be another two decades before this technique was successfully translated into a clinical procedure by Edwards and Steptoe following their recycling and recombination of several lineages of technique as well as their tenacious "forward march" into unknown territory. Like Pincus, Edwards was at least as interested in the development of new techniques as what they would reveal about the underlying biological principles they were intended to explore, and like Chang he was particularly interested to exploit the possibilities of IVF and embryo transfer in mammals for a wide variety of research purposes. Indeed, like many of the embryo transfer pioneers who preceded him, including both Chang and Pincus, Edwards was adept in exploiting the somewhat chaotic overlap between the actual and potential uses of embryo transfer for agricultural applications, as a research technique to address basic questions of mammalian reproduction and development, and as a potential clinical tool (the latter initially envisaged, as mentioned earlier, as a contraceptive device).

From *Inovulation* to IVF

Following his initial training in agricultural science in Wales, Edwards moved to Conrad Waddington's bustling interdisciplinary Institute of Animal Genetics in Edinburgh as a doctoral student, where he was surrounded not only by high-quality experimental science but by the superb facilities provided by Waddington's generous funding. Here he was inspired by a film produced by Alan Beatty titled *Inovulation* demonstrating a new method of cervical embryo transfer in mice, resulting in the birth of viable offspring. Sitting at the back of the lecture theater, Edwards recalls, "I became more and more excited. . . . There and then I knew what I wanted to do as a PhD student and who I wanted to supervise me" (Edwards and Steptoe 1980: 20). Having completed his PhD research by inducing chromosomal changes in mouse embryos, Edwards set off to California to embark on a new project in reproductive immunology, returning to a position at the National Institute for Medical

Research in Mill Hill, north London, in 1958. Here too his interests fluctuated: "I flitted from laboratory to laboratory in the UK and the USA, changed scientific and medical partners in a way unmatched in any barn dance" (37). Still motivated by his early work stimulating mouse egg development using gonadotrophins, Edwards resumed his embryological work at Mill Hill, only to discover that the in vivo maturation of mouse eggs in culture solution had already been confirmed by Pincus at Cambridge a quarter of a century earlier. And not only in mice, as Pincus had also successfully cultured human eggs. Initially disappointed ("I sat in the Mill Hill Institute library momentarily depressed; the novelty of my discovery had suddenly worn thin," 40), Edwards soon reevaluated his discovery (or rediscovery) in more favorable terms. "As I drove home to Elstree I pondered, 'Was it so sad?' It was encouraging in practical terms. Human eggs, according to Pincus would ripen outside the body and become ready for fertilization" (40).

In order to explore these practical (now translational) frontiers, Edwards needed to make contact with clinicians. Extending the interdisciplinary barn dance about which he was already somewhat uncomfortable, Edwards was to find himself even more awkwardly situated in the surgeries he needed to visit to acquire human eggs for his research. Having gained the collaboration of Molly Rose, the consultant surgeon who delivered his first daughter, Edwards became a regular visitor to the Edgware General Hospital in North London, where he attended operations self-consciously "clutching [his] glass sterile pot—the receptacle for the precious bit of superfluous ovarian tissue." Here, he felt himself both a novice and out of place—on the very threshold of the path to unprecedented future human applications, and yet ambivalent regarding this proximity. "'What am I doing?,' I asked myself. 'Do I really have a place in this theatre?'" (Edwards and Steptoe 1980: 42). Similarly, his new research on human eggs, begun with "high hopes," soon "began to feel less certain." None of the eggs provided to Edwards by Rose or other gynecologists showed any signs of ripening in culture. He decided Pincus had been wrong.

> Pincus, whom I respected and whom I had met two or three times, was wrong [and] had been wrong before. His work on parthenogenesis during the 1930s, on the birth of fatherless rabbits, had failed to stand the test of time. All the same, I admired him enormously. Among the famous scientists whom I have met and come to know he still stands near the top. Pincus had helped to reshape modern life, especially for women, with his contraceptive pill. I thought then, as I think now, that he never received full recognition for his work. There are men—

pygmies compared with him—who have been awarded Nobel Prizes. Perhaps he was too controversial. . . . He was a fighter. He was gritty and outspoken. He would have made a fine Yorkshireman! (1980: 43)

Edwards was a Yorkshireman himself, and his admiring description of Pincus draws attention to many of the traits they shared. Eventually Edwards would also be awarded the Nobel Prize in Physiology or Medicine in 2010 for his work leading to the development of human IVF, which, like contraception, has reshaped modern life, especially for women. Edwards's work was controversial, and IVF would not have been successfully achieved in humans had he not been a gritty and outspoken fighter, who valued his role as a pioneer. Like Pincus, who in many ways set the prototype for his unconventional, technique-driven, iconoclastic, and unusually interdisciplinary career, Edwards was a "scientific entrepreneur," in the way Adele Clarke (after Howard Becker 1963) has applied this term to the reproductive sciences, emphasizing the extreme heterogeneity of relationships between professional worlds that must be negotiated by key actors, who require a wide range of skills, as well as the will and energy to interconnect them, in order to succeed. Like Pincus's, Edwards's career was challenged by what Clarke describes as the "enduring illegitimacy, marginality and controversial status of the reproductive sciences as a discipline" (1998: 18)—a situation Edwards met with a combination of verve, tenacity, and hard work that ultimately benefited from a generous dose of good luck.

As Martin Johnson (2011) has noted of the partnership that would develop between Robert Edwards and Patrick Steptoe, they were both outsiders to their professions and the establishment, known not only for their iconoclasm but for their ambition and talent. It can be added that theirs was in many respects a marriage of technique, beginning with a telephone conversation in 1967 about laparoscopy, and developing over the next two decades as a modern technological odyssey the adjective Promethean is not out of place describing. Along the road to successful human IVF in Oldham, Lancashire, in 1978, not very far from either Birmingham or Manchester, or the mechanical workshops of the Industrial Revolution, Edwards dug deep into the long legacy of technical innovation in experimental embryology described in this chapter, in order to rework human reproductivity to deliver a new mode of human procreation in which biology and technology were viably coupled. To this work Steptoe added the highly successful technique of laparoscopy (now the basis for keyhole surgery and many other clinical and experimental uses) while Edwards devised the means to fertilize human eggs in vitro.

While the obstacle of infertility confronted Steptoe in his practice as a gyne-cologist, it is clear that the value of IVF went far beyond the ability to assist conception in Edwards's far-reaching vision of IVF as a platform technology for everything from preimplantation genetic diagnosis to stem cell propaga-tion and tissue engineering. The confirmation of the birth of viable human offspring from this pioneering technique both inaugurated and legitimated the progressive expansion of the reproductive frontier into future applica-tions that have since made of IVF what Walter Heape, a century previously, had established through mammalian embryo transfer—namely a platform or stem technology with a life of its own.

Thus, while the legacy of Steptoe and Edwards as the medical-scientific partnership behind the first successful human IVF may remain umbilically linked to the image of the test-tube baby, and the birth of reproductive bio-medicine, it could equally be claimed that it is the transfer of the IVF platform into human use *tout court* that has proven to be of an even greater significance we have only just begun to appreciate. The meaning of this legacy is the ori-gin of *Biological Relatives*, in asking whether the logic of IVF extends beyond human procreation to other reproductive purposes. Even the somewhat sur-prising scale of human IVF's expansion worldwide over the past thirty-five years may pale in the wake of its future significance—which will not only be measured by IVF's expansion into genetic disease prevention, human em-bryonic stem cell research, and regenerative medicine, but must take into account a watershed point in the very meaning of the adjective "biological" as it becomes increasingly synonymous with technology. Reproductive tech-nology is arguably a pivotal point of (con)fusion for the anxious contemporary question of what kind of kinship or relationality shared biological substance establishes, and what kind of mechanics reproductivity comprises, responds to, or delivers. These are not questions that can be answered in the lab unless it is the conflation of human experimentalism and human evolution that are considered to be the laboratory writ large in which the mechanisms of fron-tier reproduction will continue to be characterized over time.

But this future might be better charted by careful study of the past than by more open-ended speculation, and it is thus the lived relationship to early IVF that is the focus of the following chapters. In order to understand the condi-tion of being after IVF, or biologically relative, it is necessary to examine yet another dimension of this process, in order once again to view it from a differ-ent angle. For if, as I have suggested, the kinships of technology that engender IVF must be understood as relational—uniting tools, objects, concepts, prac-tices, and people—so too does their union reveal a new technology of kinship, and a new biology. Indeed, this is the point of IVF—its goal is to produce new biological relations through technology, and thus a new future for reproductivity, as kinship both through and as technology. As we shall see, the biological relations established through new reproductive technologies depend on genealogies not only of scientific technique but of even older social technologies. In the next chapter, then, we turn to yet another stem or platform technology—the social and cultural organization of human reproduction as kinship that has an equally elaborate set of exact mechanisms, if a somewhat different set of tools. As we shall see, this apparatus also fuses the biological with the technical—and indeed has done so for much longer than IVF.

FOUR Reproductive Technologies

In the previous chapter, the workings necessary to take reproductive substance in hand in order to characterize and remake it were explored in the context of embryology. This chapter turns to the examination of gender and kinship as technologies not only in order to demonstrate how they are necessary in order for IVF to work, or that they are also remade through IVF. By examining the exact mechanisms and elementary structures of IVF through the lens of kinship theory, this chapter suggests once again that this technique is not exactly what it seems in part because it changes what is being reproduced, by producing an imitation that is both similar to and different from the original forms on which it is based, modeled, or after. Like chapter 3, this one argues that IVF is not only biologically reproductive but technologically reproductive as well, and thus constitutive of a distinctive form of regeneration in which these two processes are combined to make new people.

As Alfred Gell notes in his discussion of technology, it is not only "inadequately understood" as tool use, but must include within its definition the sum total of social relationships that make knowledge and technique possible, thus ultimately comprising all "the necessary conditions for cooperation between individuals in technical activity" (1988: 6). But what is technical activity? Gell identifies a basic level of technical activity to provide food, shelter, clothing, manufacture, and tools. He includes language and communication in this category, which he classifies as "Technology of Production." However, as he notes, human societies are particularly notable for their tendency to "go to extreme lengths to secure specific patterns of matings and births," adding that infant socialization is conducted in "a technically elaborated way" and that human beings are "bred and reared under controlled conditions that are technically managed, so as to produce precisely those individuals for whom social provision has been made." As a result, he emphasizes, "the reproduction of society is the consequence of a vast amount of very skilled manipulation" and this technical system "include[s] most of what conventional anthropology designates by the word kinship," a term he paraphrases as "Technology of Reproduction" (Gell 1988: 7).

As Gell states, "the whole domain of kinship has to be understood primarily as a technology. . . . The patterns of social relationships we identify as 'kinship systems' are a set of technical strategies for managing our reproductive destiny via an elaborate sequence of purposes" (1988: 7). This chapter goes somewhat further to suggest that the understanding of kinship, as well as gender and sex, as technologies is not fully captured by the positing of a role for technology as managerial or strategic—although this provides a useful starting point. If, as we saw in chapter 3, technology is not only added to, or even grafted into, living substance, but becomes a new kind of living substance as a result, then technology is more than managerial. It is less additive. The work it does is more substantial, and its relations are less divisible than even Gell's encompassing definition suggests. Technology is more "world-building," to use Haraway's (1997) phrase. Arguably, this aspect of how technology works is particularly visible from the point of view of kinship, thus making it a useful perspective to graft onto those explored so far. Although the intersection between biology and technology in this chapter is rather different from that discussed in the context of embryology, it too works in ways that can be precisely charted, and the workings of kinship, as well as gender and sex, take on particularly interesting meanings in the context of IVF, where an unusually recursive form of technology transfer is ongoing—as we have already seen. An obvious question, albeit a challenging one, is to ask what relation these different models of technology, and their precise workings, might bear to one another. In the continuing spirit of a thought experiment, this question motivates my turn in this chapter to a consideration of kinship as a technology from the point of view of being after IVF.

One of the great difficulties of appreciating the operation of kinship as a technology, in both anthropology and social life, has been the intransigent question of what kinship organizes—which is conventionally imagined as the natural flow of reproductive substance. There has always been a bit of magical thinking going on in this respect within kinship theory, where on the one hand kinship emerges through the imposition of social law, but on the other hand is determined by certain universal qualities of human physiology—and indeed by the natural flow of reproductive substance that must be managed. In the same way that technological evolution has often been assumed to be automatic (if not explicitly then by default) or based on self-evident needs, so too has the evolution of kinship systems largely been explained as a process that is based on a preexisting natural mechanism with a biological purpose that requires no further explanation. The difficulties of moving beyond a naturalized model of reproductive biology, and its accompanying presumption of automatically polarized sexual difference, are both well known and widespread. The faulty logic here is the same we often encounter in explanations of technological development that simply assume it is inevitable.

What the looking glass of IVF helps to reveal is how technologies of kinship and gender, among others, activate reproductive substance, not the other way around. Indeed, IVF makes explicit how and why technologies of kinship not only organize reproduction but are reproductive substance—and thus how reproductivity is itself produced, worked up, or cultivated. This way of thinking is counterintuitive in part because natural agency is conventionally presumed to precede social, or technological, management—as if biological reproduction is a process that will occur regardless, or even by itself, as it were. However, this automatic reproductive model is exactly what the existence of IVF contradicts: if biological reproduction acted by and for itself, IVF would not be necessary. In vitro fertilization is intended to achieve reproduction in "a technically elaborated way," as Gell put it, employing "a vast amount of very skilled manipulation" (1988: 7). As we saw in chapter 3, reproduction came to be understood experimentally through technologies designed not only to manage it, but to manipulate the reproductive process—and indeed to fundamentally reshape its actions by controlling and redirecting them. Significantly, it is precisely this history of transforming biology into a technology that gives rise to clinical IVF—arguably experimental embryology's most successful translation. Because IVF is dedicated to the project of forcing reproduction, its genealogy lies in the acquisition of technological control. This is the point of view from which IVF engenders biological relativity—an identity between biology and technology that makes it impossible to determine where the one begins and the other ends—and as we shall see, this is also the perspective from which IVF can be seen to be modeling, and extending, how kinship functions as a technology not only of reproduction but of production as well.

The story that is retold in this chapter—whereby a presumed biological base to kinship, gender, reproduction, and sex came to be understood instead as a technology—foregrounds a parallel between the elementary structures of IVF and the experimental life of kinship, sex, and gender in culture, as it were. However, the effort is also to push the overall argument about IVF a bit further—by asking once again what IVF models, and what it substantiates or reproduces as a way of life, a kind of life, or a way of living the remaking of life. How does IVF model the future of kinship as a technology (or the future of technology as kinship)? Arguably, what IVF reveals, both as a reproductive model and as a technological path, is the extent to which human reproductive substance has always been activated in more complex technical ways than may heretofore have been made so explicit. If this technicality is the condition for reproductivity, then technology is more than merely a means—it is shared reproductive substance.

One of the main reasons this question matters is because it allows us to see how much more than the prospect of miracle babies is reproduced through IVF, and the future of kinship it substantializes. As is argued in the next two chapters, and as has been discussed already in chapter 1, the rapid and extensive expansion of IVF technology over the past three decades cannot simply be explained by either its success or its popularity—not least as these two criteria contradict each other. Either the use of IVF has expanded rapidly because it is popular in spite of having a less than 50 percent success rate, or its popularity and success rely on something other than its disappointing take-home-baby ratio. Put differently, the rapid and widespread expansion of IVF technology cannot be explained by its popularity as a reproductive technology unless it is successfully reproducing something other than offspring. In vitro fertilization may be popular, for example, because the pursuit of success is important regardless of the odds against it, or it may be that the pursuit of IVF offers something else, or because at least being seen to try to procreate is preferable to doing nothing. These possibilities lead to others. If biological reproduction (like kinship) is not simply driven by an automatic transgenerational flow of reproductive substance—if, as Gell claims, it must be organized and managed through complex technical strategies—then is there a degree to which it is the implementation of such strategies for their own sake that explains, in part, why IVF is so popular? While this might seem almost absurd from the point of view of the ostensible goal of IVF (to make babies), this chapter reviews the important reasons why the pursuit of biological offspring should not be presumed to be as obvious a goal as it might seem. We can also go further than this and ask whether the success of IVF is, at a very fundamental level, simply reproducing an active relationship to technology, full stop. Perhaps IVF is not only about managing or improving biological reproduction, but is itself a means of producing other things, other relationships, other values, or other identities. Surprising though it may seem, for example, there is a great deal of evidence to suggest that what IVF organizes and enables are parenthood and kinship identities that can be achieved without having babies.

As we shall see in this chapter, most theories of kinship have presumed it must be based on something else—it must come after nature, or as a result of biology, for example. Yet the alternative possibility that kinship could have been invented simply for itself is strongly implied in much of this same literature—particularly that of Lévi-Strauss, who, like Gell, strongly emphasizes free play and creativity and primarily describes kinship as a language. The most significant flaw in the arguments of Lévi-Strauss concerning the origins of kinship derive from the offensive and unnecessary argument that it is women's natural reproductive capacity that gives rise to the exchange of women, and that it is competition over this good that necessitates the first social law of exogamy, inaugurating the transition from nature to culture. But these are also his most unconvincing claims, since why should a self-acting, but gendered and sexed, reproductivity lie at the base of human social life, initially manifest as the exchange of women, and what explains this premise? The origin of this self-acting model of fecundity as a gender-specific good, and the mute intransigence of this premise—not only in the work of Lévi-Strauss, but in much of social and political thought throughout the twentieth century—lies in the fact that, unlike kinship, sex and reproduction have been viewed as "merely biological." Until recently, the exact mechanisms of sex and reproduction have simply not been theorized because they are presumed to be too obvious to require explanation.[1] Thus they have been ignored. In vitro fertilization is interesting not only because of the degree to which it makes the activation of reproductive substance so vividly explicit, but because of the further questions this revelation foregrounds—or indeed forces into view. For example, to what extent is IVF a successful conjugal technology despite its failures as a reproductive one? Similarly, might it be a highly successful technology for the reproduction of gender identities and gender roles regardless of its reproductive outcome? Is it, as Gay Becker (2000) suggests, a technology that allows for the reproduction of a trying identity, a striving-after identity, or even a means of reproducing a class identity? These are important questions to ask because if it is the case that people feel they must undergo IVF in order to be seen to be trying everything, who is this trying for and what is it in aid of? If it is for the alleviation of personal distress in the face of a failed, or spoiled, identity, then is IVF a technology for identity repair? Is this what IVF technology is after in the sense of why it is pursued by so many—who are perhaps not only seeking a technology of reproduction, but technologies of gender and sex, or the arrangement of successful conjugality? Is IVF a technology not only for making babies but for making kinship, or repairing it, in the wake of a breach in the expected automatic flow of reproductive substance? Put most broadly, to what extent is IVF a technology for producing new types of identity and sociality not only in addition to, but sometimes instead of, making babies? If IVF substantializes a new ground state of reproductivity, and if this is why it exists, does this form of reproduction come into being, like kinship or writing, simply for itself? If this appears too simplistic an explanation for the origins of IVF, it is worth recalling that the idea that kinship systems essentially reproduce themselves for themselves is taught to undergraduates as one of the elementary structures of both social emergence and social life.[2]

In sum, is IVF a technology that has never been reducible to the pursuit of successful reproduction in the strictly biological sense of the term?[3] Yes, clearly, IVF is used to provide much-wanted children for couples whose infertility prevented them from having biological offspring of their own—and this is clearly part of the reason it exists at all. And yet such a goal is more complex than it might appear, as well as being only part of the story. As with most goal-oriented applications, the objective is never entirely self-evident to begin with and is always supplemented by additional effects, even when it is achieved. This overdetermined quality of IVF technology has been the subject of considerable attention from feminists, and rightly so as IVF is a technology with more complex and often paradoxical consequences than its apparently self-evident function suggests. In contrast to the idea that IVF is a simple, essentially mimetic, technology directed at obvious ends, and that it is increasingly popular despite its shortcomings simply because these ends are so hugely desirable, exists the possibility that IVF is neither simple nor simply mimetic, and that neither what it is reproducing nor how it works are obvious at all.

Experimental Kinship

In one of the very first anthropological analyses of new reproductive technologies, published in the early 1990s, Marilyn Strathern described them as experiments and invited her readers to "ponder upon how to think about experiments being conducted in a real system that is regarded as *both* a biological *and* a social one" (1992b: 3). Such an intervention, she suggested, would be likely to have far-reaching effects, since "ideas about kinship offered a theory, if you like, about the relationship of society to the natural world": "Having sex, transmitting genes, giving birth: these facts of life were once taken as the basis for those relations between spouses, siblings, parents and children which were, in turn, taken as the basis of kin relations. Incorporated into such a reproductive model were suppositions about the connection between natural facts and social constructions" (Strathern 1992b: 5). Fittingly, Strathern's favored adjective to describe the separate and distinct but overlapping logics of the hybrid reproductive model grounding English or Euro-American kinship thinking is "merographic"—a term she explains in relation to the embryological term "meroblast" (1992a: 204n).[4] "Merographic connections," as they are habitually used in the English-speaking world where IVF was invented, work to connect plurality and singularity at once—conserving the distinctiveness of the domains that are brought into conjunction, while emphasizing the plurality of connections that can be made in this way. Thus, for example, as Strathern explains: "Culture and nature may be connected together as domains that run in an analogous fashion insofar as each operates in a similar way according to laws of its own; at the same time, each is also connected to a whole range of other phenomena which differentiate them—the activities of human beings, for instance, by contrast to the physical properties of the universe" (1992a: 73). The English penchant for merographic thinking ("putting things into context") can most simply be described as making "a connection from another angle" (1992a: 73), and this conceptual mechanism is especially useful for generating new perspectives as separate domains are exchanged, or transferred, thus changing the background against which parts can be characterized.

What Strathern wants her modern readers to note is how this mechanism introduces an inevitable plurality into the process of defining even those things that are imagined to stand for themselves—such as a biological fact. In vitro fertilization can be used as an example, since it can be thought of as part of either a biological or a technical process. In social practice, it is indeed a characteristic and even regular feature of the world of IVF that people constantly switch back and forth between these two points of view, or inhabit them simultaneously as convergent, if also distinct, perspectives. Moreover, it is precisely the experience of inhabiting multiple contradictory frames of reference at the same time that in part accounts for the distinctiveness of the IVF experience, and its inherent ambivalence. And this is also Strathern's point about merographic thinking—the fact that different domains of knowledge can be exchanged draws attention to the instrumentalism by which contexts of interpretation are altered and recombined, so that, for example, IVF can be seen as just like biology, or as a form of technological control.

In vitro fertilized embryos fit easily within a merographic model of facts that belong to multiple and transferable logics, or orders. More than just plural or hybrid, the research objects produced within contemporary scientific study in fields such as synthetic biology, regenerative medicine, and tissue engineering are classically merographic in the sense that the logics of their parts belong to several distinct but overlapping wholes. The logic of experimental embryology precisely relies upon epistemological transfers of this kind, through which biological components come to be understood by moving them around, and by resituating the same phenomena within different technological or biological orders or wholes. That these transfers produce effects is the whole point of this kind of empirical science, which it substantializes in the form of entities like Spemann's push-me-pull-you salamander. Similarly, recombining these parts to make new wholes, such as artificial embryos, cybrids, and cell lines, might be called a merographic technique that substantializes, or implements, a merographic conceptuality. Strathern's description of English kinship in *After Nature* is remarkably accurate to describe the principles informing this style of investigation. "Each order that encompasses the parts may be thought of as a whole, as the individual parts may also be thought of as wholes. But parts in this view do not make wholes. . . . Thus the logic of the totality is not necessarily to be found in the logic of the parts, *but in principles, forces, relations that exist beyond the parts*" (Strathern 1992a: 76, emphasis added). Indeed, it may be in the contemporary biosciences where Strathern's point that it is a habitual feature of the modern English mind-set to think merographically is uniquely applicable. She refers to it as "the English view that anything can be part of something else." As she explains, the "very fact of trying to put something into context is a merographic move." Not surprisingly, since it applies not only to English but to modern, post-Enlightenment thought, this principle describes experimental science, and in particular developmental biology, very accurately since it is all about recombining parts into new wholes. Hence the "whole" human genome can refer to a complete genetic sequence of a species, as in "the human genome," the genetic constitution of an individual (Craig Venter's genome), and a technological project (as in, "the human genome was sequenced in 2001").

Descriptions of genetic function likewise refer to code, information, messages, transcription, copying, mutation, sequencing, writing, splicing, programming, multiplication, language, libraries, architecture, grammar, beads on a string, spaghetti, and the alphabet. This is precisely the plurality merographic connections enable, through which metaphor and metonymy are conjoined. Similarly, the names that are given to the protein sequences that comprise genes, alleles, mutations, or markers belong to different conventions of scientific description according to how they are measured, marked, or mapped—and according to which techniques are used.[5] The postgenomic sciences connect these distinct domains merographically because they rely on multilayered understandings, which simultaneously invoke plural and divergent conventions of explanation, yet remain coherent because they are partial. Merographic thinking, then, is not only habitual but necessary to contemporary science, where it is important that a word like "gene" is neither too specific nor less real because such key concepts and analogies are only loosely attached to their objects. Like the biology the word "gene" is used to analyze, the term itself must retain a plasticity that allows it to be intercontextual.

The fact that merographic thinking is reproductive (in the sense of always generating new connections) takes on an additional dimension when it is employed in a reproductive context such as IVF. Here, and as we see further in chapter 5, merographic connections are used, in part, to instrumentalize reproductive substance—to equip it to function, or to put it in motion to reveal its mechanisms. Merographic thinking is not merely metaphorical. The substitution of an instrumental technology (IVF) for the process of biological reproduction (sex) in the name of producing future biological offspring (kin) is achieved through a translational merographic move, connecting what is imagined as substance (nature) to agency (culture). Merographic thinking, in other words, is part of the conceptual equipment necessary to make IVF both thinkable and doable, indeed to make it workable at all. This is one reason why new reproductive technologies such as IVF provide a context for especially thick descriptions of how reproduction is understood to work, or how it is imagined to be made to work, or put to work, by the technologies that make it workable.[6] This is also how IVF becomes the stage on which reproductive aspirations become newly generative, prolix, and explicit through their new connections. Merographic thinking is part of what makes the IVF platform work so well—and thus how it becomes so successfully reproductive.

Of the many reasons it is useful to revisit the feminist critique of the anthropological model of kinship as part nature, part culture, three are particularly relevant to this chapter and have determined its shape. Merographically, perhaps, this chapter makes a connection from another angle to the same questions examined in the previous chapters concerning the intersection of a biological model of procreation with a technological model through which it is reengineered (IVF). To the extent that this intersection is the viable union, or coupling, IVF confirms and reproduces in the form of viable offspring, it is worth noting that IVF also, therefore, literalizes the merographic connection between biology and artifice as a kinship connection—that is, through ties of substance achieved through cultured-up procreation. As Charis Thompson (2005) has shown, it is the way the biological relation that is the goal of IVF is taken apart and put back together in the process of producing it that can be traced so explicitly through this technology — a process she describes as "strategic naturalization." In this sense, and just as Strathern originally observed in her analysis of kinship in the context of new reproductive technologies in the early 1990s, IVF and assisted reproductive technologies more broadly introduce a new dimension to kinship — by providing new biological relatives that simultaneously make explicit new definitions of them (social, scientific, legal, ethical, cultural) and new mechanisms (technological, artificial, man-made) through which they are made. This is how new categories of biological relatives have come into existence ("gestational mother," "egg donor," "IVF twin," "saviour sibling," etc.), but also how the very idea of a biological tie has been relativized — in both senses of the term. The results, argues Strathern, are not only "a new ambiguity about what should count as natural" and a new distinction "between social and biological parenthood" (1992b: 19); in addition, IVF reveals the mechanics of how reproduction is composed and organized in order to be activated, acted upon, or realized in the making of kin and kinship. The contingency of biological reproduction is exposed, Strathern suggests, in the very process of forcing it to work. "The more facilitation is given to the biological reproduction of human persons, the harder it is to think of a domain of natural facts independent of social intervention" (1992b: 30). Here, again, we see a demonstration of how the merographic mechanism of this reproductive model becomes more generative through its contingency (it produces more kinds of biological relatives).[7] Indeed it is contingency that activates the merographic mechanism.

I return at the end of this chapter to the role of technology in Strathern's merographic thought experiment. The reason such a question arises is itself doubly assisted by developments in feminist theories of gender and kinship during the 1980s, in ways that pose yet another technological trajectory to ponder upon. This chapter anticipates the next, where I argue that a review of the feminist analysis of women's experience of reproductive technology raises the somewhat counterintuitive question of whether IVF is a technology of making sex that both underserves and exceeds the goal of making babies. In the discussion below, this question is "prequelled" by reviewing how gender and kinship come to be theorized as technologies of sex within feminist anthropology, in contrast to the use of this term by Foucault. A possibility I explore, in part relying on Strathern's earlier work in *The Gender of the Gift* (and leading up to her famous claim that Melanesian babies don't come from women), is that far from "taking away the very concept that made kinship itself a distinctive domain" (i.e., a priori natural facts), or making it "harder to think of a domain of natural facts independent of social intervention," IVF and assisted reproductive technologies simply deliver merographic conceptuality in the form of new biological relations as technologies. I suggest that this may not be so much a departure from kinship thinking but, as Strathern argues, its original form.

The approach in this chapter draws primarily on feminist anthropological debates about kinship, gender, and reproduction, and, like the previous chapter, redescribes a conceptual evolution indigenous to a specific field of investigation. The story told here is thus part of the history of science, narrated through the development of new techniques to explore the exact mechanisms of reproductivity. Like chapter 3, this one is also composed of a series of case studies, episodes, and snapshots. It begins by revisiting Gayle Rubin's crucial early theorization of the sex/gender system before moving on, in a more or less chronological fashion, to the feminist anthropological engagement with structuralism and the work of Lévi-Strauss. In the middle section I give careful consideration to the feminist anthropological critique of the nature-culture dichotomy, despite the already vast literature available on this debate, because I have a particular point in mind about its relation to the emergence of the gender-as-technology argument, most closely associated with the work of Judith Butler. The discussion here, although also covering much familiar ground, is aimed to elucidate the ways in which sex is mechanized, not only to produce a reciprocating set of linkages to chapter 3, and the rest of this book, but to explore further the meaning of biological relativity. This merographic use of the mechanical analogy is intended to emphasize points of overlap or connection between these arguments. It is the question of what these connections reveal, and how to reveal them, that determine the mosaic form of this book as a whole. If, then, the following discussion appears either to retrace familiar ground for some readers, or to introduce completely new terrain to others, that is in part because its aim is not traditionally synthetic but deliberately formal. My aim is to identify and connect the repeated elucidation of specific forms—namely the exact mechanisms by which sex is technologized not only through IVF but through the systemic apparatus of gender and kinship technologies.

The Sex/Gender System

In her landmark contribution to feminist anthropological theories of sexual inequality in the mid-1970s, Gayle Rubin introduced the term "sex/gender system" as part of her call for a "political economy of sexual systems" to explain how "particular conventions of sexuality are produced and maintained" (1975: 165). "The Traffic in Women: Notes on the 'Political Economy' of Sex" draws inspiration from Marx and Engels both in its model of social reproduction and in its diagnostic method of reading Freud and Lévi-Strauss as feminism's Ricardo and Smith, who "see neither the implications of what they are saying, nor the implicit critique which their work can generate when subjected to a feminist eye" (Rubin 1975: 159). Whereas Marx had a robust method of political critique but took no account of gender, sexuality, or sex (Rubin argues), Freud and Lévi-Strauss each outline a "systematic apparatus that takes up females as raw materials and fashions domesticated women as products" (1975: 158) but offer no critique of sexed subordination. "What we need is a political economy of sexual systems. We need to study each society to determine the exact mechanisms by which particular conventions of sexuality are produced and maintained" (1975: 177), Rubin memorably concluded, in an essay that inverted much of the feminist legacy that inspired it by arguing that gender and kinship are technologies for producing sexuality and sex, not simply organizing them.

Rubin defines the sex/gender system twice in her article. Initially she offers a "preliminary definition" of it as "the part of social life which is the locus of the oppression of women, of sexual minorities, and of certain aspects of human personality within individuals" (a definition that is explicitly meant to denote something like Marx's underdeveloped concept of social reproduction, but note the early emphasis on individual sexual personality). "For lack of a more elegant term," Rubin describes this social mechanism as the "sex/gender system," which she defines as "the set of arrangements by which a society transforms biological sexuality into products of human activity, and in which these transformed needs are satisfied" (1975: 159). Shortly afterward she offers a second definition: "Every society has a sex/gender system—a set of arrangements by which the biological raw material of human sex and procreation is shaped by human intervention and satisfied in a conventional manner, no matter how bizarre some of the conventions might be" (1975: 165). Both definitions begin with Marxist references—to products and raw materials respectively—and both emphasize that the "set of arrangements" is structural and systemic. The first definition ends with a quasi-functionalist reference to the satisfaction of certain basic needs, whereas the second definition instead emphasizes conventions—one of the most frequently used terms throughout Rubin's essay.[8] "Biological sexuality" in the first definition becomes "the biological raw material of human sex and procreation" in the second. The mechanism in the first sentence—how society transforms biological sexuality into products—is altered in the second, which refers to the way human intervention shapes biological raw material.

These variations usefully illustrate both the enormity and the difficulty of the numerous interlinked tasks outlined and tackled in Rubin's prescient and still influential essay, in which she attempted to "sketch some elements of . . . the genesis of sexual inequality" (1975: 158), but also, and perhaps more notably, forcibly challenged the ways in which this problem had come to be defined. The essay is thus dedicated, in proper Marxist fashion, both to the conceptualization of apparatus and to the apparatus of conceptuality. The difficulty of defining what "sex/gender system" refers to is one that Rubin is herself eloquent in diagnosing, both in the writings of the male theorists she rereads, and in feminist politics. Like Shulamith Firestone, she is concerned with the missing domain most often referred to as social reproduction: she wants to expand its scope and to characterize its products more completely in order both to encompass the production of sexual difference and to reverse the standard account of where sexual inequality comes from (e.g., a set of biological sex differences that are given in nature). Thus it is Engels from whom Rubin takes her main inspiration—arguing, exactly like her predecessor Firestone (1972), that we need a new and more comprehensive version of *Origins*. However, it is precisely a model of the production of sex or gender difference that Engels lacked (as, for that matter, did Firestone), and thus it is the production of sex and gender that Rubin seeks to explain—a task that leads her to the analysis of kinship.

Underlying Rubin's effort to retheorize kinship as a mode of producing a sex/gender system, and the sex/gender system as a form of political economy, is her persistent frustration with the view that it is mere biology—or "animal biology" as she calls it at one point—that is the source of women's subordination. This was, of course, a primary concern of feminist anthropology in the 1970s (as it has been throughout the history of feminist thought). The feminist effort to root out the persistent biologism within various anthropological accounts of social structure had, since the mid-1970s, taken several tracks, but with varying degrees of success—often (paradoxically) reconfirming the intractability of animal biology rather than dislodging it. Hence, for example, in her landmark essay "Is Female to Male as Nature Is to Culture?" (first published in *Feminist Studies* in 1972 and later republished in the edited anthology *Woman, Culture and Society* [Rosaldo and Lamphere 1974]) Sherry Ortner equated the denigration of women ("the universality of female subordination," 69) not with "biological determinism" (which "almost anyone in anthropology" would agree had "failed as an explanation," 71) but with "the framework of culturally defined value systems" (i.e., social conventions) within which the biological differences between women and men "take on a significance of superior/inferior" (71). In other words, woman is not closer to nature, but she is *perceived* to be through a cultural apparatus that produces this effect. She is not biologically inferior, but her association with biological reproduction excludes her from equal authorship of cultural, political, and social institutions. In other words, her inferiority is derived not from a biological function but from a grammatical one.

Ortner's influential argument took advantage of the main attraction of structuralist anthropology identified by Rubin, namely that it "places the oppression of women within social structures, rather than in biology" (Rubin 1975: 175). However, like many other feminist anthropologists in the 1970s, Ortner struggled to leave behind the generic and habitual biologism that lies at the foundation of the human sciences and remains broadly commonsensical today. Like Simone de Beauvoir, on whose work her analysis is closely based (and whose famous passage on male transcendence she quotes at length; 1974: 75), Ortner continually returns to the very "biological differences" between women and men her theory ostensibly set out to challenge. Here, in contrast to the plastic biology we encountered in chapter 3, is the rigid universal biology of so much social theory, always already imagined as preset to a binary sexual dimorphism that is determined by its reproductive function. It is this "physiological contrast between male and female" (Ortner 1974: 75) defined by the reproductive function, or, as Ortner interprets it, "women's greater bodily involvement with the natural functions surrounding reproduction" that cause her to be universally "seen as more a part of nature than man is" (76).

Within structuralism, as is discussed further below, this same model of reproductive biology similarly plays a dual role as both a sign and a condition. It is the difference between the two that provided the wiggle room for early (1970s) feminist critiques of biological determinism such as Ortner's. What makes structuralism attractive to Ortner is the replacement of biological facts by a social mechanism. In many ways, Ortner is reading Lévi-Strauss exactly as he intended to be read, as a theorist of the "exact mechanisms" out of which kinship originates. Where Rubin sees a biological trap, Ortner sees a handy device. Ortner cites the famous passage in the closing chapter of *The Elementary Structures of Kinship* in which Lévi-Strauss explains why "the rule of exogamy" is "the only means . . . of avoiding indefinite fission and segmentation which the practice of consanguineous marriages would bring about" (Lévi-Strauss 1969: 479). Such fragmentation would, he claims, create "so many closed systems or sealed monads which no pre-established harmony could prevent from coming into conflict" (479). Ortner cites this same passage still further, in which Lévi-Strauss makes the crucial claim that "the risk of seeing a biological family become established as a closed system is definitely eliminated [by the rule of exogamy]: the biological group can no longer stand apart, and the bond of alliance with another family ensures the dominance of the social over the biological, and of the cultural over the natural" (Lévi-Strauss 1969: 479, cited in Ortner 1974: 78). Adding that this is the same structural mechanism that accounts for women's universal subordination, Ortner reaches her signature conclusion that "if the specifically biological (reproductive) function of the family is stressed, as in Lévi-Strauss's formulation, then the family (and hence woman) is identified with nature pure and simple, as opposed to culture" (197: 79). It follows that "men are identified not only with culture, in the sense of all human creativity" but are seen as "the 'natural' proprietors of religion, ritual, politics, and other realms of cultural thought and action" (79). Crucially for Ortner, this is a mechanical (structural), not a biological, problem.

Having deciphered the workings of the machinery, Ortner logically proposes how it might be reverse engineered. Thus she adds an important qualification concerning the role of reproductive biology in relation to gender inequality. In contrast to the Lévi-Straussian diktat that their reproductive biology ensures that women "in general represent a certain category of signs" that are "destined to a certain kind of communication" which "like words, should be things that were exchanged" (Lévi-Strauss 1969: 496), Ortner argues women might as easily be valued as the source of culture for the same biological reasons.[9] After all, it is women who socialize infants, guiding them from nature into culture in their role as nurturers ("it is she who transforms new born infants from mere organisms into cultured humans, teaching them manners and the proper ways to behave" [Ortner 1974: 79–80]).[10] In the home, she is also "a powerful agent of the cultural process [by] constantly transforming raw natural resources into cultural products . . . which could easily place her [according to Lévi-Strauss] in the category of culture triumphing over nature" (Ortner 1974: 80).

Again, it is the grammar, not the biology, that needs to be changed. The system can be rewired, hacked, reassembled. True enough that this counterargument reinforces a biological model of sexual difference and does nothing to challenge the prominence of reproductive biology as a determinant (indeed, it is not intended to). But Ortner is hardly unaware of the shortcomings of Lévi-Strauss's biologism (in sum, that exogamy is essential to human survival because it mandates the systematic exchange of women). Arguably, she very nearly implies that his biological models are redundant to his argument altogether. What she is pointing to is his compelling depiction of the elaborate technology of kinship through which the human is not only born but made (a depiction that has long been part of structuralism's appeal to many, including Rubin). Ortner rightly questions the presumption that simply because women are deemed the "valuables par excellence" (Lévi-Strauss 1969: 481) in this system that "the emergence of symbolic thought must have required that . . . women themselves are treated as signs, which are misused when not put to the use reserved for signs, which is to be communicated" (496).[11] Thus, although Ortner has been criticized for claiming that "the secondary status of woman in society is one of the true universals, a pan-cultural fact" (1974: 67) and that "it is simply a fact that proportionately more of woman's body space, for a greater percentage of her lifetime . . . is taken up with the natural processes surrounding the reproduction of the species" (75), her argument nonetheless anticipates the later theorization of sex as technological.

Both Ortner's original article (1972) and the volume in which it was reprinted (Rosaldo and Lamphere 1974) remain paradigmatic set pieces for an important avenue of feminist anthropological models of gender subordination during the 1970s. Despite their own inscription at times within a biologized discourse of gender and sex (and often reproduction in particular), these approaches drew on the utility of structuralist approaches in order to challenge biological determinism by locating the source of gender asymmetry in the symbolic grammar, or cultural mechanics, of kinship systems, thus relativizing the cultural importance of biology—if not biology itself. The potential to denaturalize, to de-essentalize sex, sexuality, and reproduction is very close at hand in these arguments that approach the making of sex mechanically (or "technologically," to use Gell's term). Indeed, as Rubin emphasizes in her analysis of structuralism, it offers "an acute, but condensed, apprehension of certain aspects of the social relations of sex and gender" in which kinship is understood as a mode of production "in the most general sense of the term: a molding, a transformation of objects (in this case, people) to and by a subjective purpose [that] has its own relations of production, distribution, and exchange, which include certain 'property' forms in people" (Rubin 1975: 177). However, Rubin is both more cautious than Ortner in accepting Lévi-Strauss's methods and conclusions, and more focused on what his theory leaves out. She is most similar to her French colleague Monique Wittig in doubting the entire premise of *The Elementary Structures of Kinship*.[12] Rubin diagnoses a different mechanical problem than Ortner: it is not that the tool has to be used differently; it has to be improved. Indeed, and as she is among the first to suggest, Levi-Strauss's structuralist anthropology is most revealing of what it lacks, namely a more precise account of the exact mechanisms by which sex and gender are organized and produced:

> If Lévi-Strauss is correct in seeing the exchange of women as a fundamental principle of kinship, the subordination of women can be seen as a product of the relationships by which sex and gender are organized and produced. . . . There is an "economics" of sex and gender, and what we need is a political economy of sexual systems. We need to study each society to determine *the exact mechanisms* by which particular conventions of sexuality are produced and maintained. The "exchange of women" is an initial step toward building an arsenal of concepts with which sexual systems can be described. (Rubin 1975: 177, emphasis added)

Stark Categories

While she accurately perceived their potential utility as tools for analyzing sex and gender, Rubin also characterized structuralism and psychoanalysis as "the most sophisticated ideologies of sexism around" (1975: 200). Citing Derrida's diagnosis of Lévi-Strauss's ethnocentrism, she warned of the danger that "the sexism in the tradition of which they are a part tends to be dragged in with each borrowing" (1975: 200).[13] Rubin's critique of Lévi-Strauss and her concern about the pitfalls of his method (a problem indexed by Ortner's algorithm) was echoed by the response within feminist anthropology to much of the structuralist project during the 1980s, which focused in particular on the unexamined link between binary sex categories and reproductive biology. In a direct response to Ortner's arguments (as well as those of Edwin Ardener [1972] concerning "the problem of women" and Nicole-Claude Mathieu's [1973] "Homme-Culture et Femme-Nature"), *Nature, Culture and Gender*, edited by Carol MacCormack and Marilyn Strathern, was published in 1980, launching an important decade of feminist anthropological theory with a critique of these three terms. From page 1, the editors have Lévi-Strauss in their sights along with his system of "stark categories" standing in "wooden opposition" as if confirming "an ultimate human code"—"a single basic structure of binary thinking underlying all human mental functioning and behaviour"—through which to "understand the whole of human behaviour despite its manifest diversity" (MacCormack 1980: 1–2).[14] As MacCormack points out, this entire hypothesis pivots on an illusion. In place of argument stands the phantom of biological automatism. "One of the great difficulties with Lévi-Strauss's structuralism," she argues, "is the nature of the link between these unconscious functions of the brain and the 'reality' structuralism is meant to explain," especially since "Lévi-Strauss locates fundamental structure at the deep level of unconscious function, and gives it an ontological status, or existence, of its own" (3). In a potent opening chapter to the volume, she draws on the critiques of structuralism within anthropology (e.g., Leach 1970) to argue Lévi-Strauss cannot logically have it both ways—he cannot say the human mind is neurologically hardwired to produce binary categories, and also argue it is this same "natural" mechanical capacity that drives the emergence of human beings out of a state of nature into the definitively artificial state of culture (MacCormack 1980: 4). Like the rest of culture, the grammar of these "stark categories" is made not born, she insists.

Thus MacCormack proposes a counterarchaeology of these stark categories within Anglo-European thought, arguing that they uncritically reproduce narrow cultural traditions and beliefs, such as "the faith of industrial society that that society is produced by enterprising activity" (1980: 6) and the belief in the moral necessity of progress.[15] These received ideas, she continues, are the offspring of "a historically particular ideological polemic in eighteenth-century Europe" reinforced by "nineteenth century, evolutionary ideas [that] provided a 'natural' explanation of gender differences" (7). MacCormack reminds her readers that these same categories were closely associated with the emergence of modern gender roles, and that as early as the mid-eighteenth century "a well established bio-medical tradition observed and defined humans, hardening the conceptual division between unique feminine and unique masculine attributes," thus reinforcing "a biological determinism [that] 'explained' women [while] men were more defined by their social acts, [which is] an attitude of enquiry which persists in some present-day literature on gender" (21). Only the persistent ethnocentrism of Western anthropologists could explain the repeated use of such a highly specific metaphysics to explain the workings of other societies, whose own indigenous categories have nothing in common with the ruling epistemological orthodoxy of English abstract nouns, she concludes.

MacCormack's critique of the narrow historical and philosophical pedigree of the reified concept nouns set out in the first three chapters of *Nature, Culture and Gender* is succeeded by a series of regional case studies combined with historical chapters, such as that by Ludmilla Jordanova exploring the rise of the medical professional in the late eighteenth and early nineteenth centuries. Reminding her readers of the importance to the nascent medical profession of securing control over women's reproductive capacity, Jordanova emphasizes "the historical importance of science, medicine and technology" to the reification, or "hardening," of gender stereotypes and "the promulgation of myths of femininity" often based on the "naturalness" of their childbearing function (1980: 64). In particular, she explores the historical processes through which pregnancy became the object of intense clinical surveillance and medical fascination in the eighteenth century, describing the emergence of a gendered epistemology of the body, as well as the sexualization of scientific knowledge, through which the penetrating gaze of the male physician or anatomist is recapitulated as a form of male heroism and sexual conquest. Jordanova's work, alongside that of other feminist historians in the 1980s, began to revise the historical question of how gender has been shaped by modern science into one that asked precisely the reverse—that is, how modern science is gendered, or how it has been sexed. In this way, Jordanova is among the first to document "sexual vision"—the production of biological facts to order, as it were, not only confirming a naturalized gender binarism but exaggerating it and embedding it in a way of seeing that becomes an institutionalized conceptuality, or indeed convention.

Nature, Culture and Gender concludes with Marilyn Strathern's chapter, "No Nature, No Culture: The Hagen Case," focusing on gender categories in Melanesia. Here, the opening arguments of her coeditor, MacCormack, are ethnographically reprised to demonstrate the limitations of Western philosophical models and concepts, by arguing that among the Hagen

> there is no culture, in the sense of the cumulative works of man, and no nature to be tamed and made productive. And ideas such as these cannot be a referent of gender imagery. . . . These two domains are not brought into systematic relationship; the intervening metaphor of culture's dominion over nature is not there. On the contrary, insofar as gender is used in a differentiating, dialectical manner, the distinction between male and female constantly creates the notion of humanity as a "background of common similarity" (Wagner 1975:118–19). Neither male nor female can possibly stand for "humanity" as against "nature" because the distinction between them is used to evaluate areas in which

human action is creative and individuating. . . . Representations of domination and influence between the sexes are precisely about ways of human interaction, and not also about humanity's project in relation to a less than human world. (Strathern 1980: 219)

In this passage, Strathern not only argues that, as her title suggests, there is no meaningful referent for the signifiers "nature" or "culture." While critiquing the basic premise of Lévi-Strauss's argument (as well as Ortner's, and much of social anthropology), she is nonetheless borrowing from the logic of structuralism more broadly—and of post-structuralism—in her emphasis on gender systems as mechanisms or devices for producing difference. This emphasis on culture as technology is what allows Strathern to begin to challenge not only the binary opposition of nature and culture but the static definition of these categories, as if they automatically partitioned social life into separate domains (an argument that was strongly affirmed by the structural-functionalism of Radcliffe-Brown). As Strathern points out, even within Western societies, "there is no such thing as nature or culture. Each is a highly relativized concept whose ultimate signification must be derived from its place within a specific metaphysics. No single meaning can in fact be given to nature or culture in western thought: there is no consistent dichotomy, only *a matrix of contrasts*" (1980: 177, emphasis added).

Elementary Structures

The effort to extract the analysis of nature, culture, and gender from a static binary technics was accelerated by related shifts within 1980s anthropology at large, in particular the auto-critique of the discipline's colonial heritage and the embrace of more literary or hermeneutical methods, often drawing on post-structuralist insights (Clifford 1983; Fabian 1983; Spivak 1987). A new definition of structure as process, or even as event (as in ritual), and as partial (as in language) was taking hold and, within social anthropology, was giving rise to more diverse and explicitly contingent accounts of cultural forms (Clifford and Marcus 1986). Unlike a previous era in which the Africanist paradigms of British structural functionalism favored attention to lineages, descent groups, and the politics of corporate property and rank, new influences, such as Melanesian ethnography, were more focused on exchange systems, as well as gender, sexuality, and personhood. Similarly, the shift away from descent theory and toward structuralist anthropology (alliance theory) favored the "linguistic turn" toward interpretive or symbolic anthropology, championed by figures such as David Schneider, Clifford Geertz, James Boon, and Roy Wagner. Both Paul Rabinow and Marilyn Strathern were to become prominent figures in this tradition, also associated with what Donna Haraway describes, in her account of gender theory in this period, as "the disaggregation of metaphors of single systems in favor of complex open fields of crisscrossing plays of domination, privilege, and difference" (1991: 140).

At the same time they were critiquing them, however, feminist anthropologists also continued throughout the 1980s to retool established anthropological theories such as structuralism for the study of gender through a process of extended deduction. Thus, in the same way Rubin (1975: 179) follows Lévi-Strauss's deductions "even further" than he himself does, in order to diagnose, for example, both the arbitrariness of his assignment of sex "value" and the need to account for institutionalized heterosexuality, so too does Sylvia Yanagisako read David Schneider's (1984) influential critique of kinship theory several steps beyond his original conclusions in order to draw further feminist insights.[16] Schneider, like many anthropologists, was critical of Lévi-Strauss's biologism, although he also tracked this tendency across much anthropological theory, and especially the study of kinship. He claimed that anthropological theories of kinship in general relied on a base-superstructure model whereby social meaning was "added to . . . some real or putative set of biological, reproductive relationships" (Schneider 1984: 56). Schneider cited Lévi-Strauss as a paradigmatic case, pointing to his a priori reliance on the "limit of elementary structures which lies in the biological possibilities" (56, citing Lévi-Strauss 1969: xxiii) as an example of an underlying biological model of the real natural facts upon which all kinship is ultimately seen to be based: "always it is the genealogical grid, a construct modelled on the presumption of actual biological relations, that underlies the *sociocultural product called kinship*" (56, emphasis added). Schneider argues not only that this view of kinship is no more than a conventional scholarly doctrine, but that it is colonial, Eurocentric, out of date, unscientific, and illogical. He furthermore claims that while there is "virtual unanimity in defining kinship in terms of reproduction" (1984: 193), there is no attempt to justify why this is so, leading him to conclude that "kinship has been defined by European social scientists, and [therefore] European social scientists use their own folk culture as the source of many, if not all, of their ways of formulating and understanding the world about them" (193). The self-acting reproductive mechanism imagined as the base of "the sociocultural product called kinship," he argued, indexed a modeling problem caused by groupthink.

In a Rubinesque extension of Schneider's critique, Sylvia Yanagisako pointed out that the claim that "the genealogical grid" is based on the bio-logical facts of sexual reproduction indexes yet another important folk model, namely that of the sex-gender distinction: "Our model of the natural differ-ence in the roles of men and women in sexual reproduction lies at the core of our studies of the cultural organization of gender, at the same time that it constitutes the core of the genealogical grid that has defined kinship for us" (1985: 1). In their subsequent volume proposing a unified analysis of gender and kinship, Yanagisako and Jane Collier provided a lengthy diagnosis of the role of conventional idioms of natural sex within the anthropological litera-ture on kinship:

> Gender assumptions pervade notions about the facts of sexual repro-duction commonplace in the kinship literature. Much of what is writ-ten about the atoms of kinship (Lévi-Strauss 1949), the axiom of pre-scriptive altruism (Fortes 1958; Fortes 1969), the universality of the family (Fox 1967), and the centrality of the mother-child bond (Good-enough 1970) is rooted in assumptions about the natural characteristics of women and men and their natural roles in sexual procreation. . . . Above all, we take for granted that they represent two naturally differ-ent categories of people and that the natural difference between them is the basis of human reproduction and, therefore, kinship. (1987: 32)

Primary among these "natural characteristics of women and men" is the fact that women bear children, a fact that is "interpreted as creating a universal relation of human reproduction" (Yanagisako and Collier 1987: 33). Like Mac-Cormack and Strathern (1980) before them, Yanagisako and Collier go on to claim that this "folk model of human reproduction" (35) is ubiquitous, and has even "become a convention in much of the feminist literature" (33). They point out that the sex-gender distinction "mirrors the attempt of the kinship theorists reviewed by Schneider to separate the study of kinship from the same biological facts" (33), and go on to suggest that moving beyond the folk model of reproduction would involve submitting "the 'biological' facts them-selves" to investigation, insisting on a more precise account of the "patterns of action" evident in "social events and relationships" (42).

Curiously, however, Yanagisako and Collier do not cite Rubin's (or Fire-stone's) interest in this question, nor do they pursue in any detail what a more rigorous questioning of "the 'biological' facts themselves" might involve. In-stead, following Bourdieu, they advocate a form of analysis that has since come to be known as "practice theory," based on a context-specific, dialectical model of how people are historically shaped by the meanings and structures in which they are embedded, and how they experience, understand, and re-shape these same social forces. At a remove from the vigorous feminist debate concerning precisely "the natural characteristics of women and men and their natural roles in sexual procreation" occurring in other arenas of feminist scholarship during the 1980s, Collier and Yanagisako gesture toward, but do not substantially pursue, the investigation of what "questioning the 'biological' facts themselves" might actually involve. In the early 1980s, this investigation had only just begun to be undertaken (most notably by Haraway 1978a, 1978b, 1979, 1981, 1984, 1985; and Keller 1982, 1983).[17] Even at the heart of feminist anthropological efforts in the 1980s to theorize gender and kinship outside of "the 'biological' facts themselves," the intransigent hold of an imagined self-acting biological mechanism at the base of cultural technics was slow to give up its grip on the mental equipment of its interrogators.

Cross-Sex Persons

Strathern's contribution to *Gender and Kinship: Essays toward a Unified Analysis* (Collier and Yanagisako 1987a) was, like its other chapters, initially written for the 1982 Bellagio conference on which the anthology is based. "Producing Difference: Two New Guinea Highlands Kinship Systems" picks up in some senses where she left off in 1980, by exploring gender and kinship not in terms of what they are but rather what they do, and in particular how they enable detachment as well as connection (Strathern 1987: 272–273). This analysis presumes "a matrix of relationships to which people belong but from which they can also detach themselves"—an instrumental contrast that Strathern argues can be activated through concepts of gender, so that gender becomes "a vehicle for conceptualizing differences in the qualities of kinship attachments" (1987: 274)—again a kind of social technics or cultural grammar, but this time theorized as agency. She thus claims not only that there is no single ordering of gender, and no underlying biology that defines it, but that instead gender and kinship categories are productive instruments that are consciously manipulated by actors for a variety of specific instrumental purposes, and through a wide range of transactions—from gift exchange to ceremonial food production. Instead of women being exchanged like words, it is words that are exchanged to make gender in this account. Mobile gender categories, in other words, are vehicles, devices, or mechanisms put to work in the activation of other relationalities. As Strathern points out, the partibility of identity is an assumed feature even of the kinship systems described by structural functionalists such as Radcliffe-Brown and Fortes, who emphasize that "different components of the person's makeup are visible in the different ties he or she has with others" (Strathern 1987: 275). She adds to this model, however, more substantial emphasis on individual agency by tracing the exchange relations that produce recombinant, transient, and multiple gender and kinship identities, and by demonstrating how the manipulation of "an assemblage of roles" (297) is the basis for producing new persons. In contrast to Western models of "the 'person' as an already existing natural entity" (297), Strathern focuses on the amount of explicit manipulation required to manufacture a specific identity or relationship—a process she describes as a technology of reproduction.

In a closely related argument developed in the same period (although published earlier), Strathern applies these principles more explicitly to the Lévi-Straussian problem of marriage exchange, or what is also known as alliance theory. Published in 1984 in the *Annual Review of Anthropology*, Strathern's analysis of marriage exchange in Melanesia was both a tribute to the increasing importance of Melanesian ethnography and a contribution to feminist attempts to provide a unified account of kinship and gender. In her review, Strathern introduces a critique of the categories "woman" and "nature," and the presumed significance of "the biological facts of human reproduction" that receives fuller treatment in *The Gender of the Gift*, published four years later. In her technically precise reworking of the perennial question of traffic in women, in 1984, Strathern initially sets about analyzing the question of "what 'exchanges' involving and accompanying marriage are about" by using this question as a foil to the many unexamined Western presumptions it reveals (about subjects and objects, gifts and commodities, men and women, society and the individual, etc.).[18] Emphasizing the enormous variety within Melanesian societies practicing marriage exchange, Strathern notes the persistence of "an analytical problem," namely that there is no stable comparative basis within these systems to determine what, exactly, is being exchanged, or by whom. The highly varied marriage transactions, she argues, defy even the complex typologies for which anthropological comparison is renowned. Among the Tor of lowland Irian Jaya who practice sister exchange, bilateral cross-cousin marriage (including first cousins) produces dual organizations, but without named groups such as moieties.[19] There are no bride wealth exchanges, but flutes are exchanged among men to trace their connections to heirs and in-laws through matrilines. Among the Mae Enga of the New Guinea Highlands, affines are the major category of exchange partner among men who trace their connections patrilineally—wives being regarded as exogenous to the patrilineal clan body, but important to ceremonial exchange related to illness, death compensation, or marriage. Among the Kaulong of

New Britain, by contrast, exchange is based on bilateral affinal ties, while residence is organized by cognatic descent. Ceremonial exchange works in opposition to marriage, as it is linked to production, rather than reproduction. And so the list continues of organizational forms that put existing anthropological categories of marriage exchange through the proverbial Cuisinart.

As Strathern notes, such intense regional (and often proximate) variation belies conventional anthropological classification of societies based on types of marriage exchange, forms of kinship systems, or corresponding rules that govern exchange relations. Instead, she suggests, the analysis of marriage exchange requires a complex decoding of sex and gender differences as mechanisms for producing substance: "Differences between the sexes generally provide *a code* for the conceptualization of difference as a ritual or political fact" (Strathern 1984: 50, emphasis added). In other words, "A number of societies discriminate social categories according to the rubric of internal sharing and external exchange, and the gender coding of mediating links invariably underwrites the conceptual divide. *These idioms feed into those of shared substance.* They become an aspect of theories about conception and the constitution of persons and the extent to which persons may be seen as the product of differentiated others" (50, emphasis added, references removed). Strathern refers to this "differentiated bestowal of substance connections" as a means by which "categories of kin thus negotiate social identities *through the exchanges they set in motion*" (50–51, emphasis added). The way in which differentiated substances are transacted and recombined enables connections to be made and identities established, as well as changed, and thus re-activated. The work of activating these substantial connections is evident, for example, in the making of same-sex, cross-sex, androgynous, and pansexual categories of persons, things, and actions as well as recombinant and pluralized means of reproduction. "We can argue that categories of persons 'pass around' sexual attributes among themselves," Strathern suggests, through a traffic that is via gender rather than "in women" (52). This reproductive model not only suggests a different kind of social machinery from that imagined by Lévi-Strauss, who takes biological sex and gender identity as givens that do not need to be explained, but proposes a different mechanism, namely of production or manufacture through recombination and transaction.

From the point of view of the identities and relationships that are defined by the frequent transformation of things into people, and people into things, as well as the transubstantiation of food, wealth, and bodily substances in the constitution — or achievement — of personhood, it is difficult to interpret the exchange of women in straightforward terms, since "woman" becomes a more unstable and shifting signifier. It is not even the case that the very substance of gender has been mechanized, in this view (because gender has no substance in this model), but rather a mechanics that is substantialized as identity (which is the product). Here, gender has become a very different kind of structural mechanism—for which substance is never a primary or originary essence, but rather a product, or means. Identity is no longer unitary, in this view, but made up of adjustable components that can be reproduced anew. From this perspective it makes no sense to imagine woman as a singular, or global, identity—because gender only ever exists as an effect of composition. It is thus impossible even to conceive of the exchange of women, because it is the wrong way around: a woman can only be the outcome of exchange as composition. There is no prior, defining, essential substance on which the identity "woman" can simply be based. The idea that femaleness or sex are at some level merely biological is unthinkable.

This observation implicitly posits that marriage exchange is productive of the very conditions to which it is conventionally seen as a response, namely the biological facts of sex. As Strathern expresses this insight more pointedly: "If 'women' are not the only items which circulate in marriage exchanges, what then is being conveyed in those aspects of their person seen as exchangeable?" (1984: 65). The shift here is precisely away from the idea of the prior substantial person whose given attributes determine a fixed identity (e.g., male) and toward a model of the production of persons and identities through relational, transactional, and intentional labor. Only in a Western system of thought in which biology is understood as an essential, a priori, ontologically and globally defining condition can women become a stable category of goods substitutable for wealth, raw material, or precious and scarce resources, while also becoming a category from which no individual woman can ever escape. Such a premise, Strathern suggests, is unscientific—as logically unsound as the Victorian theories of the primitive horde from which this naturalized, quasi-evolutionary model of natural sex is derived. In sum, a wholesale rethink is required: "we cannot assume how women's fertility will be valued [for the purposes of cross-cultural comparison] any more than we can assume that marriage arrangements concerning women are fundamental to processes of social regeneration" (1984: 65). Strathern concludes, "Frameworks for kinship analyses which turn on the allocation of women in marriage select a particular relation as critically regenerative. This selection hides the very difference between systems whose self-modelling sets up marriage exchanges as symbolically regenerative and those which eclipse or subsume marriage or deny it centrality in the reproduction of 'society'" (66). Like

Rubin, Strathern argues that it is only the self-modeling premise that women have a value that stands for itself, and that this is why they are the transactees rather than the transactors in marriage exchanges, which allows marriage exchange to be understood as the exchange of women by men. As she demonstrates, this is not an assumption that can be empirically verified through cross-cultural comparison. Instead, she shows that gender is the product of labor, of activating a cultural apparatus that involves working it, and thus comprises a form of productivity.

From Being to Doing

These themes were significantly expanded in Strathern's 1988 publication *The Gender of the Gift*, in which, as its title suggests, she presents both a new theory of gender and a new model of exchange. Throughout this paradigm-altering work, gender is variously depicted as a form of action, a product, a medium, a code, and an aesthetic—in sum, gender is theorized as an instrument, mechanism, device, or means.

At the heart of this ambitious project were two core contributions. One, following Rubin's invitation, was a much more precise theorization of the exact mechanisms connecting social reproduction, political economy, and the sex/gender system—albeit no longer cast in any of these terms. Her second major theme was how meaning systems could be analyzed differently within social theory, and she sought to demonstrate how conceptual categories actively constitute their objects, and thus perform a constitutive role as the animating mechanisms of social life. Whereas Strathern's most prominent contemporaries, such as Schneider, had helped to bring about a shift away from structures of function toward structures of meaning, Strathern extended this further to encompass mechanisms of meaning—or indeed meaning as means. The work of Schneider, Geertz, and others had pushed anthropology toward the study of culture and thus symbolic systems, drawing inspiration from the work of both Talcott Parsons (who taught both Schneider and Geertz) and by extension Weber (rather than Durkheim, whose concept of organic solidarity strongly influenced functionalism). At the very outset of *The Gender of the Gift*, Strathern makes clear that her theory of gender is not an attempt to explain synchronic structures of social organization, but a means of introducing a new method to analyze symbols, concepts, principles, and knowledge categories as processual strategies or techniques. As we have already seen in her critique of the traffic in women model, a crucial distinction for Strathern is that "the basis for classification does not inhere in the objects themselves but in how they are transacted and to what ends. *The action is the gendered activity*" (1988: xi, emphasis added). This move from substance to technique marked a decisive shift away from an analytical model based on how social groups functionally cohere in order to produce a whole (social organization) toward a model of the production of difference. Strathern's model eschewed the analogy of either organism or system, and instead drew attention to the disparate connections out of which relationships are composed, animated, and manipulated and through which persons are made, activated, or worked into being.

Although throughout her synthetic and comparative account of Melanesian models of conception and procreation Strathern makes clear that there are enormous variations in the means by which bodies are gendered, including cross- and transgendering, and that ideas of innate shared substance, a naturalized or quasi-biological model of impregnation, or individualized notions of possessing a self are more often than not unhelpful projections based on Western models of reproduction, it is not until the close of the book that she introduces a section titled "Mothers Who Do Not Make Babies" (1988: 311). Since her book is in many ways a response to Rubin, and thus both to Lévi-Strauss and to feminism, her alternative account of reproduction can also be read as a critique of both structuralist anthropology and much feminist theory:

> In my description of the gift economies of Melanesia I have, of course, found it useful to refer to "the person" as an objectification ("personification") of relationships. In so far as people turn one set of relationships into another, they act (as individual subjects) to turn themselves into persons (objects) in the regard of others. They objectify themselves, one might say. . . . Melanesian women cannot be analyzed as commodities in men's exchanges for the obvious reason that these societies do not constitute commodity economies. The negative can take an alternative form: Melanesian women do not make babies. (Strathern 1988: 314)

In contrast to the Western tendency to presume that motherhood is self-evidently a natural fact, "relations do not have such an automatic existence" in Melanesian society, claims Strathern. It is relations that are reproductive, she emphasizes, not simply biology: "children are the outcome of the interactions of multiple others" (1988: 316). Biological capacity is not absent from this model, but it must be coupled with specific mechanisms for producing and arranging persons in order to "make babies." Making babies, to paraphrase Charis Thompson (2005), requires not only "making parents," but much else besides. Biological reproduction in this view is the outcome of a multiplex composition: it does not happen "by itself." Despite himself, Lévi-Strauss implied much the same thing: the making of viable parenthood is the prerequisite for the making of viable offspring. Similarly, his work can be interpreted to be claiming that it is the making of social cohesion that is the prerequisite for both making parents and making babies—just as it is the prerequisite for making language, making art, or making an axe. It falls to Strathern only to point out, then, that birth is the moment at which the multiple prior acts constituting the child are made known and revealed: the simple fact that women can be seen to give birth is only revealing of the penultimate act in a chain of events that can no more be described as primarily biological than as primarily temporal, primarily spatial, or primarily human (Strathern 1988: 316–317). Contrary to de Beauvoir, the assumption that femaleness always stands in immanent relation to the already-produced nature of society can be reversed: "Melanesian social creativity is not predicated on a hierarchical view of a world of objects created by natural processes upon which social relationships are built. Social relations are imagined as a precondition for action, not simply a result of it" (321).

The argument that women do not produce babies is not a refutation of a biological component of reproduction, but it offers a significant reconfiguration of how biological reproduction works. From this perspective, for example, it is evident that reproductive substance is not automatically reproductive. The various components involved in the generation or reproduction of persons must be made, secured, composed, and activated in order to make babies. As IVF similarly, and tellingly, demonstrates with equal clarity, eggs and sperm can only become reproductive within a specific composition and under carefully managed conditions—indeed, only after other preconditions are met in an ordered sequence, and only by these means, which are themselves not always sufficient. In the same way that the reproduction of persons can never be merely biological, mere biology can be induced to become reproductive only via other means. It is these means that produce the conditions of reproductivity: indeed they are reproductivity itself.

Technologies of Gender

The shift away from the taken-for-grantedness of the relationship between sex, gender, reproduction, and kinship toward a fuller account of the "exact mechanisms by which particular conventions of sexuality are produced and maintained" (Rubin 1975: 177) was not only facilitated by feminist anthropology. This was the same period that revealed what Evelyn Fox Keller has described as a "double shift in perception" characterizing feminist accounts of sex and gender: "First, from sex to gender, and second, from the force of gender in shaping the development of men and women to its force in delineating the cultural maps of the social and natural worlds these adults inhabit" (1992: 17). This double shift is also evident in the work of numerous feminist biologists in the 1980s including Ruth Hubbard (1990), Lynda Birke (1986), and Anne Fausto-Sterling (1985)—who recast the question of the biology of gender into one that addresses the gender of biology. Their critiques of the category "female" were aided by the challenge to the category "woman" that gained momentum during the 1980s from a wide range of sources, most notably black and postcolonial feminist theorists and feminists of color such as Alice Walker (1983), Cherríe Moraga and Gloria Anzaldúa (1981), Hazel Carby (1987), Hortense Spillers (1987), Gayatri Spivak (1985), and Audre Lorde (1984). Feminist post-structuralist accounts of gender from feminist literary studies and feminist film theory inspired a new, explicit attention to gender as a technology, most elaborately in the work of Teresa de Lauretis (1984, 1987). Early versions of what has become queer theory appeared also at this time, including Rubin's (1992) later essay "Thinking Sex," and in the work of Eve Sedgwick (1990), among others. These efforts to significantly retheorize gender received powerful synthetic expression in Judith Butler's (1990) *Gender Trouble*, which took direct inspiration from feminist anthropology to recast the relation of sex to gender, or biology to identity, in what remains one of the most influential accounts of the production of sex to emerge from within twentieth-century feminist theory. Disputing the seemingly commonsense view that "being female constitute[s] a 'natural fact'" and arguing instead that such "foundational categories of identity . . . can be shown as productions that create the effect of the natural, the original and the inevitable" (Butler 1990: x), Butler proposed a model that, like Strathern's, radically repositioned "the biological facts of sexual reproduction" as an effect of gender categories, rather than the reverse. For Butler, sex categories (male and female) comprise "a discursive formation that acts as a naturalized foundation" (1990: 37), and she describes *Gender Trouble* as a project designed to expose the circularity of "that felicitous self-naturalization" (33). Like Strathern, Butler defines gender as the product of deliberate artifice: "the repeated stylization of the body . . . within a highly rigid regulatory frame that congeal[s] over time to produce the appearance of substance, of a natural sort of being" (33). Gender thus becomes the substantialization of technique.

Butler, like Strathern and Ortner, is also concerned with the mechanization of sex. From the point of view of the production of new persons, both gender identity and its organization into sexual activity are logical preconditions for biological substance to be put to work reproductively. In this model, biology is not sexual by itself, just as biological substance is not reproductive on its own. Butler thus follows a path similar to that set out by Yanagisako and Collier in their assertion that "the next phase in the feminist reanalysis of gender and kinship should be to question the assumption that 'male' and 'female' are two natural categories of human beings whose relations are everywhere structured by their biological difference" (1987: 7). Arguing for an approach that locates the production of difference within a broader social context, Yanagisako and Collier suggest that "instead of asking how the categories of 'male' and 'female' are endowed with culturally specific characters, thus taking the difference between them for granted, we need to ask how particular societies define difference" (35).

Butler's contention, though pointing in a different direction toward contemporary identity politics, likewise interrogates the presumption that "there is a natural or biological female who is subsequently transformed into a socially subordinate 'woman,' with the consequence that 'sex' is to nature or 'the raw' as gender is to culture or 'the cooked'" (1990: 37). In a direct reprise of MacCormack and Strathern's (1980) arguments in *Nature, Culture and Gender*, Butler claims that "the analysis that assumes nature to be singular and prediscursive cannot ask, what qualifies as 'nature' within a given cultural context, and for what purposes?" (1990: 37). In addition, Butler presses forward Yanagisako and Collier's prediction that "having recognized our model of biological difference as a particular cultural model of thinking about relations between people, we should be able to question the 'biological facts' of sex themselves" (1987: 42).

Using embryological mechanisms as her example, Butler turned to reproductive substance to illustrate her point in *Gender Trouble*. In a section examining scientific accounts of the "master switch" of sex determination, Butler traces the production of binary sex in cases of ambiguous persons, whose chromosomal and morphological sex diverge. Asking why a binary order must be imposed on these "incoherent" sexes, even when they clearly demonstrate its nonbinary existence in nature, Butler concludes that "cultural assumptions regarding the relative status of men and women and the binary relation of gender itself frame and focus the research into sex determination" (1990: 109). In other words, it is the presumption of gender difference that produces the mandate for the discovery of binary biological sex, not the reverse. In a critique of this circularity that parallels that from within feminist anthropology, Butler concludes: "The task of distinguishing sex from gender becomes all the more difficult once we understand that gendered meanings frame the hypothesis and the reasoning of those biomedical inquiries that seek to establish 'sex' for us as prior to the cultural meanings that it acquires" (1990: 109). Here, then, is another example of how sex is made, as well as a case of how gender is a technology of revealing, or of bringing forth. The work involved in reimposing sex binarism upon nondimorphic biological sex confirms the determinism of the former in lieu of the latter—making of sexuality what Butler, following Foucault, refers to as an "ambivalent product" (1990: 134). Indeed, this demonstration exactly reveals the mechanisms through which technologies of gender are used to make sex. Thus, echoing Yanagisako and Collier's (1987: 32) complaint that "the standard units of our genealogies, after all, are circles and triangles about which we assume a number of things," Butler maintains that it is "only from a self-consciously denaturalized position [that] we can see how the appearance of naturalness is itself constituted" (1990: 110).[20]

The significance of Strathern's work on new reproductive technologies discussed at the outset of this chapter, published shortly after *Gender Trouble*, takes on an important additional dimension in relation to the emergence of a more explicit theorization of gender as a technology in the work of Butler (1990), de Lauretis (1987), and also Haraway (1991). A crucially important feature of Butler's argument, like Haraway's, is its turn toward bioscience and its lack of concern with biological determinism. It is at the juncture of these crucial feminist debates in the 1980s, where the effort to undo gender meets the project to debiologize reproduction, that a new feminist engagement with technology gains momentum. Coincidentally, this new technological turn, epitomized by Haraway's cyborg politics, takes place at exactly the same time that IVF is finally successful in humans. It is thus not surprising that the feminist debates rehearsed in this chapter are accompanied by an equally large literature on new reproductive technologies, to which I turn in chapter 5.

Conclusion

As noted at the outset of this chapter, neither the origins of technology nor its progress over time can be equated in any simple way with the use of tools, or for that matter the development of tools to meet needs, but must instead be viewed, as both Marx and Gell argue, from the perspective of the social relationships that make knowledge and technique possible to begin with. As we have seen, this is also the argument of Lévi-Strauss in his theorization of kinship as a technology—an elementary structure that not only organizes but produces and activates reproductivity in a particular form, or forms. From this point of view, the traditional distinction invoked by Gell between "Technology of Production" and "Technology of Reproduction" overlooks the important point that reproduction, like gender and kinship, must also be produced: it is not simply there to be presumed as a self-acting force. Similarly, although one of the reasons Marxist theory neglects the mode of reproduction—the means by which the laborer reproduces himself or herself—is that reproduction is assumed to flow automatically, as it were, we can see from the point of view of gender and kinship theory that a prior mode of production is required to activate reproductivity, or to put it to work. As we shall see in chapters 5 and 6, this process is neatly repeated, and modeled, by IVF—for which biology is not a necessary prerequisite on its own but must be conjoined with technology. Indeed, as a looking glass, this is exactly what IVF reveals.

However, before moving forward, it is useful to pause briefly to look back, and to ask, for example, how these arguments about gender and kinship as technologies might be used to understand the history of embryology differently. One very striking feature of the concept of automatic reproduction so prevalent within social theory, where it is seen to function naturally as a global biological phenomenon underpinning social life (and prior to it), is how differently reproduction is theorized from the point of view of embryology. Somewhat ironically, it is from the standpoint of being closest to biological reproduction that ideas of the natural are most irrelevant. There is nothing merely biological about biology in a stem cell lab: stem cells, like in vitro embryos, are artifactual. Indeed, from the point of view of experimental embryology, the entire point of analyzing reproductive substance is to explore its mechanisms by coupling it to technology—by making technology work to reveal these mechanics.

But arguably the history of embryology demonstrates something else as well, which is that in activating reproductive substance technologically—in order to study or analyze its characteristics—the definition of technology also changes, for as we have seen in chapter 3, the substance itself becomes a tool. Returning to Strathern's definition of merographic thinking, we can see that this relay between substances and tools is somewhat curiously reproduced as a naturalized form of conceptuality. And as Strathern emphasizes repeatedly, what is familiar about merographic thinking is its connections to kinship. Hence, what Engels described as the frontier between the organic and the inorganic in the context of the hand and tool is also a line that is constantly crossed and recrossed in the context of what Strathern calls kinship thinking—a context she argues is both preeminently hybrid and distinctively postindustrial. "It has become routinely thinkable in the post-industrialism of the late-twentieth century . . . to make play with juxtaposing images of the organic and inorganic. . . . The one does not imitate the other so much as seemingly deploy or use its principles or parts. . . . The parallel lies in kinship thinking. Kinship systems and family structures are imagined as social arrangements *not just imitating but based on and deploying processes of biological reproduction*" (Strathern 1992b: 3, emphasis added). This point, about how kinship thinking itself routinely relies on a traffic, or play, between substance and tool, points to a very different sense in which IVF functions as a kinship technology: it is not only a technology that is used to produce kinship (biological relations) but a technique that substantializes the merographic mechanics of how kinship is routinely thought (its conceptual technology). Among the many things IVF can be seen to model, then, is the naturalness of the relationship between substance and tool, after which logic it is fashioned, and thus reproduces.[21] Tellingly, Strathern, like Butler, argues that the deployment of imitation is the mechanism by which substance and tool are linked and routinely recombined as parts and wholes. This too is a process IVF models neatly, while also curiously undoing the very logic on which it is based (i.e., to repair the nature it imitates).

We can go further with these questions (weaving our needles in and out, backward and forward through the liana to hold all the straws together), by pointing out how closely IVF resembles the arguments put forward by Butler concerning technologies of gender. Indeed, IVF stages or performs exactly the same process Butler describes through which substance is stylized to produce the appearance of "a natural sort of being" (1990: 109), thus also substantializing a naturalized origin that then appears as if it were prior to the cultural expectations it confirms. Moreover, as we shall see in more depth in the following chapters, this stylization applies to the making of parenthood identities (and those of gender, kinship, and sex) in the context of IVF, as well as to the making of babies. If, as this book argues, we will better understand IVF if we presume it is not merely a single-purpose, obvious clinical procedure servicing a self-evident goal or need, but instead a more complex unfolding technology that serves a more diverse set of purposes, then its exact mechanisms need to be more fully characterized, just as those of gender and kinship have been.

However, before returning to the question of the extent to which IVF is not only modeled after nature but indeed after received models of gender and kinship, there is another question that will detain us in chapter 5, which is that of what happens to women or gender after IVF. In turning to the question of how IVF is lived as a way of life, I begin in chapter 5 by reviewing the extensive feminist debate concerning the social implications of IVF and other new reproductive technologies that took place in the immediate wake of the birth of Louise Brown. I then turn to the feminist focus on IVF as a source of a defining ambivalence concerning both reproductive technology and reproductive politics—a focus that anticipates much of the contemporary concern about the frontier of new biology more widely. As we shall see, IVF serves in these debates once again as an instructive demonstration, or model, of a wider process—in this case of the political response to technologies that challenge the very naturalisms they are seen to serve. Here once again the biological relativities that follow in the wake of IVF's success are very evident and thus, with the added advantage of hindsight, provide us with another context in which to explore what kinds of futures for gender, kinship, and technology are implied by IVF's recent present.

FIVE Living IVF

So far in this book we have considered the general questions raised by IVF in a pair of broadly reflective overview chapters (1 and 2) and have followed the exact mechanisms of technologies for making sex in two subsequent chapters on experimental embryology and kinship theory (3 and 4). This chapter extends this sequence of frames by turning to a rereading of the feminist debate over reproductive technologies in the 1980s and the initial empirical studies of "living IVF," which are explored from three distinct points of view. The first encounter is between IVF and feminism, the second between IVF and women, and the third between IVF and gender. These encounters move us into the realm of the social life of IVF and allow us to analyze IVF not only as a technology of living substance, but a technology that is lived as the remaking of life.[1] They also allow us to consider the question concerning technology in relation to the politics of reproduction and gender, or sexual politics. Needless to say, this is such a vast and complicated encounter it is surprising that it is ever viewed as a specific one — that is, as one that largely or even exclusively concerns women, women's rights, or women's reproductive rights.[2]

Like chapter 4, this chapter also revisits the feminist literature of the 1980s, during the period in which IVF began to become much more widespread. My aim is not only to suggest how we might engage with these debates differently with the benefit of hindsight, from the vantage point of being five million miracle babies later and in the midst of the "biotech century." Following on from the discussion of technologies of substance in chapter 3, and technologies of gender, kinship, and sex in chapter 4, this chapter foregrounds the question of technological ambivalence in the context of living IVF. Undoubtedly one of the major themes of the feminist debate over IVF, technological ambivalence has a parallel meaning in the context of feminism, where both IVF and gender (and sex and kinship) are analyzed as technologies that split both subjects and political movements. This splitting, however, is not the routine hybrid or plural conceptuality described by Strathern in chapter 4, nor is it the "ambivalence of modernity" described by Zygmunt Bauman or Ulrich Beck. It describes instead the tension graphically illustrated in the large corpus of work on women's reproductive agency, identity, and choice, especially in relation to various technologies, from abortion and contraception to prenatal screening, in which increased choice becomes a very double-edged bargain (Petchesky 1984). Finally, this chapter seeks to show how ambivalence characterizes the feminist debate in another, not unrelated, recursion of content and form: while often represented as polarized (which in many respects it was), the feminist debate over new reproductive technologies (NRTS) is, from another angle, better described as consistently equivocal across the so-called radical-feminist versus socialist feminist divide. Importantly, moreover, the most significant shared ground within an otherwise divided debate was its pivotal focus on women's experience of IVF.

All of these aspects of IVF make it an "ambivalent topic" for feminism, and this chapter explores this ambivalence politically as well as somewhat autobiographically. As Haraway (1991) notes, ambivalence is itself a double-edged sword. While ambivalence is associated with discomfort, powerlessness, indecision, and uncertainty, Haraway also points out the political danger of assuming that "clear-sighted critique grounding a solid political epistemology" is the only alternative to "manipulated false consciousness." Indeed, she claims, "ambivalence toward the disrupted unities mediated by high-tech culture" may be an important space in which to discover "new kinds of unity" (1991: 30). Holding on to ambivalence may be an important means, she argues, to acknowledge that "what people are experiencing is not transparently clear" (31) and that developing understandings even of our own personal experience requires both evolving frames of reference and collective space in which to reflect. The ambivalent and contradictory feelings engendered by many new technologies, even in their most apparently dehumanizing moments, she argues, can also be resources for new forms of political organization and social change. Citing the irony of her own historical background, "a PhD in Biology for an Irish Catholic girl . . . made possible by Sputnik's impact on US national science-education policy," Haraway argues that "there are more grounds for hope by focussing on the contradictory effects of politics . . . than by focussing on present defeats." She continues:

> The permanent partiality of feminist points of view has consequences
> for our expectations of forms of political organization and participa-

tion. We do not need a totality in order to work well. The feminist dream of a common language, like all dreams for a perfectly true language, of perfectly faithful naming of experience, is a totalizing and imperialist one. In that sense, dialectics too is a dream language, longing to resolve contradiction. Perhaps, ironically, we can learn from our fusions with animals and machines how not to be Man, the embodiment of Western logos. From the point of view of pleasure in these potent and taboo fusions, made inevitable by the social relations of science and technology, there might indeed be a feminist science. (31)

Building on Haraway's insights, this chapter makes two main arguments about the tensions within feminism concerning reproductive technologies in general, and IVF in particular, as well as the ambivalence of the IVF experience identified within repeated feminist studies of how women experience this technology. The first builds on Charis Thompson's (2005: 56) observation that the reason why NRTs have provided "the perfect text" for feminist theory is because of the extent to which they condense so many of the social, economic, and political stratifications that affect women's lives and selves, while also foregrounding the tension between accommodation to the status quo and resistance. Like Thompson, I also suggest that IVF models technologies of gender, kinship, and sex and that it has become a defining concern of contemporary feminist theory because of this isomorphism. This implies, however, that the feminist analysis of IVF is potentially applicable to technology more broadly — and this is the second argument this chapter explores in more depth. Both of these perspectives are intended to emphasize what the feminist analysis of IVF has revealed about the process of navigating complex technological change — particularly when the technology is biological. This, of course, is a much more prominent question today than it was when many of the first feminist accounts of IVF and NRTs were written in the 1980s. The main purpose of this chapter, then, is to illustrate how this body of feminist work has gained increasing relevance as some of its implications have become more pointed in relation to present-day concerns about biology as technology. In contrast to the conclusion drawn by some that the 1980s feminist debates about IVF and NRTs were overly pessimistic, too descriptive, politically failed, divisive, ineffective, or problematically dependent on the category "woman," I suggest instead that they generated a number of useful insights into the condition of being after IVF that continue to be relevant to the "tool future" of biology more generally. In particular, as I hope to show, these debates generated models of technology as identity and documented the profoundly ambivalent relationships with, to, and through technology that have increasingly widespread relevance to understanding how the remaking of life is lived in the age of biological control.

A Formative Debate

Even measured against the extraordinary output of feminist scholars during the 1980s, across virtually every academic discipline, the feminist debate over new reproductive technologies stands out as one of the most prolific to emerge during this formative period of contemporary feminist thought. Like the debate over pornography, to which it is often compared, it was frequently acrimonious and often caught between a politics of accommodation to existing (unequal, sexist, male-dominated) power structures and the attempt to change them. Likewise, the feminist debates on NRTS in the 1980s vacillated between prioritizing a distinctively sexual or gender politics and developing more complex, situation-specific, intersectional political strategies. In part, the debate over NRTS was about feminism itself. But at the same time, these debates also charted very new ground and grappled with many issues we are facing today decades before they came to more widespread prominence (egg donation being but one example). As this chapter suggests, the feminist analysis of IVF was also the first to examine not only how biology becomes a technology, or an identity, but how the transfer of new reproductive and genetic technologies into the human ("into man") could be studied, how the implications of this transfer could be analyzed, and how its politics could be characterized while NRTS became much more widespread. The feminist emphasis on personal experience — on "the personal as political" — was central to its critical stance toward NRTS and IVF — and its careful attention to the affective politics of the ambivalent engagement with technology. Consequently, these debates offer central insights that are, if anything, even more relevant thirty years later to the broad and pressing questions posed by contemporary bioscience and biomedicine. I suggest in this chapter that these insights take on particular significance in the wake of the five millionth miracle baby because the feminist debate over NRTS was primarily concerned with IVF — now a technology that has an applied human history of nearly half a century, and yet still a technology that is poorly understood and undertheorized for exactly the reasons Raymond Williams (1990) diagnoses for technology in general, namely that it may seem as though we already know what its effects have been. As feminists were among the first to demonstrate, the logics of IVF are not as obvious as they may seem.

It is no exaggeration to say that thousands of books and articles have been written by feminists on reproductive technologies—old and new—mostly from the 1980s onward, and including the first empirical studies of the experience of IVF.[3] Artificial insemination, surrogacy, surgery, and hormonal enhancement of fertility, as well as contraception and abortion, can all be counted as forms of technological assistance to reproduction, or what are known as reproductive technologies. But it is the rapid expansion of IVF, and its evolution as a technological platform for genetic as well as reproductive intervention, that gave rise to increasing concern about NRTS from the 1980s onward. Building on the legacy of the women's health movement, and a burgeoning interest in what has come to be known as science studies, feminist scholars were among the first to begin to seriously engage with the implications of bioscience and the new genetics through the lens of reproductive biomedicine. Whereas the concerns of bioethics originated in a wide range of practices, from organ donation and euthanasia to informed consent and genetic screening, feminists were particularly concerned from the outset with the encounter between NRTS and women's bodies—a tellingly dominant concern in feminist debates over IVF. Similarly, whereas it was the advent of the new genetics that dominated much social science research on the rise of the biosciences in the 1990s, the earlier period of feminist research with which this chapter is concerned prioritized reproductive biomedicine and NRTS.

Like most feminist debates, the expansive debate over NRTS has been the subject of conflicting interpretations reflecting the ambivalence that is as endemic to feminist politics as it is to the experience of being female. In addition to being a divisive topic, producing what Margarete Sandelowski (1990) memorably termed "fault lines in the sisterhood," the feminist debate over NRTS is also often characterized as neglected. Writing in one of the most influential discussions of the ethics of IVF in 1995, the British theologian Anthony Dyson remarks that it is nothing less than "astonishing that most of the contemporary literature on IVF virtually or wholly ignores the feminist arguments" (1995: 6). He goes on to note that this neglect is particularly lamentable given the quality and depth of this body of scholarship: "In contrast to the highly individualistic arguments employed in much of the literature on the NRTS, the feminist writers have developed a significant body of social ethics instead—a social ethics which must also be reckoned as political to its very core" (6). Dyson devotes an entire chapter of his book to the feminist critique of NRTS and IVF in order to give them "pride of place" in contrast to their conspicuous absence elsewhere: "Surprisingly, very few of the books and articles about IVF make any reference at all to the feminist challenge," he notes, adding, "As far as my reading goes, feminists are correct in observing that none of the male-centred criticisms of the NRTS, be they conservative or radical, has opposed the technologies because of what they do to women" (43).

Inadequately recognized for their scholarly contributions at the time of their original publication, and mainly remembered for their bitter disagreements afterward (if they are referred to at all), the feminist literature on NRTS recapitulates the difficulties faced by feminist theory and women's studies in general as marginalized research areas. The theme of the divisiveness of feminist debates on this topic is ubiquitous, even within much of the retrospective feminist literature, although it is worth pausing to ask why this is the case and how the term is being used.[4] The common, and pejorative, use of this term refers to the creation, sometimes deliberate, of unwanted or unhelpful divisions, as in causing disagreement or sowing discord. But it is hardly surprising that feminist critiques of NRTS would be the cause of disagreement. A more productive way to interpret the deeply felt divisions within feminist debate is as a measure of serious and committed critical thought, generating the diversity of perspectives that is not only intrinsic to either intellectual or political struggle, but often considered to be indicative of their quality.[5] To the extent the feminist debate over NRTS opened an important space in which to mobilize a less normative set of responses to IVF than those that have emerged, for example, from bioethics (e.g., "reproductive autonomy"; Robertson 1994), it has not so much been a matter of speaking truth to power as of "speaking ambivalence to progress."[6]

I was actively involved in the early feminist intellectual and political mobilization in response to NRTS, and this experience partly shaped my scholarly interest in IVF and my PhD research on this topic between 1986 and 1989 — so this chapter also has an autobiographical element. Since I experienced at close hand the conflicts within feminism concerning NRTS, in my twenties during the 1980s, I remain reluctant to dismiss their unsettling emotional consequences as either missing the point or as a regrettable side effect of political struggle. Such conflicts, I learned, are the political point: they taught me that the effort to remain ethically and politically responsive to the pressing questions posed by NRTS is bound to be a demanding, and sometimes painful, process. We should expect to feel uncomfortable about the issues raised by IVF and NRTS, as well as biomedicine and biotechnology more widely, as discomfort is one of the surest signs that an important ethical and political problem is nearby. Confusion and conflict are not diminishing forces: they are indices of engagement, and crucial sources of political insight and creativity, as well as thought and speech and writing. In the same way that it is short-sighted to read the feminist debate over NRTs merely as inconclusive or un-resolved, so too is it misguided to expect to resolve the question of biology as technology, or questions concerning the future of NRTs, genetic engineering, cloning, or stem cell research. One of the reasons for writing this book is my concern that the very process of having become more comfortable with IVF and its related technologies suggests the need to rethink their histories more carefully and more radically. As many ethnographic and medical studies are now asking, it may also be necessary to question whether IVF actually even is as comfortable as it seems. But I return to these questions later. For the time being, the question this chapter explores is what can be learned from the history of feminist debates over NRTs in the 1980s, particularly concerning IVF, and specifically from the divisions this topic generated. As I hope to demonstrate, these perspectives constitute a neglected resource that richly rewards revisiting, and should become more incorporated in contemporary teaching as well as dialogue about the future of biological control.

Early Feminist Primers

Two anthologies published in the early 1980s, *Birth Control and Controlling Birth* (Holmes et al. 1980) and *The Custom-Made Child?* (Holmes et al. 1981) were the first feminist volumes to focus attention specifically on reproductive technology following the birth of Louise Brown in 1978.[7] But it was not until the mid-1980s that this literature began rapidly to expand. 1984 saw the publication of *Test-Tube Women: What Future for Motherhood?*, a feminist anthology aimed at a popular audience edited by three feminist scientists (Rita Arditti, Renate Duelli Klein, and Shelley Minden) and containing thirty-three short contributions from a range of feminist perspectives. In 1985, Boston-based feminist journalist Gena Corea published *The Mother Machine: From Artificial Insemination to Artificial Wombs*, the first major feminist monograph addressing NRTs, also aimed at a popular audience, and in which NRTs are denounced as tools of patriarchal oppression. In 1986, the first academic book by a feminist social scientist, *The Tentative Pregnancy: Prenatal Diagnosis and the Future of Motherhood*, was published by New York sociologist Barbara Katz Rothman, presenting the results of her major study of amniocentesis, and promoting the effort to provide a more supportive environment for women using this technology. In these groundbreaking feminist books the major themes that have come to dominate feminist debate over NRTs more or less ever since are already evident. A brief look at these influential volumes is thus a useful place to begin.

Test-Tube Women, perhaps the best-known feminist text on the subject of NRTS, illustrated in its very composition the tensions between feminists that would define the fault lines of this field. The anthology opens with a forceful editorial introduction in which "the *real* message for women" (Arditti et al. 1984: 5, original emphasis) of reproductive technology is voiced as a call to resistance ("we are *all* at risk of becoming *Test-Tube Women*," 6, original emphasis). However, the various chapters contained in its 482 pages are significantly less unified in their assessments—offering a wide and diverse spectrum of feminist perspectives on everything from lesbian motherhood to cloning. In contrast to the unequivocal editorial insistence on the urgency of opposing new forms of biological subordination through male-controlled reproductive technology, *Test-Tube Women*'s contributors offer a disparate array of personal, political, and theoretical responses to the question of "whether we as feminists should endorse [NRTS] or [whether they are] just one more way to keep women subordinated to male control" (1). In spite of all the reasons to be cautious about NRTS expressed by the various chapter authors, there is little by way of consensus about what to do about them, other than to network, share information, monitor developments, and remain skeptical. Moreover, the strategies on offer appear contradictory—ranging from the argument that "new reproductive technologies may be the key to more functional ways of raising children" (Breeze 1984: 397) to the claim that NRTS exemplify the reification of manmade femininity (Raymond 1984: 433). The anthology is thus a primer in more than one sense: it contains not only the early seeds of feminist analysis of NRTS, but expresses in its very structure, in the contrast between the certainty of the editorial call to arms and the far less unified responses from its assembled foot soldiers, the profound ambivalence that would continue to characterize feminist debate and activism in this area.

The contrast between Corea's (1985) and Rothman's (1986) now-classic studies of NRTS is equally revealing of the scope of feminist division on this subject (as is the contrast between Rothman's early and later writings). In her contribution to *Test-Tube Women*, Rothman emphasizes the paradox of NRTS in terms of how they complicate the meaning of choice—a theme that has come to define almost all of the most important work by feminist social scientists on reproductive technology since. On the one hand, she argues, NRTS such as prenatal screening undoubtedly enable more, and in some instances much better, reproductive choices for women. They could in this sense genuinely be described as assisting women technologically. However, NRTS also transform the experience of both reproduction and reproductive choice for women, and in many ways diminish it, thus potentially leaving women worse off than they would have been without such choices, or assistance, to begin with.[8] Rothman thus argues for a continuing emphasis on the need for information and choice, while at the same time maintaining a critical political stance toward the contexts of such choices — much as her influential colleague Rosalind Petchesky (1984) advocated in the context of abortion, which she described, paraphrasing Marx, as a choice women must fight to protect, even if it is not one that is made on their own terms.

It is, of course, also paradoxical if women come to feel pressured by feminism into choosing not to choose, by avoiding the technology altogether. As Rothman concludes her chapter in *Test-Tube Women*: "We must not get caught into discussions of which reproductive technologies are 'politically correct,' which empower and which enslave women. They ALL empower and they ALL enslave, they can be used for or against us" (Rothman 1984: 32–33).

These claims are further elaborated in Rothman's meticulous, original, and still highly relevant study of women's experience of amniocentesis (*The Tentative Pregnancy*, 1986, originally titled *The Products of Conception*, 1985). Using interview data from consultations with 120 women, half of whom underwent amniocentesis and half of whom refused the procedure, Rothman provides a detailed account of the ways in which prenatal screening and diagnosis dramatically (and often traumatically) transform the experience of pregnancy. Her title refers to one of her major empirical findings, namely that a majority of the women in her study who underwent amniocentesis embodied their emotional and technological ambivalence by suppressing the physical sensation of the first palpable fetal movements (quickening) until after the test results had been revealed (often well into the fifth month of pregnancy). Striking as such empirical findings are in themselves, what makes them particularly compelling in Rothman's text is her sensitive and restrained handling of the often hesitant voices of the women whose articulate accounts of embodying ambivalent progress form her book's essential core.

A very different approach to the question of NRTs is provided by Gena Corea (1985), a highly accomplished investigative journalist, whose account of NRTs in *The Mother Machine* is dominated by the theme of male technological control over women's bodies. Here, it is the producers rather than the consumers of NRTs whose candor reveals a disturbing portrait of what Corea describes as the sinister background to the emergence of the reproductive service industry. In her often surreal and disturbing interviews with men whose names are as seemingly Dickensian as their motives (e.g., Dr. John Seed),

Corea is keenly sensitive to language—quoting at length the "technodoc's" descriptions of "bombing" ovaries with fertility drugs to produce "ovulation to order" (1985: 109); "recruiting," "harvesting," and "capturing" as many ova as possible from their women patients; sending embryos into outer space (116); and enabling "the biological manufacture of human beings to desired specifications" (133) to create a super-race (314). In tone, as well as content, Corea (whose chapter "Egg Snatchers" is placed back-to-back with Rothman's in the opening section of *Test-Tube Women*; Corea 1984) could not be more explicit in her warning that NRTs should be opposed root and branch, and have nothing to offer women. Whereas for Rothman reproductive technology is essentially neutral and can have some benefits for women, depending on how it is used, Corea draws on the work of Canadian sociologist Mary O'Brien (1981) to argue that these technologies are inherently patriarchal, manifesting a primitive male drive to control women's reproductive capacity. According to Corea, who also draws on Margaret Mead, Adrienne Rich, and Susan Griffin, reproductive technologies are, like gynecology and obstetrics, not only products of a patriarchal society but the materialization of patriarchal male desires. They are thus, inherently and irredeemably, tools of patriarchal oppression that turn women into raw material and reproduction into a market. In Corea's account, patriarchal technology is endowed with purpose, direction, motivation, and goals. Her analysis emphasizes the seamless coherence of patriarchy in the form of its technologies, which substantialize the aim of patriarchal control by extending its reach. In vitro fertilization is part of a historical process that culminates in the establishment of "The Reproductive Brothel," "The Capture of Maternity," and "The Defeat of the Womb," which are the titles of chapters 14, 15, and 16 of *The Mother Machine*.

Rothman argues precisely the opposite. In her account, reproductive technology is not inherently patriarchal—indeed it is not inherently anything; it is merely an avenue of possibility, creating new opportunities including the possibility of progressive social change. She writes, "I am not claiming that the technology is itself harmful. I think that the new technology of reproduction offers us an opportunity to work on our definition of parenthood, of motherhood, fatherhood and childhood, to rethink and improve our relations with each other in families. Freed from some of the biological constraints, we could evolve better, more egalitarian ways of relating to ourselves and each other in reproduction. The technology is a promise, beckoning us with new possibilities . . . giving us new control" (Rothman 1986: 3). These contrasting accounts of NRTs thus not only offer opposite solutions, but present radically different versions of "the question concerning technology." Rothman and Corea not only advocate opposing tactics, but rely on divergent models of the relationship between biology and technology. Whereas for Corea NRTS embody and manifest a biological male drive to control women, thus comprising in themselves the very substance of patriarchal succession, as well as its means of reproduction, Rothman suggests that technology offers a path to overcome "biological constraints" and to change patriarchal definitions of kinship and family. In one vision is a technology at one with its patrilineage — indeed a technology that intensifies male control of the very substance of patrilineage by gaining a firmer hold on biological reproduction (Corea's chapter on cloning is subtitled "The Patriarchal Urge to Self-Generate"). In the other is a view of the potential of technology to create alternative kinship structures and new definitions of family — a plastic technology that offers a path to greater flexibility and freedom by releasing the "constraints" imposed by biology. In one version, then, technology extends a biological (male) drive to perpetuate a patriarchal lineage through reproductive control. In the other, technology potentially gives control back to women themselves.

This, of course, is a familiar political dilemma — in terms of not only women's subordination (can the master's tools dismantle the master's house?) but technology (does mechanization improve the lives of workers even though it can oppress them?). Referring back to Rothman's earlier warning against polarizing the debate ("We must not get caught into discussions of which reproductive technologies are 'politically correct,' which empower and which enslave women. They ALL empower and they ALL enslave, they can be used for or against us"), it is also clear that these positions can be read as either oppositional or complementary — or even as dialectically related. The one can be seen as the more cautionary version of the other, or they can be seen as irreconcilably polarized positions — Rothman being pro-NRT and colluding in their routinization, whereas Corea outlines a more oppositional anti-NRT strategy that risks the dangers of becoming caught in a judgmental stance that defines other women's choices as complicit with patriarchal control. A key element of this contrast, as mentioned above, are the models of technology and biology being employed by each author — including the relationship between these two terms.

The Expansion of Debate

If Rothman's and Corea's positions in the mid-1980s provide a clear illustration of opposing feminist analyses of NRTs, in the two most influential early monographs on this topic, the opposite can be claimed of the two most widely cited feminist publications that quickly succeeded them. Two feminist anthologies that were seen by many to solidify the distinction between radical and socialist feminist responses to NRTS were published in 1987. However, neither volume quite fit these categorizations, and upon closer inspection it is clear they have far more in common, particularly on the question of women's agency to resist male dominance, but also, somewhat more surprisingly, on the issue of women's experience of IVF as a form of "ambivalent progress." *Made to Order: The Myth of Reproductive and Genetic Progress*, edited by Patricia Spallone and Deborah Lynn Steinberg (1987) is, like *Test-Tube Women*, an anthology introduced by a powerful editorial stance that does not exactly match its contents. Similarly, *Reproductive Technologies: Gender, Motherhood and Medicine*, edited by Michelle Stanworth, although offered as an alternative to "the view that reproductive technologies represent a vehicle for men to wrest control of reproduction from women" (1987: 4) by providing a "fresh appraisal of reproductive technologies," fails to deliver such a coherent set of contents. Indeed, despite claiming that "the authors in this volume firmly reject . . . the particular feminist reading which sees in these technologies an unmitigated attack on women" (1987: 3), Stanworth's anthology contains numerous statements that explicitly support and even strengthen the interpretation of NRTS as an attack on women.

Thus, in the very first chapter, for example, the influential feminist sociologist and reproductive activist Ann Oakley, while critical of the "reproductive brothel" model that is central to Corea's work, nonetheless foregrounds the persistent exploitation of women within male-dominated medicine, and especially gynecology and obstetrics, for the past two centuries. Indeed, as Oakley makes clear in her chapter titled "From Walking Wombs to Test-Tube Babies," her main argument is not intended to oppose the feminist claim that women are treated as "biological systems manipulable in the interests of patriarchy," claiming instead, "Just as sex can become a commodity when men and women exploit the idea that women are sexual objects for men, so reproduction becomes a commodity when women become reproductive objects" (Oakley 1987: 51). Far from opposing "the particular feminist reading which sees in these technologies an unmitigated attack on women," Oakley argues, just like Corea, that although doctors are not necessarily consciously or deliberately motivated to "control the lives of women" through reproductive technology, there is nonetheless "quite a lot of evidence that [this is] the *effect*" (1987: 50) of their introduction into clinical practice. Indeed, despite Stanworth's claim to the contrary, Oakley argues that Corea's "reproductive brothel" accusation (drawn from the work of Andrea Dworkin)[9] accurately characterizes the rise of NRTS as both a market and an industry based on increasing male control of women's reproductive capacity. Contrary to her editor's stated intentions for the volume, and even her own account of her position at the outset of her chapter, Oakley endorses Dworkin's model of NRTS as a "total mode of control," which, she argues, "illustrate[s] the contrast between reproduction before the use of modern medical technological management and [the situation] after this system was established [by demonstrating that] centralized control by a powerful medical elite claiming expert technical knowledge *is a more effective and total mode of control* than a decentralized non-professional non-technological mode" (1987: 51, emphasis added). The problem with arguments such as Corea's and Dworkin's about patriarchy and male control of reproduction is thus not that they are too radical, according to Oakley. She precisely does not reject, as her editor Stanworth (1987: 4) would have it, "the view that reproductive technologies represent a vehicle for men to wrest control of reproduction from women." Indeed, Oakley interprets the introduction of NRTS as achieving precisely this end, arguing that they intensify the objectification of women as "walking wombs" and "mindless mothers" (points she highlights in the title of her chapter). As we shall see, Oakley's concerns, along with those of many of her cocontributors, have even more than this in common with the feminist camp to which they are allegedly opposed.

Rosalind Petchesky, another contributor to the Stanworth volume, is similarly unwilling to entirely reject the patriarchal paradigm, also despite her own claims to the contrary, beginning her famous essay "Foetal Images: The Power of Visual Culture in the Politics of Reproduction" with a quotation from Hélène Cixous describing the exclusion of maternity from the patriarchal unconscious: "[Ultimately] the world of 'being' can function to the exclusion of the mother. No need for mother—provided that there is something of the maternal: and it is the father then who acts as—is—the mother. Either the woman is passive; or she doesn't exist. What is left is unthinkable, unthought of. She does not enter into the oppositions, she is not coupled with the father (who is coupled with the son)" (Cixous, quoted in Petchesky 1987: 57). This is also the article (first published in *Feminist Studies* the previous year) in which Petchesky memorably develops the astute political observation that "the current leadership of the anti-abortion movement has made a conscious strategic shift from religious discourses and authorities to medico-technical ones, in its efforts to win over the courts, the legislatures and popular 'hearts and minds.' But the vehicle for this shift is not organized medicine directly but mass culture and its diffusion into reproductive technology through the video display terminal" (1987: 58). Describing the increasingly sophisticated use by the U.S. right-to-life movement of visual images of the unborn fetus to mobilize antiabortion sentiment, Petchesky argues these campaigners were "enlisting medical imagery in the service of mythic patriarchal messages" by producing a "baby man" who is also a spaceman-astronaut—"an autonomous, atomized mini-space hero" (64). These representations—in effect the outcome of a coupling together of ultrasound and fetal imaging (NRTS) with television, film, and other media—have become increasingly influential in the effort to separate fetal and maternal bodies, she suggests. "As a result, the pregnant woman is increasingly put in the position of adversary to her own pregnancy/foetus" (65). These patterns, Petchesky argues, in turn "direct the practical applications of new reproductive technologies more towards enlarging clinicians' control over reproductive processes than towards improving health (women's or infants'). Despite their benefits for individual women, amniocentesis, *in vitro* fertilization, electronic foetal monitoring, routine caesarean deliveries, ultrasound and a range of heroic 'foetal therapies' (both *in utero* and *ex utero*) also have the effect of carving out more space/time for obstetrical 'management' of pregnancy" (64). Thus, while Petchesky criticizes "feminist cultural theorists in France, Britain and the United States" who have argued that "visualization and objectification . . . are specifically masculine" for relying on forms of "essentialism," she nonetheless concedes that the "prevalence of the gaze" is indeed a reflection of "the deep gender bias of science (including medicine) [and] of its very ways of seeing" (68). Similarly, while she is critical of the feminist arguments of Nancy Hartsock, Mary O'Brien, E. Ann Kaplan, and others who "link patriarchal control over reproduction to the masculine quest for immortality" (71), she somewhat confusingly places a quotation by one of the leading feminist cultural theorists in France (Cixous) as the headnote to her chapter (see above). She is explicitly critical of the "reductionism" of "war against the womb" feminists, singling out her cocontributor Ann Oakley's work, and citing Oakley's reference to "specific forms of the ancient masculine impulse 'to confine and limit and curb the creativity and potentially polluting power of female procreation' (Oakley, 1976, p. 57: cf. Corea, 1985a p. 303 and chapter 16; Rich, 1976, chapter 6; Ehrenreich and English, 1978; and Oakley, 1980)" (Petchesky 1987: 71). But if the lengthy list of citations provided by Petchesky to support this critique of Oakley's reductionism were not enough evidence of the complexity of feminist positions on NRTS, and the difficulty of assigning pro- and anti-NRT sides, Petchesky's subsequent criticisms of *The Mother Machine* raise still further questions about the extent to which the feminist debate over NRTs was itself marked from the outset by the same ambivalence it often described.

It would, of course, be a mistake to place too much importance on the all-too-common practice of lumping various feminist arguments together into typologies and caricaturing their contents under somewhat hackneyed labels, for this is in general how many political and intellectual positions are fought. Too much academic literalism is undoubtedly out of place in interpreting Petchesky's accusation that "works such as Gena Corea's *The Mother Machine* and most articles in the anthology *Test-Tube Women*, portray women as perennial victims of an omnivorous male plot to take over their reproductive capacities. The specific forms taken by male strategies of reproductive control, while admittedly varying across times and cultures, are reduced to a pervasive, transhistorical 'need.' Meanwhile, women's own resistance to this control, often successful, as well as their complicity in it, are ignored; women, in this view, have no role as agents of their reproductive destinies" (1987: 72). While recognizing the primary point Petchesky is making here about the limits of essentialist arguments, it is worth following her claim a bit further to see what this reveals about the fault lines described by Sandelowski (1990). Petchesky's main complaint in this passage is a familiar one — that the overvaluation of male power leads to the undervaluation of female resistance. However, neither *The Mother Machine* nor *Test-Tube Women* are particularly good examples to illustrate this problem, since they are both products of feminist activism, and are thus examples of feminist resistance. Neither *The Mother Machine* nor *Test-Tube Women* ignores women's resistance to patriarchal control — they are precisely dedicated to furthering it and constitute acts of resistance in themselves. To understand Petchesky's complaint, and indeed to comprehend the ricochet of cross-shots aimed at various forms of determinism, reductionism, and essentialism in these debates more widely, it is necessary to engage the deeply ambivalent relationship to NRTs somewhat further.

FINRRAGE

Like the Stanworth anthology, Patricia Spallone and Deborah Steinburg's 1987 anthology, *Made to Order: The Myth of Reproductive and Genetic Progress*, contains a wide mix of feminist responses to NRTs in which both their dangers and potential benefits are explored. The association of *Made to Order* with radical feminism, and *Reproductive Technologies* with socialist feminism, while convenient and conventional, is nonetheless difficult to defend on the basis of analyzing the actual contents of these two anthologies in more detail—which quickly reveals that their contributors, like those in *Test-Tube Women*, are distinctly ambivalent. Contrary to its association with an essentialized version of radical feminism, *Made to Order* contains more "traditional" socialist perspectives, such as Farida Akhter's chapter describing the coercive use of wheat relief in Bangladesh to attain sterilization targets and Maria Mies's critique of corporate capitalism in her chapter "Why Do We Need All This?" Above all, what stands out from this anthology is that, like *Test-Tube Women*, its idiosyncrasy and wide inclusiveness reflect its close proximity to feminist political activism. Unlike most Anglo-American feminist publications from this period, *Made to Order* is broadly international, containing contributions from feminists in India, Bangladesh, Brazil, Germany, Australia, France, and Britain as well as the United States. Clearly a publication produced by feminist activists, and deliberately written in accessible language, it contains, among other things, summaries of the development of new reproductive technologies globally in a series of twenty-one country reports compiled by the editors on the basis of their correspondence with the international network of local feminist activists involved in FINRRAGE.[10] A number of traditional empirical approaches to the study of the cultural implications of new reproductive technologies were also introduced for the first time in this volume, including comparative analysis of media coverage and public debate of NRTs, and of national and international regulatory strategies. Along with Patricia Spallone's (1989) insightful feminist analysis of genetic engineering, *Made to Order* is one of the first feminist anthologies to link the gender politics of IVF and other NRTs to those of bioscience, agribusiness, and biotechnology. Pleasingly, the anthology contains several authentic feminist manifestos, all of which disagree with one another. In sum, unlike the more conventionally Anglo-centric anthology edited by Stanworth, *Made to Order* offers an unusually international set of feminist political interventions that convincingly represent the diverse and impassioned nature of global feminist collective actions in response to the development of NRTs in the 1980s.

Above all, what distinguishes *Made to Order* is its indebtedness to new forms of "glocal" feminist political activism directed at the rise of new reproductive and genetic technologies. As its editors note, "this may be the era of biotechnology, but it is also the age of international feminism" (Spallone and Steinburg 1987: 16). The influence of UN Decade for Women activism is clearly evident in the form of the international feminist political networks mobilized to respond to the challenges posed by NRTs, including FINRRAGE, as well as networks of women health activists with links to the environmental movements, the antinuclear movement, and the effort to oppose coercive family planning measures in the Third World. Because of the vehement anti-NRT stance taken by some of its more prominent members, including Gena Corea, the "FINRRAGE position" came to be somewhat reductively associated with the "NRTS = patriarchy" stance.[11] What my own experience in FINRRAGE confirmed, however, was that, like the actual contents of *Made to Order*, this was an international network of much greater political diversity than any simple characterization of a single position on NRTS could encompass (the claims of some of its most prominent members to the contrary notwithstanding).

I began attending FINRRAGE meetings in 1986, shortly after it was formed, as part of its British contingent, comprised (like the rest of the network) of a loose network of feminists with a variety of backgrounds and interests united by a shared concern about NRTS. If the FINRRAGE position was associated with a single unified stance outside the network, its actual workings as experienced by those within it revealed a much more encompassing definition of collective action that was largely manifest as information sharing, innovative research projects, workshop and conference organization, (very long) meetings, campaigning, writing and publishing, and generally encouraging feminist debate of precisely the kind represented in *Made to Order*. Serviced by a rotating International Coordinating Group that was based in Britain from 1987 to 1989, and functioning with pre-Internet technology (dependent on Xerox and snail mail), the work of hundreds of FINRRAGE members worldwide largely consisted of packaging and circulating hand-photocopied "international packets" of media clippings and policy documents, monitoring developments internationally, organizing conferences, exchanging correspondence, and developing feminist analyses of reproductive and genetic technologies that emphasized the interconnections between bioscience and biomedicine as they affected women's rights and women's health, as well as the environment, the economy, and ethical debate.

Shared by the most prominent members of FINRRAGE, including Gena Corea, Renate Klein, Jalna Hanmer, and Maria Mies, was a well-defined position of opposition to all forms of new reproductive and genetic technology. This position was repeatedly spelled out in a number of documents, from the founding manifesto of FINRRAGE to various publications and conference proceedings (many of which can be accessed on the FINRRAGE website, www .finrrage.org). This position emphasized the male medical takeover of reproduction, the deceptive marketing of IVF and other NRTS, the experimental nature of many NRT treatments, the exclusion of women and women's interests from almost all forms of public debate about NRTs, and the need for women to become more critical of techniques such as IVF that were often depicted in heroic and celebratory terms. The accompanying FINRRAGE line was simple: NRTs should be banned.

This line, however, was unevenly shared throughout the FINRRAGE network as a whole, as is evident in many of the publications associated with FINRRAGE, such as *Made to Order*, which, like *Test-Tube Women*, begins with a forceful editorial introduction by Gena Corea, Jalna Hanmer, Renate Klein, Robyn Rowland, and Janice Raymond calling for a rejection of NRTs: "By rejecting these technologies we take a woman-centred stance. . . . We should not forget that . . . the 'technodocs' need our bodies. . . . If we deny them our bodies and speak out angrily against them in public, then perhaps they will be forced to stop" (Corea et al. 1987: 11). Following this introductory chapter, however, is a much more mixed series of feminist responses to a wide range of technologies, in which some authors openly reject the FINRRAGE line. Green activist Linda Bullard, for example, states that she has "no quarrel with the Age of Biology" (Bullard 1987: 117) while policy specialist Patricia Hynes outlines a regulatory model for new reproductive technologies based on the U.S. Environmental Protection Agency that would allow "women [to represent] themselves on policy boards and regulatory committees as the subjects of these risky technologies" (Hynes 1987: 198). Like the chapter structures of both *Test-Tube Women* and *Made to Order*, the FINRRAGE network conjoined a small group of prominent feminists who were strongly in agreement with one another to a much larger and more amorphous group of network members who held a more diverse range of views. In addition to disagreeing about the political challenges posed by NRTs, the bulk of the FINRRAGE membership also had different views about the need for a single, unified political position in response to them. For the feminists most committed to the FINRRAGE position of complete opposition to NRTs, such as the authors of the editorial introduction to *Made to Order*, a line was a line—not a bunch of lines. This group operated much like a radical cell, often portraying their work as part of a war against patriarchy. The rest of the network operated more like a post–UN Decade women's collective action, in which a very high tolerance of diversity was both a valued and an expected component of feminist politics.

The regular meetings of British FINRRAGE members I attended as a graduate student in London, Bradford, York, Birmingham, and Leeds were highly informative and full of debate. They were also fun. The opportunity to meet other feminists involved in writing, thinking, and reading about NRTs generated enormous energy and excitement. The meetings always involved the opportunity to learn about feminist activism in other parts of the world, and this internationalism was reflected in FINRRAGE conferences, which brought together feminist activists from dozens of countries. The model of local activism linked to a global political agenda was thus very fully realized within FINRRAGE, at a time when feminism was rapidly becoming a more diverse and well-organized global political movement. Fueled by the torrent of feminist publications concerning reproductive technology, including Haraway's (1985) "Manifesto for Cyborgs" and Emily Martin's (1987) *The Woman in the Body*, to name but two of the instant feminist classics from this period, the FINRRAGE network was in many respects one of the most successful and productive global feminist organizations to emerge during the 1980s. Like many such movements, FINRRAGE members struggled to articulate a single political line. As a result, there were, in effect, two FINRRAGES—one that unequivocally advocated complete opposition to all forms of NRT, and another, larger, constituency that had a broadly skeptical caution toward the rapid routinization of procedures such as IVF, but which stopped short of insisting that no women should use them under any conditions. One of the main differences between these two different constituencies—the copresence of which was obvious to any participant in FINRRAGE activities—was the invisibility to outsiders of the diversity of FINRRAGE activism, masked as this was by the FINRRAGE position or line.

Figure 5.1 illustrates the political structure of FINRRAGE as it evolved from 1985 to 1989 from an insider's point of view. As I have attempted to illustrate in this diagram, a division of both perception and politics separated a relatively small group of comparatively prominent FINRRAGE activists associated with the network's strong anti-NRT stance from the bulk of its membership, who held more disparate views, and this division predictably led to conflict. For example, while there was strong sympathy for the FINRRAGE position of complete opposition to all forms of new reproductive and genetic technologies, many activists in the network interpreted this position as strategic, or even as symbolic, rather than as strictly literal. After all, abortion and contraception are reproductive technologies, and no one was calling for a ban on their use. Even some members who agreed with the line doubted its likelihood of success, and others expressed concern that such a rigid political position significantly weakened the ability of FINRRAGE participants to gain a foothold in public debate. For many, the difference between their personal version of resistance and those that were officially spelled out in the many FINRRAGE manifestos was irrelevant to most of what went on in FINRRAGE. Like most political groups, the reality of participating in FINRRAGE meant

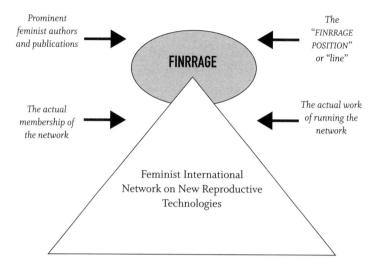

FIGURE 5.1. This insider's view of FINRRAGE illustrates the difference between how the network was perceived externally and how it appeared from within, particularly in relation to the FINRRAGE line of strict opposition to new reproductive and genetic technologies. Author's diagram.

working in small groups on specific tasks that did not require a precise definition of the network's exact aims. So while it would be inaccurate to suggest that most FINRRAGE members did not share an explicitly feminist concern with the effects of NRTs on women, and the near-complete exclusion of these concerns from public debate, it was equally true that not everyone agreed about what was to be done.

Conflicts over tactics predictably ranged from mild to severe. Some members, for example, felt it was wrong to respond to public enquiries such as that of the British government in the wake of the Warnock Report, arguing that feminist responses would only legitimize a state effort to pass laws allowing for more use of NRTs and the growth of a fertility market. Others felt a lack of response would defeat the whole purpose of FINRRAGE, which was intended to publicize a feminist critical perspective on NRTs and to expose their deleterious effects on women. More severe conflict surrounded the often-heard criticisms that FINRRAGE neglected the difficulties of infertile women, cast IVF users as collaborators with patriarchy, and naively appealed to the state for protection (in the form of calling for a complete ban on the use of NRTs). In a 1985 issue of the British feminist journal *Trouble and Strife*, infertility awareness activist Naomi Pfeffer criticized the work of FINRRAGE, claiming,

"The one voice that is never heard is that of the most directly implicated: the voice of infertile women. Because of their absence, this debate appears, from the perspective of an infertile woman, to be curiously ill-informed in terms of what it is like to be infertile, socially, medically, and emotionally" (Pfeffer 1985: 46). Shortly afterward, and in the same journal, Marge Berer, representing the Women's Global Network for Reproductive Rights, accused FINRRAGE of "imperialist dogma" that was "void of evidence" and displayed political inexperience. "To kid oneself that the state is more benevolent than science to women is politically naïve and dangerous" (Berer 1985: 33).

Tensions concerning these questions were also present within FINRRAGE and centered on various specific issues. The suggestion that FINRRAGE should take a more sympathetic stance toward women IVF users was one such issue, and the question of whether assisted conception technology could be made more "woman friendly" was another. The problem posed by the stance of complete opposition was an almost constant source of debate that sometimes led to visceral disagreements. A case in point was the decision by the Bombay-based FINRRAGE affiliate the Forum against Oppression of Women, who successfully campaigned for a law banning the use of amniocentesis for sex selection in the state of Maharashta, to support a strictly limited use of this technology to scan for fetal abnormality (largely in support of the reproductive crisis being experienced by women in the wake of the Bhopal disaster). For many FINRRAGE participants this decision was both laudable and obvious, while for others, including many of FINRRAGE's leading activists, it explicitly departed from the network's stated aims and official position by failing to enforce a complete ban on this technology.

These and other debates within the network reached a boiling point at the March 1989 FINRRAGE conference in Bangladesh, coorganized by FINRRAGE and a local alternative development agency, UBINIG.[12] Although a productive conference in many respects, and highly successful as an international feminist forum, the event was marred by a series of conflicts that led to increasing fragmentation of the network in its wake. In the autumn of 1989 the International Coordinating Group of FINRRAGE disbanded, while numerous other organizations, including the Forum against Oppression of Women, left the network. A book contract with Zed Press for the conference proceedings was canceled, and the network effectively split into those who remained part of a smaller and more politically cohesive core of radical activists (led by a new international coordinating group in Germany), and those who left FINRRAGE. Along with many other FINRRAGE participants, I left the network in the wake of the Dhaka conference, although I have kept in close touch with many of its present and former members, both in the United Kingdom and in many other countries.

Contested Conceptions

It is in many ways predictable, given my experience of the conflicts in FINRRAGE over the question of women's experiences of IVF, that I am inclined toward a different interpretation of the feminist divisions in this era than those which emphasize either radical versus socialist feminist divisions, or pro- versus anti- stances toward NRTS. My experiences led me to perceive such interpretations as too neatly polarized. Given my own interests and background, it is also not surprising that my attention was drawn to the issue that arguably unites *Made to Order* and *Reproductive Technologies* (as it united most of FINRRAGE with its opponents), namely that of the ambivalence of women's reproductive agency in general and of the IVF journey in particular. The promotion of women's reproductive empowerment and agency was not only a shared priority across disparate walks of feminist political opinion, and diverse contexts of feminist political activism worldwide during the 1980s, but also an issue that became particularly difficult, uncomfortable, and divisive precisely at the point that NRTS became involved. And no reproductive technology epitomized this difficulty more than IVF. As a result, not only in Western countries, but in India, Brazil, the Philippines, and the Middle East, the question of women's relationship to IVF became one of the most intensely fraught political questions for feminists both within and outside of FINRRAGE.

Thus, despite their other differences, and in spite of being presented as opposing feminist positions, both of the anthologies discussed above addressed the issue of IVF in strikingly similar ways. Alongside articles that were highly critical of NRTS in *Made to Order* and *Reproductive Technologies* were chapters addressing women's experiences of infertility and IVF, as well as the importance of protecting women's access to artificial insemination and other reproductive technologies that were seen to offer paths forward out of rigid normative conventions of kinship and family formation, as well as the distress of infertility. Contrary to its close association with the FINRRAGE line, *Made to Order* contains one of the first feminist analyses of women's experience of IVF by Australian FINRRAGE member Christine Crowe. As the editors note in introducing Crowe's chapter: "In the debates on the new reproductive and genetic technologies, little attention has been paid to women's experiences of infertility and motherhood. . . . Often our efforts to defend women's right to self-determination and reproductive choice have left out infertile women. . . . The availability of IVF puts our politics into a new context" (Spallone and Steinberg 1987: 15). Similarly, although none of the chapters in Stanworth's anthology directly address women's experience of IVF, *Reproductive Technologies* includes a chapter from Naomi Pfeffer, the coauthor with Anne Woollett of the first feminist guide to infertility, *The Experience of Infertility*, published by the feminist press Virago in London in 1983. Stanworth's introduction to Pfeffer's chapter closely parallels Spallone and Steinberg's introduction of Crowe's research, emphasizing (albeit in a somewhat more critical tone) "the refusal by both supporters and opponents of reproductive technologies to acknowledge the heterogeneity of infertility [which] has had the effect of further stigmatising infertile women and men" (Stanworth 1987: 6). The importance placed on a sympathetic feminist approach to women's experience of infertility and IVF in both of these opposed feminist accounts not only constitutes an important point of overlap but anticipates one of the most substantial legacies of these debates in the form of the analysis of how reproductive technologies are understood and experienced by those for whom they become a way of life.

Infertility and IVF

During the 1980s, the theme of women's experience of infertility grew significantly in importance and, once again, three of the key volumes from this era usefully recapitulate some of the main fault lines to emerge in feminist debate. Pfeffer and Woollett's 1983 guidebook was based on the authors' own experience of infertility and infertility treatment, as well as interviews with other women who shared this experience. Designed as a feminist handbook for coming to terms with infertility, it was written to provide information and advice, and to break the silence surrounding infertility. Drawing on the work of Adrienne Rich, the authors argue that both sexuality and reproduction must be reclaimed from male-dominated frameworks and values: "We believe, like Adrienne Rich, that in the realm of sexuality and reproduction, 'it is crucial that women take seriously the enterprise of finding out what we do feel instead of accepting what we have been told we must feel'" (Pfeffer and Woollett 1983: 1). In their guidebook Pfeffer and Woollett interspersed detailed medical information and practical advice with chapters describing the emotional and psychological toll of coping with infertility—very much in the tradition of earlier women's health guidebooks such as *Our Bodies, Ourselves*. Pfeffer and Woollett are not uncritical of NRTS or IVF, both of which, they argue, raise questions about the social conditioning leading women to feel childbearing is an essential part of their identity. They express concern about the extent to which IVF has been developed within a male-dominated medical profession that defines women's reproductive capacity as something to be managed and as an intrinsically flawed system (thus leading to the overattribution of infertility to the female partner, for example). They do not, however, claim that IVF is synonymous with patriarchal control, and instead are above all concerned to enable women to make their own reproductive choices, even if these may involve submitting to costly, painful, and most likely unsuccessful attempts at IVF.

Written before NRTs began to be the subject of more vociferous feminist debate, *The Experience of Infertility* successfully built on the self-help model of women's empowerment established through the women's health and reproductive rights movements of the 1960s and 1970s. That such an approach had become significantly more problematic for feminists by the mid-1980s may be one reason why no successor project to this volume was ever published. The closest candidates for such a companion volume are both, indeed, quite different from it. *Tomorrow's Child: Reproductive Technologies in the 1990s* (Birke et al. 1990), produced, like *Test-Tube Women*, by three feminist scientists, was also a Virago feminist health handbook published in London in 1990.[13] Like its predecessor, it provided up-to-date practical information about infertility, its diagnosis, and its potential alleviation through IVF and other procedures. Unlike the earlier volume, however, *Tomorrow's Child* is concerned less with women's experience of infertility or childlessness than the feminist debate about them, arguing, like Rothman (1986), against a wholesale rejection of these technologies and instead for greater accountability for their marketing and use, as well as better information for women who are considering these options. In the concluding chapters the authors call for an improved debate over the role of science and technology in society, increased control over reproductive technology by women, and more support of the use of such technology to challenge existing social arrangements of family, child care, and kinship, rather than reinforcing the status quo. In addition to being a guidebook, *Tomorrow's Child* drew on Shulamith Firestone's vision of the need for science, technology, and society to change in unison in order for reproduction to be redefined in ways that truly liberate women.

A different set of emphases and arguments distinguished *The Experience of Infertility* from Renate Klein's 1989 anthology, also published as a feminist handbook of sorts by Pandora, titled *Infertility: Women Speak Out about Their*

Experiences of Reproductive Medicine. This volume is much more similar to *The Experience of Infertility* than is *Tomorrow's Child* in its foregrounding of women's personal experience and testimony as a basis for feminist politics, feminist analysis of reproductive health, and the feminist critique of NRTS. However, *Infertility* is intended to be a condemnation of IVF and NRTS, most closely resembling the account offered by Gena Corea (with whom Klein co-authored *Man Made Women* in 1985). As in *Test-Tube Women*, of which Klein was a coeditor, an emphatic editorial introduction affirms that "the message is clear. . . . IVF is a *failed* technology" (Klein 1989: 1, original emphasis), leaving no room for equivocation. These technologies not only expose women to "dangerous health hazards" and require that women be used as "living test sites for drugs and new techniques" (1989: 2), but "often severely violate a woman's sense of dignity" (4) by invoking a "brutal ideology which sees women as mere breeders who need to be controlled" (6). In sum, and as the cover of Klein's anthology affirms: "Reproductive technology fails women: it's a con." Correspondingly, the aim of Klein's book was twofold. On the one hand she was seeking to expose the hidden truth of IVF and the reality behind the image of benevolent medicine and happy media stories (much as Corea had attempted to expose the hidden background of the science and marketing behind IVF). On the other hand, Klein sought to empower her readers "to have a *real* choice to say 'No' to conventional fertility treatments as well as IVF" (1989: 7, original emphasis).

Like Pfeffer and Woollett, Klein included in her handbook chapters covering a wide range of experiences of infertility and childlessness, as well as forms of its diagnosis and treatment. This inclusive spirit does not extend to Klein's final assessment of NRTS, however. Her book closes with a forty-five-page denouncement of NRTS that calls for immediate global legislation to ban their use, and a worldwide feminist movement of resistance to oppose their future development. It is in this context that Klein pointedly describes FINRRAGE as a network that is not so much concerned with, but opposed to, NRTS. In a passage reminiscent of more recent critics of biomedicine and biotechnology, such as Bill McKibben (2004), Klein infuses her conclusion with a passionate injunction to act before time runs out: "There is still time to stop the techno-patriarchal clock that races towards a future of people 'made to order'—an un-humanness of an unprecedented degree. It is not too late. Immature eggs cannot yet be matured. . . . The artificial womb is not yet perfected. Living women still play the most important role in the technological set-up. May the voices of the women in this book increase a movement with a strong bias in international feminist solidarity that resists the technologies and says no with passion" (1989: 289). Though largely critical of NRTS, however, few of the contributors to Klein's anthology are as certain as Klein herself about the viability of alternatives to high-tech medical options such as IVF, or the possibility of large numbers of women resisting them. To the contrary, many of the contributors suggest that despite having considerable reservations about these techniques, they remain sympathetic to women who choose them for a variety of reasons. Even some of the women most critical of NRTS on the basis of their own experience reject the blanket opposition Klein advocates. As one woman described her experience in a chapter authored by German feminist health activist Ute Winkler, for example: "I could not say to a woman that she should not try it. I can understand why she would want to go for it. So I would say to her: 'OK, it will be nasty and you will suffer.' But I would not say that she should not be allowed to try" (Winkler 1989: 100).

The dilemma described by "Inge M.," whereby she says for herself that she would never go through IVF again, indeed that she "would not like to be part of their machinery ever again" (Winkler 1989: 100), yet that she could not say to another woman that she should not try it, exposes the ambivalence of choices and choosing familiar to many areas of feminist politics. Indeed it is a statement that precisely recapitulates the feminist ambivalence toward IVF that has since come to dominate the debate over NRTS in general. Even while denouncing "their machinery" for herself, "Inge M." is reluctant to dictate other women's choices. For Klein, this presents a double dilemma since it represents not only a failure of feminist resistance but the tragedy of women's voluntary compliance with patriarchal science, thus providing the "technodocs" with "experimental test-sites" (Klein 1989: 230): "The tragedy lies in women's cooperation with the experimenters" (246), Klein laments, adding that "women taking part in IVF do not realize that, unwittingly, they contribute to this sick scenario of interfering with human reproduction" (279). According to this view, women who participate in IVF are not only victims but colluders (246). Yet although Klein argues that "there are no better spokeswomen against these technologies than women who have actually gone through the procedures, and survived" (286), such women themselves, as is made evident by their own published testimony in Klein's book, do not always endorse their editor's imperative "to be firm and advise women not to use these technologies" (287).

The model used by Klein is in fact less that of either the women's health handbook or the self-help guide than a publication in the tradition of "speaking out" against war crimes, as in the feminist tribunals of crimes against women organized around sexual violence (Bunch 1982; Russell and Van de Ven 1976). Klein is not an infertile woman herself seeking to break the silence in order to raise consciousness in a manner that will assist women to find their own path. Contrary to her avowed reliance on women's own personal testimony, which, although critical, is distinctly equivocal, Klein attempts to reframe her spokeswomen's voices as evidence of the imperative to "stop this crazy technology by saying *no*" (1989: 279, original emphasis).

Inevitably, accusations from feminists such as Klein, who describes women who undergo IVF as "addicts" who "willingly become research material" (1989: 249), were the source of concern to feminists researching the dilemma of infertility more sympathetically, such as U.S. nurse and anthropologist Margarete Sandelowski, whose interviews with infertile women patients during the 1980s led her to offer a very different interpretation of their testimony. Writing in 1990, Sandelowski warned of "fault lines" in an "imperilled sisterhood" and, specifically that "many feminist critiques of reproductive technology perpetuate and intensify the tensions that already exist between fertile and infertile women and reinforce, rather than counter, patriarchal ideas about and divisions among women" (1990: 34). She adds, "Current feminist discourse has largely focussed on the consequences of using technologies developed to remedy infertility rather than on the infertility experience itself" and that as a result "infertile women find themselves confronted with a group of feminists who suspect their motivations to procreate as strongly as they suspect the medical community's desires to create babies by artificial means" (39). To the extent that such feminist arguments interpret women's motivations to pursue IVF as "a sign of the perversity of women's socialization" (41), argues Sandelowski, echoing Rothman (1984), they are unhelpfully "pitting one group of women against another" (42–43).

Somewhat contrary to the network's anti-NRT reputation, the beginnings of a more comprehensive feminist account of the encounter between women and NRTs was initiated largely by members of FINRRAGE during the 1980s. Alison Solomon, for example, a FINRRAGE member and feminist health activist from Israel, was among the first to emphasize the importance of separating an analysis of the often traumatic experience of infertility treatment from the experience of infertility itself—a distinction, she suggested, that many feminist critics of NRTs had failed to make (Solomon 1989). Somewhat ironically, given its editorial stance, Renate Klein's *Infertility* also contains a chapter from the Danish feminist historian and social theorist Lene Koch, a member of

FINRRAGE who did not share Klein's view that the only possible response to women who chose to undergo IVF was to reeducate them. Instead, like Sandelowski, Koch sought to reeducate herself by seeking out women who had undergone IVF in order to learn from their experience. As she explains in her chapter in Klein's anthology, her research in Denmark with women who spoke to her about their experience of IVF forced her to reconsider the nature of the dilemma the technology poses, in part because of her increasing sensitivity to the reasons women are so determined to undertake it, and to succeed despite the odds.

This dilemma—which is in many ways that of "Inge M."—was taken up by an increasing number of FINRRAGE members in the 1980s, following the lead of Christine Crowe, the first feminist researcher to conduct a detailed empirical study of women's experience of IVF, which she published in 1985.[14] Titled "Women Want It" (and reprinted in *Made to Order*), Crowe's article, based on interviews with women undergoing IVF in one of Sydney's first major assisted conception clinics, explored women's reasons for desiring IVF treatment and, like Rothman's study of amniocentesis, chronicled how their understandings of such a choice could change over the course of treatment, frequently resulting in outcomes they had not anticipated. Like many feminist researchers on IVF since, Crowe provided compelling data on the extent to which IVF was as much a technology of gender, kinship, and conjugality as of reproduction. A dominant theme in Crowe's study is the role of social pressures to attempt IVF in order to complete a family and to confirm a gender identity, as well as to affirm or repair conjugality through biological reproduction—or at least to be seen as trying to establish a pregnancy.[15] As Crowe noted, "Most women expressed the feelings of being excluded from the social nexus of mothers and couples with children, not only in terms of neighbours, but with long-established friends. Parenthood was perceived to be the common experience around which friendships were maintained" (Crowe 1987: 89). Notably, Crowe also emphasized the difficulties described by her respondents of not being seen to try hard enough if they considered dropping out of IVF programs:

> Many women stated that being on an IVF program *forced them to centre their lives even more explicitly around reproduction*. They recognized the inability to attempt to accept their infertility and to come to some resolve about life plans. . . . Once a woman has decided to undergo an IVF procedure, participation in the program seems to have a life of its own. For various reasons women found it very difficult to "give up" the program. Those who had initially set a time limit to how long they would

participate, or how many attempts they would have, found it very difficult to adhere to their initial resolve. (1987: 91, emphasis added)

Such findings were important to the feminist debate about NRTs for several
reasons, not least the extent to which they revealed, even in these very first
studies, that the pursuit of IVF was not exclusively driven by the desire to
have children. As Crowe demonstrated, a fuller understanding of women's
motivations to pursue IVF revealed that being seen to try to become pregnant
through IVF could in some ways perform a role similar to actually having children—at least for a time.[16] Pursuing IVF, for example, could ameliorate the
social pressures to participate in the common experience of parenthood by
allowing women to center their lives around reproduction even if they failed
to produce offspring. In this way, IVF could be seen to enable the performance
of gender that Judith Butler would shortly be naming as a compulsory feature
of identity, and that feminist kinship theorists were already describing as the
product of exogamy—rather than its source.

Whereas earlier feminist accounts of the experience of IVF had documented women's sense of being trapped in an endless series of failed IVF
cycles, Crowe was able to offer an explanation of why this was so. Hence, for
example, Gena Corea had clearly researched women's experiences of IVF as
part of her investigation of reproductive biomedicine for *The Mother Machine*.
Her examples, like Crowe's, accurately and poignantly depicted what is particularly painful about the IVF encounter:

Nancy was one of the "lucky" women who had a successful embryo
transfer after her first laparoscopy in an Australian program. She was
pregnant. Part of her cheered, while another part cautioned that the
chances of success were small. "It was this incredible turmoil that I
was in," she explained. After about a month, she lost the pregnancy.
"I wasn't really surprised when I lost it. Some other people who I've
talked to in the program feel devastated. I didn't. I just felt real sad. I
felt grief-ridden for a while, but I didn't think about giving up." After her
second laparoscopy, while she, still sore, was recovering from surgery,
the doctor told her the eggs they had just harvested had been abnormal.
"When I went in [that] second time and my egg didn't even fertilize,
that was harder than the first time because I thought, "Well, I've lost a
pregnancy, but next time they're going to get it." There were six more
"next times"—seven operations in all—and they still had not "gotten
it" by the time Nancy was interviewed in 1981. (Corea 1985: 180–181)

Both the tone and the context of Corea's depiction of the experience of undergoing IVF reflect a single interpretation of this encounter, namely that it confirms a pattern of exploitation. "Of the thousands of women hoping to get a baby through the 200-odd IVF programs across the globe, the vast majority have been disappointed. The cycle of hopes raised (she's accepted in the program) and dashed (the doctor could not get an egg), raised (got an egg) and dashed (the egg was abnormal), raised (got a normal egg) and dashed (embryo did not implant), raised (embryo implanted) and dashed (miscarried) harms women in ways pharmacrats have not acknowledged" (Corea 1985: 180). For Corea, there is no possibility of interpreting this scenario other than in terms of the harm done by patriarchal culture and its message to women about their place. "The message comes down with the force of centuries-long repetition. The patriarchy gives us the message through games, stories, toys. Our mothers whisper it to us. Our protests preach it. Our doctors give us treatments if our ovaries or our wombs fail us. It is our cell-deep knowledge: We are here to bear the children of men. If we cannot do it, we are not real women. There is no reason for us to exist" (1985: 170).

Crowe's examples, by contrast, are more equivocally interpreted in order to reveal a more complicated struggle against these same norms of femininity. Her examples are differently inflected to allow room for resistance and to allow a more nuanced understanding of how and why people adapt themselves to circumstances beyond their control. Crowe not only illustrates but helps to explain the exact mechanisms by which people adapt themselves to choices that are not being made on terms they have chosen:

> IVF may be seen by many women with fertility problems as the last in a long line of medical procedures. . . . Some women feel they "owe it to themselves" to attempt this last possible avenue before making further long term decisions about their life. Once undergoing an IVF procedure many women find it difficult to discontinue. One woman described IVF as a "whirlpool" where hope is offered "just around the corner." The fact that IVF is possible, and its persistent lure of "next time," makes it even harder for a woman to consider life without a child born of herself. (1988: 58)

By this means, Crowe can illustrate not only why women undergo IVF, but how they attempt to protect themselves in the process. As one patient she interviewed explained: "I know it's not going to work again, but we'll try anyway. You try to protect yourself. That self-protection is very strong. . . . All you're trying to do is to cushion that emotional blow at the end" (Crowe 1988:

60). Crowe's findings further confirmed that IVF patients are hardly unaware of the fact that they are undertaking IVF in a highly unequal situation, in which medical experts are in charge, while patients are both subordinate and dependent upon their doctors for the help they are seeking. As another interviewee explained: "When we first went to see the doctor [at the IVF clinic] I was saying to my husband: 'Now, whatever you do, keep your mouth shut and be good, because this is the last chance we get'" (1988: 60).

Documenting the phenomenon later characterized by Charis Thompson (2005) as "ontological choreography," Crowe revealed that the women patients she interviewed expected to be objectified and thought their doctors were likely to be incapable of treating them other than as "uteruses and tubes": "They're technical, they're success oriented, they want to get pregnancies—that's their job . . . to do IVF and to put embryos back, and to keep doing it day after day after day, with lots of women coming through on a conveyor belt. I don't see how they can *avoid* just seeing women as objects because after all that's what they are to them . . . just uteruses and tubes. Also, they have no training in the psychological or emotional aspects. They'd be *terrified* to get into that!" (Crowe 1988: 62–63). Crowe's findings anticipate the description offered by Lauren Berlant of "cruel optimism," defined as "a relation of attachment to compromised conditions of possibility" (2006: 21). In the same way, Berlant draws our attention to "the labor of reproducing life in the contemporary world [that is] also the activity of being worn out by it" (2006: 23), so too does Crowe provide an account of an attachment to chasing an impossible baby, noting of the patients in her study that "those who had set a time limit to how long they would participate in the program found it extremely difficult to adhere to their initial resolve; none kept to their original limit." As another patient she interviewed explained:

> I've been chasing a baby ever since I was 22. You've got to draw the line somewhere. Thirty-five was going to be "it" . . . but I still feel that physically and mentally I could still have a child. For the last twelve months I've been trying to kid myself into saying that I don't care if I quit anyhow. I'd like to be in a position so that I feel freer and not subject to any manipulation, and it's not so important to me . . . but *really*, for all that twelve months it's been a struggle inside myself, and I've *never* really reached the stage where I could say I could quit. (Crowe 1988: 64–65)

In addition to illuminating the precise mechanisms by which IVF becomes a way of life, Crowe identifies not only a feminine, and feminist, dilemma, but a technological one. There are several important paths that follow from her investigations, including the question of what happens when technologies of gender and technologies of reproduction intersect. Or, to put it the other way around, are there circumstances in which the engagement with a technological quest or pilgrimage becomes a distinctly feminizing experience, for example in the psychoanalytic sense of how femininity is positively defined by subordination and lack? Is a certain kind of familiar heroism attached to the pursuit of impossible goals? Sara Ahmed makes an important point about the "relation of attachment to compromised conditions of possibility" (Berlant 2006: 21) in her account of "the promise of happiness" and what happiness comes "after":

> If we think of instrumental goods as objects of happiness, important consequences follow. Things become good, or acquire their value as goods, insofar as they point toward happiness. Objects become "happiness means." Or we could say they become happiness pointers, as if to follow their point would be to find happiness. If objects provide a means of making us happy, then in directing ourselves toward this or that object we are aiming somewhere else: toward a happiness that is presumed to follow. The temporality of this following does matter. Happiness is what would come after. Given this, happiness is directed toward certain objects, which point toward that which is not yet present. When we follow things, we aim for happiness, as if happiness is what you get if you reach certain points. (Ahmed 2010: 26)

As Ahmed notes, "we might assume that the relationship between an object and feeling involves causality: as if the object causes the feeling," when in fact the attribution of happiness to causality is often retrospective. Thus "the object of feeling lags behind the feeling" (Ahmed 2010: 27).

Berlant's attention to the inherent ambivalence of attachments to "compromised conditions of possibility" and Ahmed's account of "happiness means" are highly pertinent to the problem posed by IVF, which cannot simply be explained in terms of women being given the wrong messages or false hopes. The question of women's relationship to the promise of happiness IVF offers is both more complex and in many ways less specific to women than such an explanation suggests. To paraphrase Ahmed, if IVF offers a promise of happiness, then to follow the path of IVF is precisely to move toward that which is not yet present, and thus to associate oneself with the happiness that is presumed to follow, even if the object of feeling never materializes. This is why IVF can offer a fulfilling orientation, whether or not it delivers a "take-home baby."

A question we can now ask as a result of the long tradition of feminist studies of women's experience of IVF that began with Crowe's work—and indeed that some concerned IVF practitioners have increasingly asked themselves as IVF has become so much more widespread—is whether IVF is so popular in part *because* of its elusive and demanding requirements. Like a modern technological pilgrimage, IVF can be understood as a path that acquires moral and affective significance through the very nature of the journey as much as, if not even more than, through the fact of arrival. This is an important reason the path to IVF may be so difficult to leave despite serial failure, since ironically the endurance of so much deprivation only confirms more emphatically a dedication to the journey's objectives.

The question of IVF's complex appeal was also the subject of Canadian FINRRAGE member Linda Williams's (1988) PhD in Toronto in the mid-1980s. Exploring women's motivations for undergoing IVF, and titled "It's Going to Work for Me," Williams's research focused on why women continue to repeat IVF after failing, as most do, on their first complete cycle. Although it is in some ways a seemingly obvious question, Williams, a feminist sociologist like Crowe, provided the much-needed empirical data to account for what she described as "parenthood motivation"—an argument further developed in both Charis Thompson's (2005) monograph *Making Parents* and Gay Becker's (2000) study of IVF as a form of consumer culture in the United States. In Denmark, Lene Koch extended her study of women's experience of IVF to make another important early finding that has been repeated many times since, namely the counterintuitive way in which women's desire to pursue IVF treatment appears to increase in roughly the same proportion as their knowledge of why it is most likely to fail. "Somehow," Koch observes, "*information did not matter*" (1990: 225, original emphasis).

In her 1990 article titled "IVF—an Irrational Choice?" Koch explores the reasons for this apparent discrepancy (later a central theme in studies of new genetic choices; e.g., Rapp 1999). She makes sense of this dilemma, as her title indicates, by arguing that the reasons women want to undertake IVF, or want to continue to undertake additional cycles despite repeated failures, are not irrational but are reinforced through the unexpected physical and emotional intensity of IVF, which engenders a rationality that is specific to the rigors of undergoing the highly stage-dependent IVF protocol, as well as the need to protect oneself against its high failure rates. Like many later researchers who have investigated women's experience of IVF, Koch demonstrates the ways in which technological promise, reproductive labor, gendered identity, and individual agency interlock in the pursuit of IVF to produce a situated rationality characterized by a distinctive temporality, instrumentality, affective orientation, and self-protective mechanisms. She argues that appreciating the specificity of the "different rationality" experienced by women undergoing IVF is essential both to understanding why women want it and to building a dialogue about their decisions that is based on respect for their experience—to which they alone have access. To understand and respect such experiences, Koch emphasizes, is not necessarily to agree with the choices that led to them. However, she points out, a starting point of respect and understanding is a far more politically viable standpoint from which to openly disagree with such decisions than opposing them as either irrational or politically incorrect—never mind as culpable, illogical, or threatening to the future welfare of women as a group. In the context of feminist debate over IVF, Koch argues, "the belief that some views are 'right' and others are 'wrong' will not bring us closer to a better world for women" (1990: 231). Nor, she implied, would it lead to a greater understanding of the logic of IVF.

I began my own research on women's experience of IVF in the mid-1980s for both political and intellectual reasons, including concerns I shared with several other FINRRAGE members working on this theme. Like them, I became educated in the learning curve of the IVF experience through the generosity of women who were willing to share with me their experiences of this technique, revealing its many paradoxical and unexpected features. I learned, for example, that it was indeed possible to become a little bit pregnant while undergoing IVF, and that, just as Rothman (1986) had shown, such experiences changed women's relationships to their prior understandings of choices they had made before they began the arduous process of embodying their consequences. Hence, I discovered, the choice to undertake IVF may be made on the basis of a kind of guarantee that at least if you fail, you will have the compensatory satisfaction of having tried everything, meaning you will at least not be worse off even if you do not succeed in bringing home the much-desired take-home baby, since you will have more, not less, than what you started with (having neither a baby nor the emotional closure of having left no stone unturned). What this equation leaves out, I learned, is the extent to which IVF changes the terms of this guarantee over time. By enabling a woman to begin to experience pregnancy, for example by seeing her own eggs, seeing them fertilized with her partner's sperm, and then having potentially viable embryos transferred back into her womb, IVF ironically intensifies the very deficit it is intended to mitigate. Often, once this proximity to pregnancy is physically and emotionally experienced, the more offered by simply knowing you have tried everything is no longer enough. Thus IVF may have taken away something you did not even realize you could lose, which is even the prospect of a closure to the pain of infertility — producing an opposite outcome to the more imagined at the outset, and one for which it is impossible to be prepared.

Conclusion

Becoming a little bit pregnant is but one of many distinctive features of what I described in my 1997 book *Embodied Progress* as "IVF as a way of life," and many such insights continue to be gleaned by researchers from interviews with women and couples undergoing this procedure. Similar accounts of how reproductive technology alters the terrain of reproductive choice have been derived from what is now a significant number of sociological studies that broadly follow in Rothman's footsteps by chronicling not only the situated rationalities but the embodied logics of experiencing reproductive technologies such as amniocentesis, IVF, preimplantation genetic diagnosis, ultrasound, surrogacy, artificial insemination, or egg donation. Indeed, many of the phenomena Paul Rabinow described as "biosociality" in the early 1990s — to denote the technological remaking of biological ties, and the denaturalization of human biology as it came to be reengineered technologically — were first documented in the context of the new reproductive, not genetic, technologies. In vitro fertilization involves exactly what Rabinow described as the matrix of biosociality, "nature . . . known and remade through technique [until it] finally become[s] artificial, just as culture becomes natural" (1992: 241–242). "Biosociality," he predicted, would become "a circulation network of identity terms and restriction loci, around and through which a truly new type of autoproduction will emerge" (241–242). But although he very accurately predicted these transformations in the context of the new genetics, they had already been described and documented within the feminist literature on NRTS, which precisely chronicles the emergence of new types of identity, new relationalities, and new types of "autoproduction" (as well as family production, kinship production, and identity production) in the context of NRTS.

What Rabinow's account of biosociality leaves out is the complex texture of living an ambivalent relationship to technologies of remaking life. In contrast, this ambivalence is precisely what is so vividly foregrounded in feminist accounts of IVF. Whereas biosociality emphasizes new forms of social affiliation, and the emergence of new communities bound by a shared stake in biological redesign, the encounter with compromised possibilities that is so determining of the relationship to both infertility and its treatment is the focus of the feminist work on IVF, which reveals the isolation and exclusion that create the feeling of "having to try." In the context of IVF described by many feminist researchers, the emphasis on gendered identities adds an important dimension to understanding biosociality, as the pursuit of NRTs involves the remaking of identities, relationships, social groupings, and kinship ties. It is in this context, for example, that we can see more clearly how the familiar identity technologies of kinship and gender are not only the precursors, but also the products, of the pursuit of technologies such as IVF.

In vitro fertilization, it turns out, is a reproductive technology in more than one sense. While enabling biological reproduction, it also offers a context for the reproduction of gender norms, family values, and kinship structures. At the same time, and in the same way that it is both just like and not like unassisted reproduction, IVF provides a context in which established norms are changed. The ambivalence of the IVF encounter, at one level symptomatic of its high propensity for failure, is also, in more positive terms, a space of possibility: despite its shortcomings it may also offer a welcome source of hope, a pathway forward, a stone to turn. Embarking on an IVF quest may function as a mechanism to adapt to social conventions despite its all too common failure as a method of procreation and its relatively high risk of worsening the very problem it is intended to solve. And it is also popular because of the means it offers to defy convention, by enabling entirely new forms of reproduction to be pursued, such as egg donation, postmenopausal pregnancy, preimplantation genetic diagnosis, and gestational surrogacy. In sum, IVF, for all its newly regular status, remains a reproductive frontier. Not only a technology of reproduction, IVF is a technology of identity and subjectification. To better understand the complex appeal of IVF that began to be charted in the mid-1980s by feminist researchers, it is useful to review the data now available on how IVF both reproduces and also challenges the norms it is ostensibly aligning with, or toward. This chapter thus picks up more or less where chapter 5 left off, by developing a more detailed analysis of the feminist literature on the experience of living IVF—a literature that has continued to reveal how the embrace of IVF paradoxically becomes curiouser and curiouser during the same period it has become more regular.

IVF: A New Model of Sex?

In her meticulous and comprehensive 1993 study, Margarete Sandelow-ski provided the first major sociological account of the experience of infertility, infertility treatment, and adoption, outlining many of the patterns and themes that would come to define later studies in this field. *With Child in Mind: Studies of the Personal Encounter with Infertility* was the first monograph to chronicle many of the patterns that have since been repeatedly reported in subsequent social studies of assisted reproductive technology (ART), including my own, which was conducted in a different country and in a later period but nonetheless reconfirmed many of Sandelowski's original findings. The disruption posed by infertility to the lives of individuals and couples, the stalled life course, the pressure from family and peer groups, the experience of failed or inadequate identities, the difficult choices and decisions that must be navigated with few landmarks, and the obstacle-course nature of the IVF quest, with its underlying teleology of hope, have all emerged as remarkably consistent themes across a widely disparate set of regional studies that now span the globe.

As noted in the introductory chapters, an important question to consider in the wake of the surprisingly rapid expansion of IVF worldwide since 1978 is how to reconcile its apparently boundless appeal with both the considerable demands (physically, emotionally, financially) on those who undertake it against its equally well-known high failure rate (still well above 50 percent). These demands have been chronicled in a series of major academic studies from the mid-1980s onward that, perhaps inevitably, foreground the questions of how and why people choose and navigate IVF and other ARTs.[1] One approach to this question returns us to the role of IVF as a model, and to the IVF pioneer as a role model, for a new form of achieved parenthood that increased in prominence and public visibility toward the close of the twentieth century, and has thus come to play an increasingly large role in the parenthood narratives of the twenty-first.[2] It is with this increasingly normalized status of IVF in mind that many researchers have turned to the question of what this technique and its ilk are reproducing other than, or in addition to, children (especially given that take-home babies are more the exception than the rule). To the extent IVF is modeling a new role for technology in the context of assisting human reproduction ("giving nature a helping hand"), so too has sexual reproduction become increasingly interrelated with another form of coupling—that of biology and technology. Indeed, the burgeoning IVF industry appears increasingly symbiotically linked to a sense of crisis surrounding fertility and the necessity—or even duty—not to take biological reproduction for granted, or to ensure that it is (like other bodily capacities) prosthetically enhanced. This important context of the relativization of the biological has arguably been more fully mapped empirically in the context of IVF than any other.

The shift in cultural attitudes toward biological reproduction occurring from the 1980s onward is particularly striking in contrast to the taken-for-granted status of reproduction within much of social theory during this same period, where precisely the same process that is "taken in hand" through techniques such as IVF remains passively imagined as the self-acting mechanism at the root of social organization. From the point of view of IVF, the "universal relation of human reproduction" described by Collier and Yanagisako (1987a: 33), and the "natural characteristics of women and men and their natural roles in sexual procreation" (32) do not add up to the same "folk model of human reproduction" (35) upon which so much social theory in the past has been based. Instead, from the point of view of IVF the allegedly obvious natural value of women's reproductive capacity disappears. In stark contrast to its imagined obviousness as a motor of social evolution, IVF reveals a context in which the engine of reproduction is stalled. Indeed, in the context of IVF the driving force, the natural genealogical flow, and thus the assumed telos of biological reproduction are reversed: rather than being a physiological basis for social evolution, the automatic mechanisms of biological reproduction are in need of being kick started—or simply replaced—by technology.

After IVF, this shift in the significance of biological reproduction—its altered causality—is equally evident in popular culture, where the drama of failed reproduction is coupled to both the promise of technology and the fear of infertility—as well as to new technological horizons, such as cloning and designer babies. For the post-IVF generation of young women born in the 1980s, and now entering their thirties, both ART and fertility anxiety are now facts of life—as familiar as YouTube or Facebook. It is as if their biological clock is not so much ticking toward offspring as toward a newly routinized technological encounter. As journalist Gemma Soames wrote in the London Sunday Times in February 2009, IVF has become "as much a part of female dialogue as waxing and highlights":

> We are part of a generation raised on IVF stories—a generation more acutely aware of and educated about dodgy ovaries, potential fibroids and infertility scares than our mothers and elder sisters ever were. . . . IVF is now as much a part of female dialogue as waxing and highlights. Through magazines, celebrities, soap plot lines and mates around the

corner, we have all lived vicariously through story after tear-jerking story of failed pregnancy attempts. We all watched Charlotte from Sex and the City fail to conceive for three whole seasons. Girls as young as 18 have responded to IVF features printed in this magazine. (Soames 2009)

To the extent that feminine identity is typically characterized by its proximity to failure (a view that is strongly reinforced by the media), it could even be argued there is a close fit between the anticipation of failed reproductivity and the formation of normal femininity. It would follow, as Soames suggests, that the mere presence of so much fertility technology itself encourages a sense of potential deficit—a process made explicit through fertility fairs, advertising campaigns, and social media, while also being dramatized in popular films and TV shows. In the literature on IVF this phenomenon (we might call it the "because it's there" phenomenon) is well documented. In my own study, conducted in the United Kingdom during a period of rapid expansion of IVF in the late 1980s, one patient described the U-turn she experienced when an IVF clinic opened nearby as immediate, despite having already reconciled herself to childlessness: "Mind you, we'd forgotten, we'd said alright. . . . We'd accepted [our infertility] pretty well until the clinic opened and then you go, ah! I've got another chance. I mean you've got to take it really, you've got to have a go" (Franklin 1997: 172).

The mutually reinforcing relationship between the rapidly expanding consumer base for ART and its increasing availability as a global health service industry is substantially aided by the vagueness of the fear of infertility, a famously difficult condition to define. Fertility has always been biologically relative: it is unusual in that it is a condition that can be either individual or shared (ultimately, fertility can be achieved only by two people), and it is a highly dependent condition (on age, diet, health, and thus income, class, and race). The clinical rule of thumb is that a third of infertility is male, a third is female, and a third is combined. It is typical for infertility to remain undiagnosed (unexplained infertility) or to be only partially diagnosed—and there is often more than one source of potential difficulty. Since it does not typically present as an independent condition, the most common way to define infertility is retrospectively—as the persistence of an unexplained and unwanted nonevent in the wake of having tried to achieve conception for a specified period of time (often a year or two). It is thus perfectly possible to be infertile without ever knowing it, either as an individual or a couple, since it comes into being largely through failure, that is, through something that does not happen—or indeed something that does not happen over a prolonged period of time.

However, these are not the only reasons infertility is hard to define precisely. Many of the findings from sociological and anthropological studies of IVF suggest that it is the frequent underdefinition of infertility that has, somewhat paradoxically, led to an expansion of its diagnostic, or peridiagnostic, remit as an umbrella category. Thus, for example, the diagnosis of infertility is increasingly linked to genetic diagnoses, and thus also to the prevention of genetic disease (e.g., in the case of cystic fibrosis). Infertility can comprise everything from repeated miscarriages (which may also have a genetic cause in the form of a chromosomal translocation) to lifestyle factors (couples that commute or live apart) or incompatibility of the male and female gametes. A common cause of temporary infertility is home redecoration. On the face of it, such a wide range of factors make infertility a complex condition to diagnose, and this complexity is exacerbated by the growing awareness of infertility as a potential problem for both couples and individuals—a possibility that ART services have made more visible as they have become more prominent. Hence, for example, during my fieldwork in several ART clinics over many years I have frequently had conversations with very experienced clinicians who suspect that some of the prospective clients who visit their fertility clinics are looking for something other than a baby. The impression described by one IVF service coordinator I spoke to, based on the differences between her initial interviews with couples, and the fairly large proportion of those who did not keep their second appointment (approximately 50 percent), was that some people visit a fertility center "almost as a rite of passage," or as if from a vague sense that fertility enhancement was now somehow necessary to successful conception.

The possibility that IVF might be offering various forms of what this clinician dubbed "fertility reassurance" remained vague for her as well as for others I have spoken to who share the widespread suspicion among IVF personnel that they are not always dealing with individuals or couples who are worried they are technically infertile, but who are instead confused about the new role of technology in the business of making babies. Do they want advice about sex? Are they worried they do not know how to make a baby? Do they think technology is now necessary to have high-quality offspring?[3]

In one of the few discussions of the question of why people want to have their own or biological children, Karin Lesnik-Oberstein asks: "Even if the [new reproductive] technologies may be examined in terms of how people use and experience them, the outcome of the process seems to be seen as self-evident and obvious, beyond question: children are children" (2008: xiii). The obviousness of the desire to have children leads to the view, Lesnik-Oberstein suggests, that the choice to use reproductive technology "is merely a practical one," adding, "Any questioning of these assumptions has certainly not affected the continued expansion and use of reproductive technologies. And yet these assumptions provide the single underpinning motivation and justification for these activities" (xii).

As Lesnik-Oberstein also notes, there is a significant amount of evidence from the empirical literature on new reproductive technologies that assisted conception technologies, and the culture of which they are a part, are reproducing much more than children per se. After all, part of the answer to the question of why people want children, whether or not they are their own biological children, is what having children represents in society. It is not necessary to be an involuntarily childless person to recognize that having children is a highly normalized, naturalized, and valorized activity in society, closely correlated with the successful achievement of adult gender identities and the fulfillment of kinship obligations, particularly in relation to marriage. Given more careful consideration, it is all but self-evident that the culture of ART is rapidly proliferating not only in the face of, but by means of, a host of interlinked insecurities concerning not only fertility in its narrowest sense of the biological ability to procreate, but other anxieties related to social expectations and social roles. This, in turn, suggests that IVF is not a response to failed reproduction per se but to the social expectations that are linked to successful procreation. Arguably it is also these expectations the existence of IVF makes more visible.

These expectations return us to Gayle Rubin's question of how "the exact mechanisms by which particular conventions of sexuality are produced and maintained" (1975: 177). In the context of IVF the production of these conventions is now contextualized by, or indeed fused with, another set of regulatory norms, more akin to those examined by Marx in his discussion of the introduction of a model of progress and improvement into the history of technology. As Marx notes, the desire to significantly change, or improve, manufacturing methods did not characterize, for example, much of the history of milling machines, which remained the same for centuries before the advent of the Industrial Revolution. The expectation that science and technology should be the source of continual improvements to the quality of life, which is one of the definitive expectations of the modern era, began to be applied to biology initially through agriculture and selective breeding, and later, as I observed in chapter 3, through the promise of engineering life. In vitro fertilization is the offspring of the coupling of these two genres of expectation: that particular conventions of sexuality are produced and maintained (Rubin), and that technology can aid in this process (Marx). The Loebian ideal of mechanizing life is what enables these two trajectories to become one — that is, for the maintenance of sexual (reproductive, conjugal) convention to be assisted technologically.

Curiously, however, this marriage of technological progress with sexual convention in the context of the modern fertility market explicitly reverses the relationship between biological reproduction and social aspiration presumed in the traditional models provided by either social theory or evolutionary biology: after IVF it is no longer the case that social aspiration (initially in the form, according to Lévi-Strauss et al., of the aspiration to become social at all) follows from either the self-acting force of procreation or the desire to organize its flow in the wake of its natural occurrence (as a feature of what Rubin calls "animal biology"). In the context of IVF, it is social aspirations that activate reproductive substance, by mechanizing it, in order to make it work. Indeed, the agency here is doubly reversed: social aspirations become the antecedent of biological function, and biological function becomes a technological expectation, or even convention. At the very point, then, that the embryologist composes by hand the arrangement of reproductive substance in glass intended to achieve IVF is the moment when technologies of making sex are doubled: here, sex is remade, twice. Sex becomes a technological convention, and conventional technologies are used to make sex. Like exogamy, IVF proceeds via the conventional organization of both parties and parts guided by established principles of composition: these are its exact mechanisms.

This process is what Strathern described when she noted that it has become "routinely thinkable in the post-industrialism of the late-twentieth century . . . to make play with juxtaposing images of the organic and inorganic." This merographic mechanism is enabling, she claims, "because the one does not imitate the other so much as seemingly deploy or use its principles or parts" — it is the recombination, or mix, that is generative (facilitating in the case of IVF the remaking of sex). But the doubling of this function in the context of reproductive technology also visibly exceeds its immediate pragmatics insofar as "kinship systems and family structures are imagined as social arrangements *not just imitating but based on and deploying processes of biological reproduction*" (Strathern 1992b: 3, emphasis added). Thus, she argues, a new reproductive model is produced in the context of new reproductive technologies: "Perhaps a new ground for individual action will be this very capacity to combine desire with the appropriate enabling technology. If this is a change, then the change has occurred as result of people becoming self-conscious about values already held. When the traditional yearning for parenthood can be satisfied by 'artificial' arrangements, it is the yearning that seems natural" (1992a: 177). This new reproductive model is what is substantialized as IVF — indeed, is its origin. However, as Strathern notes, and this chapter also argues, IVF exceeds and transforms this model — in Strathern's terms it does not reproduce it exactly. The very reversal the model confirms, in which it is social aspiration and convention that activate and mechanize reproductive substance, enabling it to be taken in hand, remade as technique, and reconfigured, defines the condition of being after IVF, and thus of becoming biologically relative (or being before as well as after nature). The question of what it means "not only to imitate but to deploy" the processes of biological reproduction comes explicitly into view as a set of future possibilities via the success of IVF "in man" in the 1970s, and later as a market in fertility services. The future of kinship suggested by such possibilities is one of artificial arrangements that, partly as a result of IVF, have become not only routinely thinkable but routinely reengineerable too. What is naturalized in this new reproductive model is precisely the reverse of that which structures the history of social theory, for it is now convention that naturalizes reproduction, not the other way around.

Thus, as IVF has become a better-established and widely available consumer option, and itself a more normalized and naturalized activity, the questions of what people want from it, and what they are doing with it, have become more prominent concerns in research on IVF as well. This chapter explores the two halves of the new reproductive model introduced by IVF in two parts. In the first part, the literature on IVF is reviewed with an emphasis on how it both reveals and can be seen to alter "the exact mechanisms by which particular conventions of sexuality are produced and maintained" (Rubin 1975: 177). By exploring all of the reasons people pursue IVF in addition to wanting to have children, I ask whether its increasingly widespread use can be explained not only as a response to social expectations and conventions, but as a means of naturalizing and normalizing new means of responding to these conventions — thus paradoxically instituting a new norm of reproduction that does not necessarily involve having children. The point of this approach is not to diminish the importance of having children to people undergoing IVF, nor in particular to dismiss the profound distress IVF can produce when it fails. The point is rather to explore the exact mechanisms linking convention, technology, and biology in the context of IVF because these artificial arrangements are increasingly how the future of kinship will be shaped through identities and agencies similar to those produced in the context of IVF. Ultimately, in other words, the aim is to explore what it means for kinship to be imagined in and through technology as a context of natural achievement or the achievement of biological relations. Conversely, what does it mean for technological relations to be imagined biologically as kinship—for example, in order to form a kinship identity through a technological quest?

This is of course a very open-ended question, and in the second part of this chapter it is explored somewhat differently, through the medium of visual imagery—a perspective that is capacitated by the actual apparatus of IVF as a window onto the precise mechanisms of fertilization. If one of the questions IVF poses is how traditionally biological identities are reimagined and remade technologically—and in particular what are the exact mechanisms through which this occurs—it is helpful to explore the prominent ways in which this process is facilitated by that other crucial reproductive technology—the media. Thus, in the second part, I once again attempt to fuse the exact mechanisms of embryology with their translation into other conventions, or genres, or substances, of making sex—in this case high-profile visual images of manipulated embryos, such as those that have become routinely viewable on the evening news, in the cinema, and in advertising. The aim here is, again, limited and specific, not least as the study of the visual culture of biomedicine is an enormous field in its own right. Specifically, then, I offer a reading of IVF imagery, or public spectacle, that is intended to contribute to the effort to characterize the artificial arrangements out of which I suggest the future of kinship is already being imagined. If IVF is a lens, what can we see through it? And how can this perspective help us understand how the logic of IVF is lived?

What Is IVF After?

Strathern's prediction that after the fact of artificial reproduction it will be the yearning for parenthood that is naturalized in lieu of a biological base to reproduction is both confirmed and complicated by the now extensive literature on how and why IVF is chosen by its users. Indeed, what is seen as either natural or biological in the context of IVF appear to be among the most flexible components in a procedure than can otherwise often feel relentlessly regimented to its users. In the context of IVF it is the fixity and limits of technology, rather than biology, to which identities, hopes, aspirations, and desires must be accommodated, since they, unlike the strict clinical protocols of IVF, can bend. Thus, to the extent that IVF consumers are seeking to realize a traditional (or nontraditional) dream of parenthood, it is the dream and not the means that must be tweaked when things do not turn out as planned. It is for this reason that the context of IVF can be characterized very generally as one of highly flexible conventions coupled to a newly adjustable biology. Indeed, even the most traditional conventions and idioms, such as biological relatedness, heterosexuality, the unity of the conjugal and procreative function, or the dictates of conservative religion, can be creatively warped and woofed to make a baby, or the attempt to have one via IVF, fit in. The achievement of viable offspring via IVF appears to be an event capable of aligning even the most unconventional of situations into happy conformity with the overarching social norm of celebrating the birth of a much-wanted child.[4]

Somewhat more surprising is the finding that the alignment with convention IVF enables its users to achieve through their technological pursuit of parenthood not only can be realized without having children, but can even succeed in lieu of having them. While it might seem obvious that what people want from IVF is a take-home baby, an increasing amount of data on IVF suggest that this motivation is not always so straightforward. For example, in her PhD dissertation on IVF in Mexico, Sandra Gonzalez-Santos (2010) relates a revealing anecdote about disclosing her own voluntary childlessness during the course of her research in several different Mexican ART clinics between 2006 and 2008. Worried it might be alienating to some of the women IVF patients she was interviewing that she herself did not share their desire for children, Gonzalez was both surprised and relieved to discover that a significant number of her informants not only lauded her choice to remain childless but envied it, claiming they wished it was an acceptable option not to have children themselves. They were having IVF, they explained, because it was ultimately easier to succumb to the constant pressure from in-laws than to resist: if they could not have children they at least needed to be seen as trying to by aligning themselves with the child-oriented trajectory of IVF. These responses thus provide a counterintuitive (or not) example of women in IVF programs for whom "being seen to try" to procreate could provide an alibi for not doing so: being seen to be trying to have a baby could, to a degree, substitute for having one, at least temporarily—and possibly permanently. In vitro fertilization could even be a way not to have children (since it would probably fail), while at the same time avoiding at least some of the stigma normally attaching to such an outcome (by being seen to have tried everything), and nonetheless acquiring an achieved parenthood identity along the way.

The question of how identities are being produced and managed, or crafted, at various stages of IVF is not new, but one that has been repeatedly characterized and in some cases prioritized by researchers such as Sandelowski and Gonzalez, among others. This is the main theme, for example, of much of Charis Thompson's work, for which she has developed the term "ontological choreography" in part to describe the constantly recombinant process of identity transitioning over the course of ART treatment. This finding corresponds with another of the most strikingly consistent themes across the now rather large literature on women's and couples' experiences of infertility treatment, which is the staggering amount of labor involved in this form of activity. This aspect of the experience of unwanted childlessness featured prominently, for example, in Margarete Sandelowski's aforementioned study of 123 women and couples trying "to achieve a pregnancy":

> The amount of effort expended in negotiating the maze and in managing its dead ends . . . was staggering. The women and couples had been trying for an average of five years to achieve a pregnancy prior to their participation in these studies. Of the forty-eight infertile women interviewed in the first study, eleven women had been trying for five to ten years, one woman thirteen years, and one woman seventeen years; sixteen of them had suffered one or more pregnancy losses or infant deaths prior to entering the study. Of seventy-five infertile couples interviewed in the second study, twenty-eight couples had been trying over a five to ten year period to achieve pregnancies and two couples over an eleven to twelve year period; seventeen couples had suffered one or more pregnancy losses or infant deaths prior to entering the study and eight couples had suffered one or more adoption failures. (1993: 92)

Conducted in the mid-1980s, Sandelowski's research was the first to identify and characterize a pattern that has since come to appear noticeably dominant in the IVF literature ever since—be it drawn from interviews with women or couples in North, Central, or Latin America, Europe, the Middle East, India, China, Southeast Asia, Scandinavia, the former Soviet Union, Australia, or Africa. This is the pattern of determined, middle-class couples who desire services to provide them with children, and whose expenditure of effort, cash, and determination plays a key role in the identity formation process specific to the context of choosing ARTs. This trend toward increased investment of both time and money in technological assistance as part of the parenthood quest is increasingly accompanied by the expanded use of IVF to prevent genetic disease (via both preimplantation genetic diagnosis and savior siblings), fertility tourism, and increasing lower-middle or working-class consumption of fertility services, using limited disposable income, as is seen in parts of China. New dimensions of the IVF quest continue to be revealed, as in Marcia Inhorn's (2011) overview of diasporic Middle Eastern communities seeking to return to have IVF at home in a complex pattern of reproductive repatriation. Together, these and related phenomena constitute a new biosocial public sphere — a domain of activity characterized by the proliferation of services aimed at assisting couples to achieve parenthood, and the consumption of these services not only in pursuit of healthy biological offspring, but the new parenthood identities this sector also offers, which are sought as one of several means of being seen to meet social expectations defining successful family formation. Unpacking the motivation to pursue IVF, in other words, reveals the desire for both more than a baby, and in some cases less.

It is, for all of these reasons, important to ask a variant of David Schneider's question about kinship, namely, what is ART all about? Even if we take for granted that much of the pursuit of ART is merely practical, it is clear the quest involved in procedures such as IVF is often precisely that — a heroic struggle in pursuit of elusive goals. According to the *American Heritage Dictionary*'s definition of "quest," it is "the act or an instance of seeking or pursuing something; a search" or "an expedition undertaken in medieval romance by a knight in order to perform a prescribed feat." That IVF is deliberately chosen is undoubtedly an important feature distinguishing its clientele, while at the same time the complex motivations engendering this choice, or path forward, have been one of the most carefully analyzed and exhaustively documented topics within the ART literature. That romance features in the quest narrative is hardly irrelevant, since ART is often pursued with the explicit aim of achieving marital fulfillment or conjugal completion. Often for religious as well as personal and social reasons, couples without children may be seen as conjugally failed or even illegitimate. In Israel, as Susan Kahn (2000) demonstrates, an insufficient effort to have children may be seen as a dereliction of national historic duty, whereas in neighboring Lebanon, as Morgan Clarke observes, it may be seen as the occasion for a familial crisis of faith (as one of his informants notes of a childless couple, reprising a now-familiar injunction, "they should at least try IVF"; 2009: 159). To the extent that IVF is a search, the question must be posed of what it is a search for, which, the literature would seem increasingly to suggest, is rarely, if ever, just a baby.

It is in the answers to the question of what ART is all about that we may also be better able to begin to explain not only the enormous popularity of IVF, and its rapid expansion, but the staggering amount of work involved in pursuing resolutions to infertility. The amount of work is staggering not simply because the IVF procedure is demanding and difficult. The more complex explanation, suggested even in the very earliest studies of women's encounter with infertility and IVF explored in chapter 5, is that the amount of work is so staggering because IVF is a resolution of much more than infertility itself. Moreover, and as we have already seen, it is precisely the staggering amount of labor that can itself provide a defense against a failed or spoiled gender identity, because in trying so hard is found a means to achieve the very thing that is sought (in other words, the quest for parenthood becomes a substitute for it).[5] If IVF were as easy as "passing him on the stairs" it could not serve this function. The sense of having to try has many sources, and one of them may well be the need, or desire, to be seen to be trying. The word "quest" that is so widespread in the IVF literature also has many sources, one of which is that the experience of undergoing IVF is never entirely private. In vitro fertilization requires a constant public performance, whether its aim is to protect one's privacy or to achieve the reverse—to make a clear show of willingness to undergo anything in pursuit of a child of one's own, the eventual fulfillment of a childless marriage, the provision of much-wanted grandchildren for relatives, a greater sense of belonging to friendship networks, or simply devotion to a partner or spouse. Sociologically known as "face work," this performative dimension of IVF is increasingly visible as one of its most substantial components, and constitutes an important part of its public face as well in the now-common representations of it in popular media.

These themes are clearly brought out in Charis Thompson's insightful study of reproductive technologies published in 2005, a quarter of a century after the first feminist analyses of new reproductive technologies began to be published. Highly attentive to the question of identity formation in the context of IVF, and closely following Judith Butler's (1990) account of gender identity as a performance, Thompson notes how much of her fieldwork and interview data from IVF confirms a pattern of exaggerated gender and kinship roles stereotypically emulating those of "the ideal nuclear family" (2005: 141). This is hardly surprising, she suggests, given that one of the main ways IVF has been normalized is through its naturalization, thus challenging the "monstrous" stigma once more firmly attached to this form of building a family by "domesticating" ARTS. "A significant way to normalize the newness of the techniques [of ART] and the kinship relations and social interactions they represent is to naturalize them as much as possible. . . . Naturalization normalizes and domesticates procedures making them seem like appropriate ways of building a family rather than monstrous innovations" (141). Both male and female gender identities, Thompson argues, become "fundamental principle[s] of categorization" in the context of IVF treatment because these threatened identities are precisely what need to be reinforced in the face of infertility or unwanted childlessness, while also being the core categories around and through which treatment is organized. "Gender, both biologically and socially understood and enacted, is a fundamental principle of categorization in ARTS. Furthermore, the deficit and stigma of infertility are often experienced substantially as gender deficits and gender stigma" (119).

What is also noticeable about the temporal sequence Thompson describes, whereby exaggerated familial and gender-based stereotypes are enacted during the process of IVF, is the sense of a compensatory substitution provided by IVF itself—not only in terms of what the procedure might eventually provide, in the form of viable offspring, but through the gender-appropriate enactment of each individual stage of the IVF procedure in pursuit of such an outcome. After all, IVF is designed to precisely replicate each of the steps in the journey to parenthood, by restaging them as an extracorporeal simulacrum of the real thing IVF is imitating.[6] As Thompson observed in her fieldwork, the effort to perform gender and kinship identities more strongly as part of the pursuit of successful IVF thus constitutes part of the labor and effort involved in following this arduous quest—which is aimed potentially at having a baby, but in the meantime is also about producing appropriately gendered parenting behavior along the way. Indeed, this behavior is deliberately exaggerated in an effort to help the process to work. Tellingly, Thompson uses the adjective "hyperconventional" to describe the gender roles she observed for both women and men during her fieldwork in IVF clinics—a process for which she also uses the military analogy of "retrenchment." "As I explored gender in infertility clinics, I found that supposedly natural gender dimorphism is often invoked most strongly at those times when the natural is unstable or poorly integrated into patients' lives. Patients and practitioners retrench into hyperconventional understandings of some of these sorting binaries to stabilise and domesticate others and remove stigma" (2005: 142).

It is hardly surprising that couples seeking IVF treatment either consciously or unconsciously produce "highly scripted roles and stereotypes" of kinship, family, and gender identities in the carefully monitored, arduously clinical, and heteronormative context of IVF, where patients are highly conscious of their dependence on the medical staff assisting them in their pursuit of an elusive goal.[7] Indeed, argues Thompson, these "parodic performances of hypergender-appropriate behaviour are also sometimes used to script and navigate treatment itself" (2005: 119). At the very least, "patients going through treatment need to pass, socially and biologically, as the gender to which they have already been assigned" thus offsetting "the possibility of failure to perform hegemonic gender by those who precisely in this site must *try harder than ever* to perform and norm gender" (118, emphasis added).[8] Thompson further describes these efforts to mobilize identity technologies as if to instrumentalize, or produce, the biological process they seek to achieve, as means of domesticating the unruly and unfamiliar process they are involved in. Here too we see the direct parallel discussed in chapter 5 of inhabiting identity categories and navigating the technology of IVF.

Strathern's point that in lieu of a naturalized biological conformity to conventional expectations it is the yearning for these conventions that is naturalized instead becomes more pointed in this context. For it is not only the yearning for conformity with the demands of peer pressure, or the expectations of in-laws, that is at stake. There is also a yearning for gender conformity, and for alignment with the institutional norms of both heterosexuality and marriage. In fact, so much yearning is occurring in the context of IVF that we might rephrase Gayle Rubin's question to ask, what are the exact mechanisms by which the yearning for particular conventions of sexuality is produced and maintained? Part of the recursive answer to this question is that the widespread availability of IVF is now contributing to the reproduction, and indeed intensification, of the very desires it is intended to satisfy, thus reinforcing a paradoxical pattern that is by no means limited to this particular technology. The fact that IVF is more likely than not to fail in its primary function of making babies is part of what renders it particularly complicated, but hardly unique.

Significantly, however, and undoubtedly adding to the staggering amount of work involved in trying to make IVF work, is the fact that in addition to being the site of an understandable effort to naturalize and normalize infertility treatment, and to use it as a context for the production of conventional parenthood identities (with or without babies), the ART clinic is also home to many new and very unconventional versions of the biological facts understood to be grounding these same gender and kinship roles in nature. Women undergoing IVF, for example, need to be treated in such a manner that their hormonal systems are aligned with an egg maturation protocol that will maximize their chances of conceiving by overproducing ova. Somewhat paradoxically, this requires the induction of artificial menopause by downregulating a woman's normal cycle of menstruation (in effect, it is switched off). As one U.K. clinic explains this procedure in their online introduction to IVF:

Your pituitary gland needs to be "switched off" before you can receive drugs to stimulate egg production. These drugs stimulate the production of a "follicle." A follicle is an immature egg, surrounded by a bubble of fluid, in the ovary. These immature eggs need to grow and develop inside their bubbles of fluid before they can be collected.

If the pituitary gland is not "switched off" it may release a hormone that causes the bubbles (follicles) to burst (doctors call this "spontaneous ovulation"). . . . Turning off your reproductive hormone cycle in this way allows the doctors to have better control over the actions of your ovaries. . . .

Having your reproductive cycle turned off tricks your body into thinking it is going through the menopause. Because of this, you may experience symptoms similar to those of the menopause, such as hot flushes, headaches, mood swings, dizziness, lack of concentration, dry mouth and vaginal soreness. Don't worry—this artificial menopause is only temporary and will stop once you stop taking the drugs. (Hull Fertility Services, http://www.hullivf.org.uk/treatment/ivf/step1.html, accessed April 11, 2013)

After the old cycle is switched off, a new cycle—one that allows more biological control to maximize both the number of eggs that are surgically removed and their quality—is then induced, again using a bespoke pharmaceutical protocol to imitate a natural cycle, albeit not the patient's *own* natural cycle, but a standardized one:

You will receive drugs to encourage follicle production after your own reproductive hormone cycle has been switched off (or "downregulated"). You will need to carry on taking your downregulation drugs at the same time as you take your follicle stimulating drugs. . . .

Remember, your drug regime will be PERSONALISED TO YOU. It is vitally important that you take these drugs correctly every day, so please, please, ask if there is anything that you are not sure about. (Hull Fertility Services http://www.hullivf.org.uk/treatment/ivf/step1.html, accessed April 11, 2013)

The challenges of performing hyperfemininity while undergoing artificial menopause notwithstanding, these treatment protocols indicate the extent to which normal understandings of female biology are reconfigured in the context of IVF—so that, for example, menopause becomes a route to fertility, and thus an enabling not an opposing phenomenon in the pursuit of a successful pregnancy.[9] Thus, however personalized it may be, and however normalized it may have become, it is simultaneously the case that IVF significantly disrupts conventional understandings of biology, thus departing from a patient's prior experience of her own normal biological physicality, or natural cycles, by introducing a whole new fertility ontology to be choreographed. The double-identity demands of IVF can thus be described as exaggerating a conventional gender identity while inhabiting an unconventional biology. Importantly, this effort is accompanied (and explained) by the new reproductive model provided by ART, in which conception is highly technologically mediated, so that some of the key biological facts are no longer understood or narrated in terms of imitating natural biology at all, but in terms of its opposite — artificial biology, a kind of parallel fertility universe. This new biology — the supplementary, additional, additive biology of standardized biological control — is what must be renaturalized by women IVF patients (i.e., made to be as similar to "the real thing" as possible so IVF will work) through gender norms at the very same time it denaturalizes their own reproductive biology as they have normally experienced it in the past.[10] Here, again, the denaturalizing effects of technology replacing biology, or taking it in hand, can be met with a reverse, compensatory naturalization of reproductive desire and hope. No wonder gender norms are strengthened in the face of this confusing experience, since they are one of the only variables that remain somewhat within patients' own control.

Precisely, then, because IVF both is and is not just like what it is imitating, it requires both a normalized and naturalized compliance with conventional gender roles, and an adaptation to unconventional biology in order to achieve this end. For both women and men on IVF programs, such an ambivalent situation thus requires the kind of "double consciousness" described by feminist phenomenologists Sandra Bartky (1993) and Iris Marion Young (1990), or by Emily Martin (1987) in her account of the medicalization of the reproductive body.[11] To the extent, then, that IVF is, in Annemarie Mol's (2002) terms, a "multiple" that is reproducing more than babies, this mode of inhabiting a technological imitation of life is one of the technologies of self it also generates. It is the complex ways in which these new tactical subjectivities are embedded, or grounded, in what are often highly naturalized versions of social convention (e.g., gender) that also perform an instructive imitation — by recapitulating the reproductive model they have displaced, namely the social construction of natural facts. Here, however, and at the same time, the condition of being biologically relative is also manifest as the natural construction of social facts: social convention is naturalized as the before, to which the biological functions IVF performs come after. These, then, are the (somewhat confusing) exact mechanisms of how technologies of gender and sex are interwoven with reproductive substance in the quest to make babies. No wonder it is tiring.

Identity is not the only personal attribute to become the subject of increased tactical and adaptive labor in the context of IVF and achieved reproduction. The artificial metabolism this procedure requires is often described by women undergoing IVF as a time of suspension of their normal physicality, punctuated by unfamiliar emotional, psychological, and emotional sensations and an altered sense of self, or personality. Similar disjunctures between competing versions of the same physical events are particularly well illustrated by the way experiences of the moment of conception can be transformed by IVF, as well as the new possibility IVF introduces of becoming "a little bit pregnant." Margarete Sandelowski was the first of many commentators on IVF to notice and record the significance of what she calls "ambiguous conception" in accounts of the new biological facts introduced by IVF. Whereas, she explains, under normal (unassisted) circumstances naturally fertile couples do not experience conception as a discrete event, or moment, in the process of producing a pregnancy, the IVF process breaks conception down into distinct stages that are each part of a carefully managed, highly monitored, and thus largely observable sequence. This also means that patients are very conscious of which stage they are in, and precisely which step of each stage they have reached, the vacillating temporality of which (fast then slow then interminable, only to speed up again and slow down at the very end) is in part what gives IVF such a quest-like character for those undergoing it. This unfamiliar temporal sequence is also what allows for the novel sensation of being nearly, or partially, pregnant. As Sandelowski explains, "Infertile couples were more likely to think of themselves as in one or another phase of getting pregnant. They were, therefore, in a position to challenge the adequacy of a commonly accepted biocultural dichotomy—the either-or-ness of pregnancy—according to which a woman could either be pregnant or not pregnant, but could not be a little bit pregnant" (1993: 122).

As Sandelowski notes, the experience of conception as a lengthy, drawn-out process of stages enables a range of different definitions of pregnancy to be, in effect, individually adjusted, or personalized, by women undergoing this procedure—some of whom may experience themselves as being impregnated through the process of embryo transfer, but others of whom may (in a manner akin to the tentative pregnancies identified by Rothman [1986]) more cautiously define the start of their pregnancies in terms of successful implantation. A feature, then, of the biotechnical model of reproduction offered by IVF is that it can be described as both debiologizing and rebiologizing, offering a version of biology that is bespoke, artificial, controllable, personalized, and redesignable, while also providing essentially the "same" route to conception, pregnancy, and parenthood as that naturally experienced by fertile couples.[12] This is also why, although it is conventionally defined as an imitation of existing biological processes, IVF allows for these same physiological events to be experienced in ways that enable new biological facts to be born—such as the condition of being partially pregnant.[13]

As noted earlier, these and many similar observations throughout the feminist and social scientific literature on IVF since the mid-1980s have confirmed the extent to which IVF has become a fluid technological way of life that is at once highly strategic and completely out of control. In vitro fertilization is now a curiously familiar procedure through which a highly visible and explicit process of reshuffling the facts of life is assisted by a strategic parallel organization of natural and artificial biologies. Part of the labor involved in IVF is the dual requirement to work within both naturalized and artificial, normal and abnormal, and familiar and novel biologies simultaneously: compliance with IVF requires constant adjustment to its norms, and thus IVF itself operates as a powerful norming technology. Yet, however practiced the modern IVF consumer might be in this topsy-turvy world of artificial biology, it is hard work to make sense of its workings.

These observations in turn lead us back to the questions with which this chapter started—What is IVF reproducing? What kind of technology is it? What do people want from it? What does living IVF reveal about other technologically inflected identities—or indeed the analysis of identity as a technology? On the basis of the above discussion it appears that one of the reasons IVF becomes curiouser and curiouser, especially to those who inhabit this technology as a way of life most intensively, is because it both conventionalizes an unconventional biology and because it norms a familiar technological ambivalence. Inhabiting this world seems to require a constant workload of innovation, adaptation, and adjustment in order to reestablish conventional norms in what are often odd or strange circumstances (e.g., becoming menopausal to become fertile or becoming partially pregnant). An overriding norm for this context is thus simply labor itself—laboring through IVF to do one's best to make it work. Yet it is clearly a labor-intensive context in which much more than babies are being made. The quasi-mythic connotations of the quest for IVF, so ubiquitously commented upon in the literature, while no doubt an accurate and important dimension of the IVF experience, also point

toward some of the functions IVF fulfills as a heroic task—namely to perform that familiar oxymoron of ordinary heroism.[14] As on a frontier, it is the
overcoming of substantial obstacles that is at stake in this process of domesticating unfamiliar territory. These paradoxical, counterintuitive dimensions
of IVF have been noted by many observers, beginning with Sandelowski's account twenty years ago (in which she also tellingly describes how difficult it
may be for some couples to eventually "make the conversion" to pregnancy—
i.e., to finish their quest [1993: 91–120]) and greatly furthered by Thompson
([2005] who, as her title suggests, describes how IVF makes parents as well
as children). Similarly, Judith Lorber (1989) describes IVF as a conjugal adjustment technology that enables women to acquire more control and resources in marriage (a process she calls "patriarchal bargaining"), while Gay
Becker (2000) has documented the embeddedness of the quest for IVF in the
consumer world of the late twentieth-century ethos of the American Dream
(much as I also showed the case for consuming IVF in the "enterprise culture"
of Thatcherism in the U.K. during the 1980s [Franklin 1997]).[15]

A number of more recent studies have also shown why IVF is not so paradoxical from the point of view of gender as a technology. In her highly per-
ceptive study of "making modern mothers" in urban Greece, for example,
anthropologist Heather Paxson explains how IVF norms gender expectations
in much the same way gender conventions norm IVF. As she notes, "When
gender is a matter of personal responsibility, when mothering 'completes' a
woman's nature . . . women have a moral obligation to aspire to motherhood.
In this way women are shown to be good at being women, and good Greek citizens" (2004: 211). In Paxson's account, this work of being good at gender and
complete as a person is explicitly theorized as technological: she describes
urban Greek motherhood as a *techni*, from the Greek word *technologhia*, signifying the arts, mastery of technique, and craft. As Paxson emphasizes, *techni*
is not imagined as separate from nature, or *fisi*, as in the Anglophone tradition. Rather, claims Paxson, "Athenian women today approach motherhood
as something to be worked at, achieved, and continuously demonstrated"
(214).[16] She argues that in Greece, naturalizing is not the opposite of socializing but rather its synonym in the sense of crafting—"when customary behavior is naturalized in Greece, there is always room for strategic maneuver-
ing. . . . Naturalization in Greece does something other than suggest fixity,
inevitability, or a sense that there is nothing humans can do about the matter" (214).

Consequently, IVF is imagined as the fulfillment of a social duty to make
nature that, in the Greek context, adds heroism because, as one of Paxson's

informants describes it, "there's some procedure" (2004: 223), meaning work to be done. "They think I'm a heroine," this informant continues. "You have to want it a lot . . . to enter into a procedure and have a baby like that" (223). In the same way that IVF reveals an added dimension to maternity—maternity by special service, we might call it—Paxson argues it similarly adds to the pressure to become maternal. "The introduction of IVF," she claims,

> Helps constitute a parallel shift in how women's proper relationship to *teknopiia* [the art of maternity] is assessed: the having of children is no longer a taken-for-granted aspect of marriage that "just happens," but has become an achievement based on techniques of motherhood that are both newly proliferating and increasingly scrutinized. A notion of achieved motherhood is further constituted by a capitalist market economy (of which medical technology is a part) and the increasingly diversified participation of women in this economy as workers and consumers. . . . The substance of the nature that women must control in order to demonstrate gender proficiency is also transforming: women's need to control their sexuality is giving way to a need to control, even rationalize, a biological capacity to bring forth babies. (2004: 240)

As Paxson observes, the extension of the maternal arts to include IVF also changes the terms of gender proficiency. There is now not only more women can do to become gender proficient; there is an added level of service that can make maternity even more of an achievement than it was previously. Under such conditions, to say no to IVF is not only to decline the opportunity to become gender compliant but the opportunity to become gender heroic.

To the extent that IVF is not only a reproductive technology in the sense of producing offspring, but in the sense of being a technology of gender, or a maternal art, we can better understand its corresponding aspirational ideals and imaginaries. These may in part account for the appeal of what this technology reproduces somewhat independently not only of its actual outcome, but even of its stated or intended outcome. Were we to understand the difficulty of IVF to constitute part of its appeal, the question of what it is all about becomes one that is better understood through the lens of multiple, adjustable rationalities—which is, in fact, exactly what IVF has been documented to require of its users, consumers, and clients in the numerous accounts now available of how this technology is lived. While not in any way wanting to suggest that large numbers of people who undergo IVF do not really want children, or that it functions as much as a substitute for parenthood as a potential route to it, that it is a strategic alibi for women who do not actually want to become mothers, or that it is attractive because of its alluring mythic connotations—or even simply because it is there—I suggest that one way to read the considerable body of empirical evidence documenting the experience of undergoing IVF and ARTS is simply that their appeal is more complex and paradoxical than it might at first appear.

Drawing on the various threads woven together so far, I want to consider further the shift IVF makes most vividly explicit, which I suggest is the coupling not of egg and sperm, but of biology and artifice in the service of a new kinship norm. This new norm, as we have seen, affirms a code for conduct that is no longer naturally based on shared reproductive substance, but instead on new formations of technological agency that are before as well as after nature. An important point here is that it is within this formulation that the operation of kinship as a technology is again made doubly explicit. In vitro fertilization is at once a technology reproducing social forms and norms, and a scientific technique that replicates the imagined origin of these forms and norms, but which also re-creates this original template through the direct manipulation, or crafting, of shared reproductive substance. One of the most important points noted about this duplicity of IVF as a technology is its many similarities to technologies of gender, which share this same duplicitous pattern. Indeed, as we can see also from Thompson's (2005) work, IVF is literally a kind of procreative drag in its quasi-parodic in vitro imitation of "the facts of life." As noted in chapter 5, Judith Butler was among the first to ask of sex whether it is "as culturally constructed as gender" or indeed whether it is, in this sense, just like gender in that sex too is "tenuously constituted in time . . . through a stylized repetition of acts" that can only be interpreted through the lens of the very gender differences that the biological sexes are imagined to "ground" in natural fact (1990: 179). In this chapter so far, we have looked at how IVF establishes a code for conduct that is modeled on a technological protocol that is itself modeled on a naturalized expectation for biological reproduction, that in turn imitates the facts of life as they are imagined to exist naturally as a sui generis biological base.[17] We have also examined how the empirical analysis of IVF as a lived technology of life can be used to reveal the labor involved in the complex ontological choreography this technique requires. In this way, IVF has been used as a lens to investigate the patterns involved in living a biological life that is remade by technique—a complex pattern of subjectification that is arguably indigenous to IVF as a way of life but by no means necessarily limited to this specific technique. I turn now to the related question of how this process has been not only lived but witnessed as a live spectacle on-screen.

IVF Live

This section, which could also be titled "Virtual IVF," offers another close reading of IVF as a model of a model of a model to examine a different form of its serial recursivity—from technics into technics, culture into culture, and ART into art. As it happens, we can do this instructively and quite literally using the widely circulated imagery of the manipulation of human reproductive cells provided by IVF, in the appropriately doubled form of digital mirroring. Here we return to the question of the hand and tool raised earlier, but also to the role of another form of culture media, namely the circulation of IVF imagery in popular culture through which this technique becomes increasingly legible as itself a convention, or even genre, of remaking life. Thus, IVF reveals its made-not-born pedigree as ontological choreography through a series of now-familiar media images that provide access to the scene of being before nature—in the sense of facing it, or of being on a frontier, dedicated to assisting the flow of life through new forms of technological husbandry. In addition to being a technology of living substance and a way of life, IVF has been implanted into popular consciousness over the past three decades as a set of images and narratives depicting live embryological procedures such as fertilization, microinjection, and nuclear transfer. Part of the way IVF has become more comfortable and familiar is through a kind of mass public education in reproductive biology so that the human gamete in a petri dish now recognizably codes for a celebrated arena of technological innovation and capacity. Indeed, these increasingly familiar visual images have arguably become the dominant visual signifier of the expansion of the IVF platform over the past half century, if not for the age of biology in general. Like ultrasound imagery, with its ability to convey the live action of pregnancy as a screen image, IVF offers privileged visual access to the previously unseen events of early human life—and indeed is popularly associated with precisely this capacity. Thus, the following section turns to a different perspective on what IVF is all about in relation to its staging and performance of a new reproductive model by exploring, in visual terms, its circulation as a highly public spectacle of the remaking of sex. In order to be taken in hand, the IVF embryo, as we saw in chapter 3, must first be made available to the eye, and this process means it can be reproduced as imagery, broadcast, or downloaded from the Internet at will. Unlike in the nineteenth or early twentieth centuries, the technological means of broadcasting such images enables them to proliferate within the media-saturated technological culture of the twenty-first century. In this section, then, I revisit the question of the labor involved in IVF from a position more akin to that of Marx and Engels, as they observed, often in minute detail, the evolution of machines in front of them, and in particular the interposition of tool and hand that so distinctly marked the onset of the Industrial Revolution. However, I also turn to the interface between IVF technology and its worldwide audience, who are increasingly literate in its language of visual form, to explore how live IVF circulates as a different kind of shared technological substance, and virtual life, as an iconic spectacle of making sex.

In vitro fertilization is, of course (and among other things), a very famous technology—perhaps even a technology that to a certain extent epitomizes what a technology is imagined to be and to do, and thus also a sign of the technological (especially where it meets the biological). The difference between conception via IVF and unassisted, natural, or spontaneous conception is precisely what is celebrated by the adjectives "precious" or "miracle" commonly used to mark IVF babies as special. As Stewart Brand observes, what is also iconic about IVF babies is that despite their artificial or test-tube origins, the viable offspring of IVF are indistinguishable from regular children. This is another of the unifications IVF can be seen to perform, by linking the normal and the technological biologically. In the remainder of this chapter, I turn to the public face of IVF as a set of visual images to explore the question of how IVF has itself become conventional—a new norm of making sex that is based on a new set of exact mechanisms. The turn here, to IVF as a technology of representation, adds another crucial layer to the question of what it is doing and why people seek it out. We turn, in other words, to the way in which IVF can be interpreted as a technology of refiguration as well as reproduction through its interface with the mainstream media.

THE BABY IN THE BOTTLE

As Susan Squier (1994) points out in her analysis of the twentieth-century history of the image of the baby in the bottle, IVF technology has a powerful visual and literary genealogy that can be read, among other things, as a series of reflections on the reproductive politics of gender and sex filtered through the lens of artificial conception. Looking back to the nineteenth century, Squier points, for example, to feminist readings of Mary Shelley's *Franken-stein* and her critique of "the new male birth of fraternal contractual democracy" with its "male monopoly on political creation" as well as her "powerful critique of the newly revised institution of mothering." Together these themes have been argued to converge in Shelley's creation of "a nightmare image of scientific procreation that anticipates IVF" (Squier 1994: 14). In the early twentieth century, she argues, these themes continued to proliferate in a host of tales, fables, novels, and children's stories featuring technologies of embryology and reproduction, and the moral, scientific, and political questions they raised. From Charles Kingsley Amis's *The Water Babies* to Julian Huxley's "Tissue Culture Kings," J. D. S. Haldane's essay "Daedalus, or Science and the Future," the prolific writings of his sister Naomi Mitchison, and their close friends and colleagues the Huxleys, Vera Brittain, J. D. Bernal, and H. G. Wells, in whose writings the figures of ectogenesis, cloning, and artificial reproduction conspicuously serve as the lens through which definitions of the future, and future technologies, are both imaged and imagined. As Squier notes, these stories produced by a highly scientifically literate group of friends and kin (many of whom were closely biologically related as well as related through the study of biology) typically wove together elements from the history of embryology with science fiction, even sometimes very accurately predicting the future, as in Haldane's account of the young Cambridge undergraduate who successfully developed IVF (1924). As Squier notes, "Haldane's story of the development of *in vitro* gestation parallels the actual story of the development of *in vitro* fertilization, as told in Dr Robert Edwards's autobiographical account. Both narratives move from successful animal embryology to advances in human embryology" (1994: 71). And yet, as she points out, Haldane's story—first delivered as a lecture in Cambridge to the Heretics Society—is also couched in the language of myth, narrating the victory of Daedalus over Prometheus as confirmation that biology has become the "pivotal" science for the twentieth century (72). Thus, "Daedalus looks cheerfully ahead to a future in which the invention of ectogenesis enables the control of human reproduction, the improvement of the human species, and finally the emancipation of mankind" (73).

In the same way that Squier argues the complex interwoven plots of Haldane's vision of ectogenesis united British biofuturists, humanists, and socialists with their detractors throughout the 1920s and 1930s in a debate over reproductive technology, so too can this period be understood in Foucauldian terms as an extension of the "entry of the phenomena peculiar to the life of the human species into the order of knowledge and power [and] the sphere of political techniques" (Foucault 1990: 141–142). Except that, to be precise, it is not merely sex, or even sexuality, in these debates that serves as the "pivot of the two axes along which developed the entire political technology of life" (145), as Foucault suggests, but a more literal technologization of reproduction in the form of taking it in hand. It is artificial reproduction and ectogenesis that are pivotal in this debate about the future of the human—just as they have continued to be since.

Squier's account can help us to move more explicitly into the realm of IVF as a contemporary, twenty-first-century representational field, or what I describe as the visual logic of IVF, and in particular its role as a source of symbolic imagery coupling biology and artifice. What is notable in Squier's account is the sheer amount of imaginative reconstruction of sex, gender, kinship, and reproduction that was occurring through the lens of the baby in the bottle in this period, but also how much these debates explicitly addressed what were later described as the technologies of sex, gender, and kinship described by theorists such as Foucault, de Lauretis, Haraway, Strathern, and Butler. The conventions of sexual difference, sexual reproduction, and sexual identity, as well as sex roles and sexual practices, were all being debated during this period through the defamiliarizing lens of experimental embryology and its unusual tool kit. New possibilities of regeneration as well as recombination, in the form of chimeras, hybrids, and mosaics, as well as cloning, transhumanism, and ectogenesis, were in free play amid the questioning of traditional gender and kinship (and economic) orders in the mid-twentieth century. As in the context of IVF, cloning, and transgenesis today, these technologies are imagined at once as repair mechanisms, or enhancement devices, and as radical rewrites of the biological rule book—transgressive by their very nature, and thus both paralleling and enabling the social transformations to which they are linked. As Squier herself suggests, the history of the baby in the bottle supplies a prehistory for IVF in which this technique plays a far more radical role than its use as a "renormalizing" technology in the present might suggest. However, as she also points out, this history further suggests that a technological imitation, substitute, or even aid is by its very nature a supplement, a prosthetic, and thus a superordinating logic that, as Derrida famously claims, is never neutral.

SCREENING IVF

As argued in chapter 3, it is crucial to the history of IVF that it provided a technological platform through which reproductive substance could be both seen and handled. It is equally crucial for IVF as a representational technology that it has, in this sense, a natural visual interface with the mainstream media—among other things, it is a screen-based technology. As we have seen with the dramatic success of the iPhone, the introduction of the handheld screen was in itself an iconic moment for the history of human technologies, enhancing the hand-tool relation by intensifying its depth as well as scale. In vitro fertilization too is a powerful handheld screen window onto early life that achieves a similar, if less portable, marriage between visualization and manipulation—

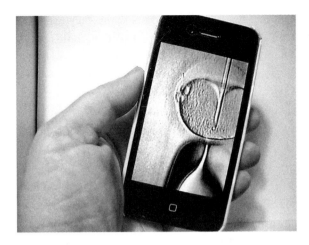

FIGURE 6.1. In vitro fertilization offers a screen window onto handheld life that is, in the age of the Internet, virtually downloadable, contributing to the mass circulation of IVF imagery, or what we might refer to as iVF. Photo by the author.

and one that is greatly amplified by the capacities of micromanipulation harnessed to digital reproduction (figure 6.1).

Crucial to the visual logic of IVF on-screen is the fact that what we are looking at when we observe a fertilized egg, or embryo, in a petri dish—or the manipulation of an egg or embryo in one of these handy chambers—is no ordinary sight. For many people, scientists, clinicians, and patients alike, witnessing a live human embryo is special. Images of early human life—be they of gametes, embryos, or fetuses—are distinctively mediagenic in that they merge highly specialized scientific imaging apparatus with intimate human biological substance. Crucially, what is also witnessed in such a spectacle is the fact that this substance, such as a fertilized egg, has been rendered newly manipulable, or ready to be, as Landecker (2007) puts it, "taken in hand." This makes of such images an especially suggestive primal scene of the new reproductive mechanics brought about by assisted conception, and it is not surprising much has been written about embryos as visual objects (Franklin 1999). As many artists as well as news editors and lobbyists have recognized, contemporary embryological imagery is a potent contact zone uniting scientific research, high-tech laboratory apparatus, biological substance, and powerful visualizing techniques with the promissory future of the age of biology. These images at once sign the beginnings of human life, to suggest both common human origins and shared human futures, while also depicting a shared technological, and uniquely human, technological legacy through the very fact of their existence in vitro (thus a second sign of beingness as human technological agency). The images thus themselves model a fusion of accumulated scientific knowledge, human reproductive substance, and technological artifice, multiply overdetermining the viewer position of witnessing ourselves, our technology, our future, and our obligations to one another. In this sense, and as the artist Suzanne Anker has poignantly suggested, the in vitro lens is also a mirror (Anker and Franklin 2010).

Importantly, and unlike other reproductive screening technologies, such as ultrasound, IVF imagery involves a form of witnessing that requires a viewer position that is after the fact of direct manipulation of what is shown. In the very fact of these images' existence is the structuring presence of the technologies that make them possible, the hands that hold these tools, the screens that display these scenes, and the logics that make such interventions both possible and desirable. The sense of being hands-on is irrevocably part of what these images display from a spectator position that reproduces the point of view of the manipulator. Thus the viewer who participates in witnessing these scenes is visually implicated in the substantive and conceptual connections they establish.[18] Hence, in addition to the practical or scientific questions posed by these primal scenes (how does life begin, what are its mechanisms, how do they work), and their special content (early human life, shared origins, potential offspring, cures for disease, etc.), there is an inevitable form of complicity in what Evelyn Keller (1996a) describes as "the biological gaze," because the very ability to witness these objects references a past intervention that has allowed us in as viewers, looking, as we inevitably must, through the keyhole science has provided for us to observe a formerly hidden domain. It is impossible, in other words, to view an image of an in vitro embryo without inhabiting the position of its handler.

The popular version of the reproductive gaze inaugurated by the fetal photography of Lennart Nilsson in the 1960s, and now manifest as the contemporary imagery of IVF, stem cells, and cloning, is derivative of IVF's history as a research tool, both in its logic and in its logistics. The taking in hand of reproductive substance made possible by and for the technologization of sex is now both familiar and quotidian in the form of still photography or clinical apparatus such as the ultrasound monitor, and also publicly broadcast live images, such as those often shown depicting micromanipulation techniques. The now increasingly common flat-screen image of micromanipulation that punctuates news items on cloning, for example, routinely displays a cell secured in place by a holding pipette on one side being penetrated by a microinjection needle, a biopsy pipette, or some other microtool on the other. This image has consequently become a powerful visual shorthand for the union of technology and biology in the name of remaking life. This familiar screen scene typically appears as a horizon, the pipette-cell-pipette fusion bisecting the

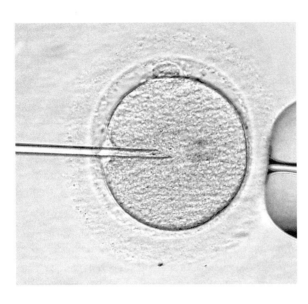

FIGURE 6.2. The ICSI procedure is now commonly viewed in many media, including Hollywood cinema, television news programs, and scientific documentaries, as a live-action sequence that explicitly displays the taking of life in hand. Reproduced courtesy of the Guy's stem cell team.

frame in an assemblage that now codes for biotechnological investigation writ large. It is this explicit image of cellular manipulation, greatly enlarged and often shown in live motion, that has inaugurated the mass witnessing of new flows of reproductive and genetic substance in a spectacle of reengineering at the ground zero of built biology. Already iconic, micromanipulation imagery is used in advertising, in corporate logos, and on fashionable club wear and CD covers, as well as being featured on the evening news, in mainstream films, and in documentary accounts of new reproductive technologies such as cloning (figure 6.2).

The image of micromanipulation shares a visual kinship with earlier iconic images uniting the logics of life and technology with the question of human obligations to the future, most notably the much-celebrated late twentieth-century images of the fetus and the blue planet (Franklin et al. 2000). Like the fetus and the blue planet images, the cell at the center of the micromanipulation image glows with a radiant light—often blue or amber—combining the ethereal beauty of life itself with the power of the bioscientific gaze. Unlike such earlier images, however, the distinctly planetary cell becomes a window onto the ability to reengineer biological interiority. With its faintly visible cumulus, or corona, the cell appears to emit vitality, or energy, as a kind of bioluminescence, but it is not floating in space. The cell is at once bounded and permeable, captive and already joined with the tools that hold it in place. Translucent, it is also somewhat opaque, with an obscure and grainy interior, lacking depth of field while at the same time the tools convey a sense of reach beyond the visible frame, or edge, of the image. Structuring the image is the shallow plane of focus, which, like the holding pipette, positions the cell securely in a flat visual field. Like a living petri dish, the micromanipulation setup handily presents a visually engaging biopic of tools that are the source of new life and poised to grasp, probe, and penetrate the cell's interior. In particular, the image of microinjection, in which a needle is shown penetrating an egg cell, recapitulates the familiar moment of conception, restaging the conventional denouement of the sexual union of egg and sperm, and thus life's beginnings (Martin 1991). Instead of the agency of fertilization being carried by the substance itself, however, micromanipulation images depict the helping hands of science as the active agents, which assume the activity formerly understood to be merely biological, self-acting, or naturally automatic. Here, then, are the new mechanics of making sex — replacing and extending biological action in the form of handheld tools.

In contrast to the still portraits of the fetus or the blue planet, the scene of microinjection is cinematic, and the movement of the micromanipulation tools is the main story these images convey and emphasize.[19] Notably, these are more evidently working screen scenes than the earlier images of inner and outer space, often linked in newsreel footage with accompanying shots of white-coated scientists at work in their labs.[20] The cell in these images is tightly coupled to its tools, engaged in a process of itself being retooled, whereby its internal mechanics will be recomposed, reprogrammed, and remade. This is the bespoke wet life of the biotechnology lab in the making — no longer the pristine, untouched, natural life of the planet or the fetus, part of whose grandeur lay in the autonomy of their inherent and ultimately mysterious life-giving properties, which exceed and predate even our most powerful means of technological creation.

The new animated digital embryological imagery also differs from earlier photographic reproductive portraiture in not being self-contained: this imagery does not remain within the frame. Whereas Nilsson's fetal portraits remain within the margins of the photograph, as set pieces that speak for themselves partly through the independence of the fetal body, the scene of micromanipulation always extends off-screen, breaking through the frame of the image along the trajectory of the handles of the microtools. These tools, and the camera, thus become the connecting substances linking the cell to the larger apparatus of the micromanipulation station and the guiding hands and eyes of its live operator. The manipulation tools are scaled precisely to cellular dimensions to create a workable fit between the microscopic object and the prosthetic hands of the operator who will delicately reconstruct it, and so they are also magnified, creating the shallow depth of field, the flat light, the blurred background, and the slow, jerky, groping movements depicted in the now-familiar genre of animated films that unite two lives through tools. These effects of scale, dimension, perspective, framing, and context reproduce the scientific gaze, its instruments, and its object—as well as its labor—exactly.

The biological relativity introduced through these images is particularly pronounced in the blurring of the tool and object they so vividly reveal. In the magnified image of micromanipulation, the aqueous environment of the cell is evident in the viscosity of its contents, and can be seen as well in the flows of substances within the hollow glass tools themselves. Like the cell, the instruments are transparent, enabling us to both see and see through this multi-layered scene of fertile coupling. In a kind of respiratory movement, the injection needle appears to inhale cellular contents for removal, and to exhale new material into the cell's interior. In this sense, micromanipulation imagery mechanically imitates a metabolic symbiosis of parts. And indeed this is precisely what is occurring. Micromanipulation takes place on cells that are typically submerged in clear sterile oil, using tiny glass tools as thin as strands of hair. The microtools are secured with small clamps that attach them to hydraulically driven joysticks that allow the manipulator to conduct various procedures, using touch as much as sight to guide his or her movements. The eyepieces are connected to a video lead that allows the manipulator to view the bed of the machine on a monitor, and to record, transmit, or display these processes on-screen. To view the contents of a cell takes a practiced eye, as there is little contrast, for example, between tiny semitransparent organelles, such as the multiple pronuclei, and the rest of the cell contents, consisting largely of cytoplasm (Franklin 2003b). It is for this reason that a color filter is often used, to aid the manipulator in identifying the various parts of the cell by increasing resolution or contrast.

For both clinical and scientific procedures, there are five basic microtools that are used exclusively for manipulating eggs, embryos, and sperm:

1 Holding pipette to fix and position the oocyte or embryo during
   a procedure
2 Microneedle to create an opening in the zona pellucida or
   shell of the egg
3 Blunt biopsy micropipette 15–16 μm in diameter for polar
   body removal
4 Blunt micropipette 25–30 μm in diameter for blastomere biopsy

5 Finely pulled micropipette of 7–8 μm inner diameter beveled to a thirty-degree angle with the tip pulled to form an intracytoplasmic sperm injection (ICSI) needle

As we have seen earlier in the clean room, additional varieties of micropipette for human embryonic cell line procedures are commonly forged by hand by softening a glass capillary tube over a burner and pulling it to form the desired width and tip. Mechanical pipette pullers can also be used, and commercially prepared micropipettes are increasingly available. Two additional instruments, a microforge and a beveler, are used to fashion specialized features of these glass tools. In addition to controlling for the diameter of the end of the micropipette, and sharpening, beveling, or flame polishing of the tip, microtools are bent to an angle commensurate with the bed of the micromanipulator, so that they can be positioned parallel with each other and with the machine. As well as precision and pre-preparation, sterility is essential to the success of micromanipulation techniques such as microinjection or embryo biopsy. For example, newly made tools may be exposed to ultraviolet radiation before use for up to twenty minutes to sterilize them, and cells are immersed in sterile equilibrated mineral oil during manipulation procedures to keep them clean. Purity has become more important to assisted conception technology as the effort to alleviate infertility has increasingly involved various kinds of genetic testing, screening, and diagnosis, and also, as we have seen, to the derivation of human embryonic stem cell (ESC) lines. The presence of male gametes adhering around the cumulus cells of the ova is potentially the cause of misdiagnosis when an embryo needs to be screened for molecular abnormalities, or contamination of a cell line.[21]

The most common micromanipulation procedure in the context of contemporary reproductive biomedicine is ICSI, now used both to enhance the purity of IVF embryos (by eliminating excess, potentially contaminating sperm) and to increase the fertilization rate of the limited egg supply by ensuring that the sperm penetrates the thick outer coat of the egg. Scenes of ICSI dominate the micromanipulation imagery made available to a wider audience, both because they are readily available, and perhaps because they replay the iconic moment of conception, involving penetration of the egg with the sperm-containing injection needle. This refiguration of the process of fertilization, however, is, like IVF in general, both like and unlike its unassisted counterpart. As the following technical instructions for ICSI emphasize, the roles of the egg and sperm are significantly altered in this version of the drama of life's beginnings:

Under control of the stereomicroscope the washed sperm are added to the drop containing 10% PVP [polyvinylpyrrolidone], to slow down sperm movement, facilitating selection of morphologically normal sperm for injection. This also minimizes sperm adherence to the glass surface once it is inside the micropipette. . . . A sperm is immobilised by gently rubbing its tail on the bottom of the dish and aspirated into the pipette, tail first. . . . Once the oocyte is brought into focus, the ICSI micropipette containing the immobilized sperm is lowered and brought into focus; once again, the fluid control and sperm movement within the pipette are assessed. Should the sperm become stuck in the pipette, it is expelled and another sperm is retrieved, or if necessary the microtool is changed.

The holding pipette is lowered and the oocyte is rotated so that a slit opening in the zona pellucida is at the 3 o'clock position. The outer edge of the oocyte is brought into focus and the sperm is brought to the tip of the micropipette. The micropipette is guided through the slit opening in the zona pellucida into the center of the oocyte, and a small amount of ooplasm is aspirated into the micropipette to ensure breakage of the membrane by slow turning of the micrometer of the microinjector. Once the membrane has been broken, the contents of the micropipette, i.e. ooplasm and the immobilised sperm, are expelled slowly into the oocyte and the micropipette is slowly withdrawn. Complete control over aspiration and expulsion are needed to diminish the amount of medium deposited along with the sperm. (Verlinsky et al. 2000: 22)

As is evident from this technical description of ICSI, fertilization in the context of assisted conception is not narrated as a journey, an adventure romance, or an epic quest, but as a difficult feat of manual control. Thus, although the image is legible as an analogy to normal fertilization, the procedure is clearly quite different in terms of both form and content. Indeed, other than the fact that a sperm ends up inside an egg, almost nothing about the means of achieving this legendary union is analogous to the conventional narrative of the exact mechanisms uniting egg and sperm. Indeed, as in the case of IVF, for which artificial menopause is a counterintuitive precursor, ICSI is in many respects the opposite of its unassisted corollary. Far from being an all but automatic natural process ensuring the flow of reproductive substance across the generations, these images depict a skilled manual feat of precision microengineering. Deliberately prevented from being either self-acting or automatic, the union of the gametes emerges instead from the delicate labor of manual assemblage. Formerly imagined as unstoppable, the sperm cell is firmly taken in hand by the micromanipulator: first it is immobilized, then immersed in ooplasm, and expelled into the egg—its tail having been cut off to make it more easily manageable and cleaner. No longer a heroic gamete-Olympian, the sperm must be brought under "complete control."

What is just like normal conception in the context of ICSI remains its purpose, namely the unification of egg and sperm—thus activating the process of fertilization leading to potential biological offspring. From the point of view of the continuity of biological relations between parents and offspring, the logic of ICSI is identical to that of unassisted conception. Consequently, according to the familiar kinship pattern of bilateral descent, through which the offspring inherits an equal amount of shared substance from both parents, ICSI is isomorphic with the standard model of unassisted conception. However, it is arguably a different union than that of egg and sperm which defines the visual and technical logics of these images, namely the merging or fusion of substance and tool, and tool and hand. The ICSI coupling, then, comprises several interrelated pairs: egg and sperm, camera and screen, tool and hand, viewer and manipulator, and substance and tool. The reproduction of this screen scene via the mainstream media adds yet another level to the logic of these images too, as it is the images themselves that now provide a shared cultural frame of reference for witnessing the remaking of sex—or even a shared culture medium for understanding them. This layering of techno-logics—whereby ICSI might be viewed on television, for example—in turn introduces a new convention of witnessing the exact mechanisms of reproduction live on-screen, so that one technology of reproduction (TV, iPhone, Internet, etc.) encompasses another (ICSI).

What is on display in such a spectacle is thus not only the logic of IVF, but the biological relativity implicit in making biological relatives. The relativity of the biological to the technical could hardly be made more explicitly visual than in the scene of microinjection, in which substance and tool engage in the complex intercourse of merging with a purpose. Beyond the frame, beyond the invisible hands, beyond the camera and its monitor, beyond the lab are all of the other surrounding elements of this composition through which it makes sense to even a casual viewer. But like IVF, the sense it makes may be superficially obvious in ways that obscure what is implicitly contradictory and even queer about such images. For in addition to everything legible and ordinary about their logics of biology, kinship, reproduction, technology, progress, and hope (among others) are the counterlogics such a scene has the potential to suggest or imply.

Conclusion

It is in the convergence between the prevailing logics and conventions of biological kinship and those introduced by new reproductive technologies that IVF, ICSI, and their ilk open up the space of biological relativity that remains to be charted as the age of biology unfolds. There is no reason not to assume that the remaking of nature as technique will remain largely compatible with the logics of unassisted nature, or natural procreation, or of the automatic flow of genealogy—nature has long been cultured, after all, and as we have seen even maternity is an art. Nature and biology are highly plastic categories, and kinship has long been the idiom to describe how they are worked, cultured up, and mediated. As we have also seen, the logic by which biological kinship is understood to create a natural tie, or a biological relation, is highly dependent on specific forms of labor, including the crafting of substantial connections. In Charis Thompson's term, natural facts are used strategically. Thus, we do not need to imagine that either the ambivalent aspects of living IVF or its paradoxical logics necessarily displace earlier models of biological reproduction or biological kinship. They are ambivalent precisely because they include these logics as well as others. However, we can observe all the same that the new context of biological relativity that is introduced by conception after IVF adds new dimensions to conventional understandings of reproduction and biology—reproducing these conventions, to use Strathern's term, inexactly. This new doubled or contingent biology has become one of the iconic spectacles of the twenty-first century, while at the same time, like television and airplanes before it, a regular fact of life.

The way in which these new dimensions of reproductive experience stretch the frame of existing conventions is both paralleled and demonstrated in the imagery that has accompanied the rise of IVF over the past thirty years, and specifically the rise of micromanipulation imagery, in its very explicit staging of the mechanization of reproductive substance. If micromanipulation has become an increasingly recognizable visual shorthand for the fusion of tool and substance, and if ICSI introduces a new figuration of conception that is more strongly defined in visual terms than in narrative ones, what are the consequences of these shifts for understandings of the facts of life? Or what we might call iVF? How do these new images interact with older, more established representations of reproductive substance, such as the traditional egg and sperm narrative? How do they display, or model, the work of making IVF work? If micromanipulation is a source of new, mainstream, public, and popular images of the workings of sex, by working it up, as it were, what is the iconography to which they belong? In sum, how do these new images re-signify reproductive substance, and what is the visual grammar they bring into being?

For example, one of the most important grammatical or indexical changes these images both suggest and confirm is the introduction of a new genealogical model, in which it is not only reproductive substance, but its directionality, orientation, or flow that is redesigned. In the familiar tree models of natural history, so favored by Darwin and still a basic tool of genetics today, reproductive flow is always one way. It is also always brachiating and bilateral, but contained, and limited, in its irrevocable path. This arboreal pattern of biological flow is superseded in micromanipulation images both by new conduits for the transmission of substance in the form of tools, and the possibility of open-ended dissemination. These hollow glass straws are the new conduits of micromanipulated life. Extending beyond the frame, the microtools point not only to the newly manipulable cellular interior that is their object, but to the termination of the conventional genealogical model (so familiar to kinship studies) that was their predecessor. The rotation of life's regenerative axis to a horizontal position correspondingly reorients the genealogy of flat-screen life, detaching this scene from its former genealogical trunk, and leaving it literally open ended. The new stem of life in the flat-screen world of cultivated human cells is the deconstructed inner cell mass — the source of totipotent cells that can be endlessly amplified and redirected into bespoke regenerative lines. In the context of flat-screen life, genealogy is an open door.

The visual grammar that holds the micromanipulation image in place, then, is not derived from the logic of sex or genealogy belonging to natural history, but rather to modern scientific technique. It might be difficult to find a more explicit visual representation of Rabinow's (1992) claim that life "will become technique" in a manner that reverses the order of Darwinian evolutionary time and telos, by making culture the origin of biology. The fact that the cells on the bed of the micromanipulator are submerged in culture medium reminds us of the etymological roots of the term "culture" in cultivation, that is, in the art of technique. What micromanipulation imagery provides is the kind of horizon-altering perspectival shift described by Barbara Duden (1993) in relation to fetal photography — offering an instrumental reframing of reproduction as technology. This is how micromanipulation imagery has become, in Duden's words, "part of the mental universe of our time" (1993: 1) in its depiction of the production of new life in ways that are detached from the orders and logics of living things that have structured far more than biological categories in the past.

It is the relativity of these former biological categories that IVF arguably makes more visible—both in its use as a clinical procedure, and as a research tool in science. To describe IVF as a technological platform has a literal meaning in relation to micromanipulation imagery that is both technically and metaphorically apt (as is the common description of the micromanipulation table as its bed). The mental universe in which both IVF and flat-screen life are legible—their grammar—is increasingly widely shared, and help to contextualize the question of why IVF is so popular in spite of all its difficulty, and why it is so curious despite having become more regular and normal. The same logic that makes IVF useful for clinical purposes—as a tool to aid in the overcoming of the obstacle of infertility—applies to the remaking of biology as technology more generally, and thus also to the newly conventional visual logic of micromanipulation, with its vivid depiction of taking human reproductive cells in hand. To the extent this logic also grounds a new understanding of technology as biology, through the recomposition of reproductive substance, so too has it already reshaped the future of how kinship can be both imagined and made.

SEVEN

Frontier Culture

As the introduction to this book outlined, IVF can be understood both as a technologization of substance and as a substantialization of technology, and thus as a lens that allows us to reconsider the meanings of both technology and biology. By tracing this argument through a series of frames, and drawing on a range of theorists to examine IVF as a stem technology, I have asked how we might understand the retooling of reproductive substance and its institutionalization as both new kinds of making life and new ways of living the remaking of life. As chapters 5 and 6 have suggested, there are many ways to investigate the condition of being after IVF, including the perspective offered by experiencing it directly as a patient or provider, and the more distant, but increasingly explicit, encounter with it in mainstream popular media as a representation, and now generic imagery, of embryo retooling as an open door. In both of these cases, which I suggest have important structural parallels despite their differences, the retooling of reproductive substance appears, among other things, to exceed the frames of existing understandings of sex, biology, kinship, technology, and even life itself. At the same time, I have also argued that the logics of IVF both belong to and extend familiar ideas and conventions associated with reproduction, science, and technology, as well as parenthood, the family, and kinship. In my previous work (Franklin 1997) I have used the idiom of hope to describe this convergence between the known and the unfamiliar, suggesting, as many others have also done, that the discourses of both hope and progress act as powerful forces extending reproductive technology, and the biosciences more generally, continually into unknown territory — or out of the frame. As noted in chapter 3, this is why both reproduction and technology are often envisaged, celebrated, and defended as frontiers, and why those who inhabit this territory, be they clinicians, scientists, or patients, are similarly described, and may experience themselves, as pioneers.

However, it is worth returning to the concept of the frontier once again, and for the same reasons it was discussed earlier in this book—namely, its analytic value in staging and refiguring from another angle the question concerning technology for which it is often an analogy. As noted in chapter 3, the frontier is a familiar but strange concept—at once describing a border between states and open-ended, unknown terrain. It at once provides an idiomatic figuration of opportunity and reward, and, in the discourse of the New World frontier at least, recalls a place of reversion, lawlessness, mutability, and conflict. Contradictory as well is the dual association of frontier life with movement and settlement, catastrophe and rebirth, wilderness and domestication. It is both an idealized concept and a temporary place or setting. Both practically and ideologically, the frontier signifies exploration, and thus transition, as well as conversion. The forward, or facing, orientation of the exploratory frontier idiom has its temporal equivalent in futurity: it is encountered by going forward.[1] But by definition the frontier is eventually left behind in both time and space.

What is left behind in the advance of the frontier line, or the edge of the frontier, is a zone of hybridity, in which settlement and domestication are entangled with the unknown or wild elements—a mix of agencies, entities, and forces. The labor of the frontier is one of ordering and imposing control, often imagined as seeding the growth of civilization through technologies of cultivation, epitomized by agriculture, which pave the way for a more elaborate social infrastructure. In this chapter, I begin by returning to the concept of the frontier in order to revisit the question of how this idiom models, or mirrors, technological evolution or progress. Drawing on recent anthropological and archaeological theory, I borrow from models of agriculture and domestication as frontier zones to suggest yet another perspective on the endless frontier of technology. In turn, this brings us back to the question of technology as evolution or natural history—for in all of these contexts (and perhaps especially that of domestication) explanatory models have shifted toward more hybrid, contingent, nonlinear accounts of interaction (Haraway 2008). Such a shift, I suggest, is consistent with what we might expect from the frontier idiom— with all of its magical conversion abilities—and also, if perhaps less obviously, of science, and in particular embryology.

As well as being important to what is changing within the biology lab, where the role of tools increasingly troubles the frontier between the organic and the inorganic, the analogy to frontier culture remains a useful trope for considering what is going on outside the lab as well, in the border zones of waiting rooms and clinics. The second part of this chapter thus returns to the in-between of the IVF–stem cell interface. Crossing over to the IVF side of the hole in the wall connecting the stem cell lab and the assisted conception unit (ACU), I follow the development of a permanent art installation inside the clinic produced by photographer in residence Gina Glover. This major installation of artwork, *The Art of A.R.T.*, represents the IVF encounter from both patients' and clinicians' points of view. Something of an ethnographer herself, Glover in her installation offers a visual logic of IVF that is an alternative to that described in chapter 6, as yet another window on the topsy-turvy world of IVF. One way to interpret her installation, I suggest, is as frontier bioart.

It is here, in an encounter with an artist's depiction of the future of kinship that is also the rendering of an encounter with the reproductive frontier, that I want to sketch some of the ways we might imagine a sociology of technology that is more robustly sociological — that is, which offers us a more fully sociological model of technology and technological change. As we have seen, the hole in the wall of the lab is itself a frontier line of sorts, not only demarcating a space of pioneering science, but dividing the space of frontiering between those who inhabit one kind of work space in the ACU, and another where reproductivity itself is being explored and domesticated. Always a problematic idiom, and not necessarily one whose mock heroism we want to reclaim, the frontier concept is nonetheless useful, I suggest, as itself a kind of artifice — a representational apparatus that performs a distinctive kind of work converting meanings. In other words, the idiom of the frontier is itself a conceptual tool. In this chapter I suggest that it can be used to investigate what is going back and forth through the hole in the wall, and indeed why the hole is there at all.

Frontiers of Knowledge

On the cover of the 1925 American Library Association pamphlet *Frontiers of Knowledge* is reproduced an engraving of a man reading a book at a desk under a starry sky.[2] Looming above him is the headless, winged statue of Nike, the Olympian goddess of victory, the remains of which were found in Greece in the late nineteenth century, and are now prominently displayed at the Louvre in Paris (figure 7.1).

This American frontier image combines classical antiquity and European culture, set against the backdrop of the universe, with the figure of a reader,

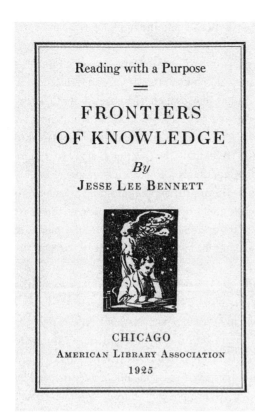

Reading with a Purpose
=
FRONTIERS
OF KNOWLEDGE
By
JESSE LEE BENNETT

CHICAGO
AMERICAN LIBRARY ASSOCIATION
1925

FIGURE 7.1. The cover of Jesse Lee Bennett's pamphlet is illustrated with an engraving of a frontier thinker seated before the headless statue of the goddess Nike famous from the Louvre. Behind them is the universe, starry sky, or open void. Jesse Lee Bennett, *Frontiers of Knowledge* (Chicago: American Library Association, 1925).

or thinker, in the foreground. Written by Jesse Lee Bennett, a journalist and popular writer, *Frontiers of Knowledge* is aimed at a general audience and intended to explain the origins and functions of knowledge and to make it more available to all. A practical guide, and part of a series titled Reading with a Purpose, it is dedicated to "those who, wishing to educate themselves over a lifetime, desire a broad perspective of the whole field of knowledge" (Bennett 1925: 5). In his brief didactic treatise, Bennett uses the idiom of the frontier both as an analogy to knowledge, and as a synecdoche for American pragmatism and self-improvement. He writes, "There are now only a few unexplored parts of the earth on which we live. But there are such great unexplored portions of the universe that the little world of knowledge we now possess must rather be thought of as a clearing in a wilderness with frontiers steadily advancing into the mystery of what mankind does not yet know than as a complete thing like our planet" (1925: 17). At once a concrete geographical comparison intended to convey the difference between an expanding clearing in the wilderness—of unknown proportions—and the finite, known, and complete size of planet earth, Bennett's analogy is also more abstract, and magical, in its invocation of the "mystery" into which frontiers advance, against the realm of "what mankind does not yet know." In this description, the conventional movement of the frontier (steadily advancing) appears as a self-acting force of expansion, set against a void (the universe), while simultaneously the frontier is also depicted in terms of actual historical events, manual labor (clearing), and human progress. Developing the frontier analogy in a more explicitly American vein, Bennett continues: "Today the frontiers of knowledge appear very, very far removed from the simple questions which originally sent intelligence ranging far afield seeking answers, just as the coast of America seemed very remote from the little villages where the sailors of Columbus grew up and from which they set out to see what lay beyond the western horizon" (31).

This analogy, between frontiers of the mind and exploration "beyond the western horizon" recalls the blurred line between what Gell (1988: 8) called the "merely real" and the imaginative reach of exploration, while seamlessly also inserting Old World civilization into the New World trajectory made famous in Frederick Jackson Turner's depiction of westward expansion on the American frontier as manifest destiny—the same idiom later invoked by Roosevelt, and now ubiquitous in science policy in Europe and many other parts of the world. Like Roosevelt and his advisors, whose inspiration may well have come from writers such as Bennett, *Frontiers of Knowledge* proposes an inexorable advance of civilization in the wake of such heroic American pioneers as Daniel Boone. "Only a few people were out on the frontiers of civilization with Daniel Boone; only a few people were near Peary at the North Pole or with any explorer or adventurer in wild, remote places. But today great cities exist in the place which was a frontier in the time of Daniel Boone. Soon airships will be going regularly across the North Pole" (Bennett 1925: 31).[3] At work in this generic description of manifest destiny and the inevitable march of progress are the familiar coordinates of time and space associated with the frontier—its forward expansion in the past transforming over time into a settled place in the here and now of the contemporary, epitomized by the rise of cities out of what were once "wild, remote places." Prominent in this passage, however, is also an account of modern technology—analogized to the progress of "great cities" by reference to what has become taken for granted, or regular—in much the same way Stewart Brand refers to IVF babies having become more regular over time. Thus the analogy of the frontier that was initially a depiction of space becomes one of time—"the place which was a frontier" having vanished, its very existence having been eclipsed by the transformation its advance has brought about.

The logic of these analogies may be so familiar as to appear in need of no further comment, so established is the frontier narrative still in the account of the growth of human civilization, technological advance, and scientific progress. However, it is precisely the magical logic of the frontier that invites further scrutiny because of its deeply paradoxical composition—a mix of historical fact, nationalist fiction, mythic allegory, and colonial propaganda.[4] The problem here is similar to that often described for the evolution of technology—that of mistaking the consequences for the cause, as if airplanes evolved by themselves. This is the intransigent problem Habermas describes as the "thesis of the autonomous character of technical development" and dismisses as "prescientific" (2010: 174). Also known as technological determinism, the attribution of an autonomous character to technical advances is further denigrated by Habermas as a ruse: "in the end," he asserts, such an attribution ultimately "serves to conceal preexisting, unreflected social interests." After all, as he notes, "the pace and direction of technical development today depend to a great extent on public investments: in the United States the defence and space administration are the largest sources of resource contracts" (174).

The extensive debate over the extent to which Marx attributed too much neutrality to technology and not enough politics to the evolution of technics (other than the interests of the ruling classes and the needs of capital) has long remained unresolved in part as a result of this either-or approach to the question of technological autonomy.[5] What the idiom of the frontier and the "self-propelling" model of technology have in common, in other words, is the neglect of their specific mechanics—or as it may turn out, their organics. As Raymond Williams (1990) also points out, it is as if the only critical question to be asked of either of these idioms, or of the manifest destiny ethos that suffuses both of them, is whether they are, as Habermas puts it, "a mere extension of natural history" (2010: 87).[6]

Indeed, both Marx and Engels did conceive of technology as an extension of natural history—so much so that Bernard Stiegler (1998: 2) suggests Engels's account of the coevolution of tool and hand "troubles the frontier between the organic and the inorganic" to such an extent that it all but constitutes a new theory of life itself.[7] Such a view invokes yet another model of the frontier, as well as of natural history, which is in Stiegler's account reimagined as a genealogy of technics. Whereas for Habermas mere natural history implies a lack of explanation, or even a convenient deceit, another approach can be arrived at by assuming that natural history itself is undertheorized. Thus, as noted earlier, when Marx cites Darwin's model of the evolution of organs in order to explore the increasing differentiation of tools and technique, he need not be read as either naturalizing or neutralizing technology, but instead as proposing a more complex mechanism for technological development, as well as for human evolution—indeed that these are at one level isomorphic.

It is no surprise that the models of both the frontier and technology (as well as evolution) most similar to those of Marx and Engels have long been found in both archaeology and anthropology—where for over half a century the human-tool relation has been theorized, to repeat Engels's language, as a frontier.[8] The frontier model of the archaeologist of early agriculture today, for example, is likely to be more similar to contemporary nonlinear, symbiotic accounts of evolution, domestication, or speciation than earlier, quasi-Darwinian narratives of human emergence driven by steady cultural or technological advance, such as those of Lewis Henry Morgan (1877), Leslie White (1959), or Lewis Binford (1965).[9] Paralleling developments in science and technology studies more widely, the analysis of human technological development advocated by anthropologists such as Pierre Lemonnier favors not only the view that "techniques are first and foremost social productions" (1993: 2) but that "the logic and coherence of . . . technological knowledge . . . are not related solely to the physical phenomena that are set in motion by a particular technique. Social representations of technology are also *a mixture of ideas* concerning realms other than matter or energy" (3, emphasis added). Thus, for example, in his account of early agriculture (neolithicization), the archaeologist Marek Zvelebil argues against any simple equation of technological development with cultural or economic change. Summarizing the view that has increasingly come to dominate the effort to model both local and general patterns of agricultural experimentation in the evolution of settlement culture, Zvelebil emphasizes the importance of complex interactions rather than functional causality:

> Ostensibly, the transition to farming is an economic process involving a shift from dependence on biologically wild to biologically domesticated resources. However, the process cannot be separated from the cultural, social and historical contexts in which it occurred. The change in economy may be a cause of, or perhaps a consequence of, changes in ideology, material culture or the social organization of participant groups, changes often referred to as neolithicization. It is not clear whether these changes were broadly simultaneous or whether, in Europe, the

shift from dependence on undomesticated local resources to agro-pastoral farming can be regarded as a signature for the sociocultural developments of the Neolithic [more generally]. (1994: 323)

To analyze in more regional specificity a process of transition (e.g., to agro-pastoralism) that is less likely to have involved singular stages or direct causes than a series of overlapping, repeated, and nonlinear events, Zvelebil employs the concept of an agricultural frontier zone to describe a context of exchange, of to-ing and fro-ing, including the cross-transfer of genes as well as of languages, material culture, and other resources. An advantage of such models, according to the author, is not only a "finer resolution" but a larger scale: "The agricultural frontier is more than a boundary. It is a far-reaching phenomenon, covering a wide geographical space, within which contacts between foragers and farmers occur, and which is occupied by communities in different stages of the transition" (Zvelebil 1994: 328). This archaeological model of the frontier as a contact zone, allowing for a much wider range of types of interactions, exchanges, and transfers, as well as a larger pool of active variables shaping technological change, typifies the shift within archaeology and anthropology generally toward a more mixed picture of the emergence of both agriculture and domestication.[10] In contrast to the progressive linear models of influential twentieth-century archaeologists, such as V. Gordon Childe (1952), who painted a picture of early farmers similar to that of Jesse Lee Bennett—pursuing avenues of progress out of their wilderness clearings toward a more civilized society—more recent theories have, for example, concluded that mobile subsistence farming may well have been compatible with livestock domestication, and that one need not have preceded the other. Indeed, it now appears increasingly likely that a wide range of strategies were employed simultaneously even within specific regions—as the very term "agropastoral farming" suggests.[11]

These shifts have been strongly reinforced by work in social and cultural studies of science, where, as the work of Haraway (2008), among others, clearly demonstrates, the idea, for example, of nature as a mixed, hybrid zone of contiguous agencies is, if anything, now the dominant approach in social theory. The identification of what the anthropologist Rebecca Cassidy describes as "porous, culturally-variable distinctions between wild and domesticated" (2007: 3) that have increasingly dominated the retheorization of agriculture and human evolution have important implications for understanding the history of technology as well. The fact that Darwin based much of his research into the concept of natural selection on domesticated animals, as well as artificially housed or contained animal specimens, becomes increasingly significant in the context of the resurgent epigenetic paradigm within developmental biology, suggesting, among other things, that, as Darwin speculated himself in his much-discredited thesis of pangenesis, the flow of inherited substance is neither strictly one-way nor entirely independent of environmental influences. (Indeed it was precisely this theory Walter Heape was testing in his original embryo transfer experiments of the late nineteenth century, prefiguring the increased significance reproductive biology has acquired in the context of remodeling developmental genetics.) In retrospect, what is so suggestive within Darwin's discredited model of pangenesis is the possibility that artificial and natural selection interact. To the extent that it foregrounds how organisms interact in the context of a technological culture, the petri-dish model of tooled life appears less and less specifically modern, and indeed more like a neolithic frontier.

Contemporary theories of biological development have been radically altered by the possibilities that learned behavior may become heritable, and that terminal differentiation can be reversed (and that human embryonic stem cells are themselves "an epigenetic adaptation to the *ex vivo* environment" [Smith 2008]). In turn, new possibilities are opened up for redesigning whole organisms and their parts — including both the generation of new cellular applications and the production of new cellular tools to enhance not only genetic but epigenetic control (Smith 2008: 453). That genes are no longer "one-way" but can be "told what to do" is reinforced by the unorthodox discovery that a relatively small number of genes can reset a cell's developmental clock, rendering it newly embryonic, by inducing pluripotency. Thus the importance, noted earlier, of the induced pluripotent stem (iPS) cell (named for the iPhone), which can now be used in many experiments that previously required difficult-to-source human embryos. The Loebian concept behind the iPS cell is that fundamental biological processes can be retooled to access a different part of their structural memory. This technology has precisely the magical reach we would expect from a frontier science that is developing new horizon applications.

This magical reach also appeals well beyond science. New concepts such as epigenetic reprogramming, induced pluripotency, and gene transfer have begun to travel more widely, and have been adopted as learning aids by leading biofuturists such as Stewart Brand, who urges (much as Firestone once did) that evolution must be "taken in hand" in the name of a survivable human future. The turn to in vitro models in Brand's influential publication *Whole Earth Discipline* thus extends his analogy to IVF discussed earlier, by annexing it to the language of molecular and synthetic biology: "Thanks to horizontal gene transfer, microbes have developed astounding skills. Tiny as they are, microbes can learn. . . . Microbes do complex quorum sensing, both within species and between species. . . . They make rain on purpose" (2010: 175). The new reeducability and skill of the complex microbe described in this passage exemplifies how such models themselves have become, like IVF, more regular. The astounding powers of these complex microbes and their potential to cross species borders appear to offer a new theory of biopower, according to which biological substances can become versatile and powerful tools in the effort to reverse engineer evolutionary change. Now that we know how adaptable genes are in taking, as well as giving, instructions, they can be retrained to make smarter tools. This is the same "biology is technology" model discussed in chapter 1, and it is the promise of this same logic that leads Brand to cite IVF as the big example of why we need to learn to live by remaking life, by tooling up biology, as it were. Alongside the work of leading synthetic biologists such as Craig Venter, Drew Endy, and George Church, Brand cites the Princeton physicist Freeman Dyson's claim "that the domestication of biotechnology will dominate our lives during the next fifty years at least as much as the domestication of computers has dominated our lives during the previous fifty years" (Dyson quoted in Brand 2010: 179). In vitro fertilization is the regularizing analogy by which these possibilities are tamed through the now familiar facts of technologically assisted parenthood.

As noted in chapter 3, Hannah Landecker (2007) has insightfully documented how "biotechnology changes what it is to be biological" in the context of cells that become "living tools." As that chapter argued, it is now increasingly evident that the working up of biology through techniques such as IVF is also changing what it means to be technological. In the increasingly quotidian crossover between the languages of natural history, evolution, and biology with those of technology, redesign, and engineering emerge exactly the same porous distinctions described by Cassidy in the context of the relationship between domestication and agriculture (distinctions that were already porous, as we have seen, in the writings of Marx and Engels, as well as Darwin). Now that biotechnology itself is being described as the object of domestication, it is worth returning to the question of what evolution and natural history refer to, exactly—for example, from the point of view of IVF.

Through the lens of the frontier idiom, we might describe the relationship between biology and engineering in the early twenty-first century as a classic example of a hybrid contact zone, primarily characterized by exchange, mixtures, and trading. Like the frontiers of old, the contemporary biofrontier is a zone of exploration, of domestication, and of prospecting for new sub-stances—now also including living tools. As in the case of the British parlia-mentary defense, twice in the last twenty years, of the nation's right to new human embryo tools to improve the health of the population, the prospect of "walking hopefully into the foothills of a gigantic mountain range" is in-creasingly seen to be of significant economic and political importance—and not only in the United Kingdom. Few national governments appear to be in any doubt today concerning the substantial economic importance of the bio-frontier—and the imperative to accelerate the domestication of new species of biotools and bioproducts for the benefit of the biopolity. The age of biology, as *The Economist* magazine has dubbed it, is today substantially manifest as the effort to domesticate biological substance by making it more technologi-cal, while at the same time this merographic analogy returns to redefine tech-nology as more biological. To describe biology as a frontier today essentially means describing it as a tool future. This view of the technological vitality of biological innovation in turn suggests a different model of kinship as it becomes substantialized not only through biological relations but through their identity with technology. If it is the case that modern human reproduc-tive substance has never been strictly biological—in the sense of being inde-pendently biological, naturally biological, or biologically automatic—since it is organized through a selective reproductive apparatus, then this biology must "always already" have incorporated the technicity of its environment (which not only humans have introduced) since—well, more or less since it started. Such a hypothesis—of a physical chemistry between the organic and inorganic that is exaggerated by in vitro life—would offer yet another looking-glass perspective out of the world of IVF, and onto its future.[12]

Cabin Fever

Given these complex imbrications linking biology and technology with the prospect of reengineering human futures, it is fortuitously apt that it is the sculpture of the Winged Victory of Samothrace that appears on the cover of *Frontiers of Knowledge*, looming behind our lone frontier everyman at his desk—as she too has a special relationship to the future of technology, as well as its perils. This sculpture from approximately 200 BC depicting the goddess Nike is thought to have been commissioned to commemorate a naval battle, and to have been installed on the island of Samothrace in Greece in such a manner as to suggest she was standing on the prow of a ship. She leans for-ward, and her missing right arm was once cupped to her missing mouth in a cry of victory, inspiring her crew to triumph over adversity. Much admired, she is considered to be one of the masterpieces of Hellenic art and one of the Louvre's greatest treasures in part because of the powerful sense of movement she conveys — not only in her posture, but in the finely wrought ruffling of her gown, as if facing into a gale. The sense of her movement into openended space is furthered by this active stance — her wings fully outstretched, as if addressing fate itself.

In addition to physical momentum, she thus evokes a sense of spirited engagement (indeed perhaps with the spirits themselves). In the imagined space ahead of her lie the obstacles to be overcome, and in her eagerness to confront them she both embodies and inspires progress. She thus evokes in her entire (sculptural) figure the magical reaching out of the frontier, the child as airplane, and the future of airships regularly traversing the North Pole. Thus her incorporation into the Rolls-Royce "flying lady," the figurine also known as the Spirit of Ecstasy introduced at the Paris motor show in 1904 and still a feature on the hood of these iconic cars. As if embodying, then, the transfer of the frontier analogy not only to knowledge, but to technological advance, as well as the military origins of this idiom, we see in this statue's role as the mascot to elite machines both the sense of hopeful inspiration and the recurring themes of conflict and of confrontation that have defined the modern technological age.

As Ulrich Beck (1992) has argued, the equation of technological innovation with progress characteristic of the postwar period, during which the frontier idiom guided the establishment of large-scale publicly funded institutions such as the National Science Foundation, became increasingly strained toward the end of the twentieth century, burdened by what Beck describes as "an anarchy of side effects" (1992: 214), and characterized by increasing political conflict.[13] Far from enjoying automatic public consensus, faith in progress becomes, in his view, something that must be enforced, thus inaugurating a countermodernity equivalent to a secular religion over which battles are increasingly fought. Unguided by democratic deliberation, and yet enforced as a government economic priority, the automatic policy of pursuing scientific and technological progress creates "a blank page as a political program, to which wholesale agreement is demanded as if it were the earthly road to heaven" (214). Unequivocal on this point, Beck identifies late twentieth-century faith in progress as an inversion of the very modernity it created. Indeed, he writes, progress "can be understood as legitimate social change without democratic political legitimation. Faith in progress replaces voting. . . . The fundamental demands of democracy have been turned on their heads by the model of progress. . . . Progress is the inversion of rational action. . . . It is the continuous changing of society into the unknown without a program or a vote" (214). In addition to the more well-known cases of nuclear power and genetic engineering, Beck describes the introduction of IVF and embryo transfer as an example of the "free pass" (207) handed over to science in the name of progress, resulting in what he describes as "an avalanche of problems" (206). In addition to the question of whether IVF will lead to "completely new types of social relationships, whose consequences cannot be predicted," he notes that "deep-frozen embryos could be stored and sold," thus "provid[ing] science with long hoped-for 'experimental objects' . . . for embryological and pharmacological research [as well as] genetic diagnosis and therapy on embryos, with all of the associated fundamental questions [including] what constitutes a socially and ethically 'desirable,' 'used' or 'healthy' genetic substance? Who will perform this 'quality control of embryos' . . . and by what right and with what standards? What will happen to the 'low quality embryos' which do not satisfy the requirements of this prenatal 'entrance examination for the world'?" (206, citations removed). Like both Hannah Arendt and Jürgen Habermas, Beck interprets the birth of IVF as a "secret farewell to an epoch in human history" that has transpired without public, political, or parliamentary consent. "How is it possible," he asks, "that all this can happen and that only subsequently the questions regarding the consequences, goals and dangers of this noiseless social and cultural revolution must be pursued by a critical public against the professional optimism of the small clique of human genetic specialists, without real influence of their own and fixated on scientific conjecturing?" (206–207, emphasis removed).

Published in Germany in 1986, and widely hailed for its introduction of the concepts of the risk society and reflexive modernization, Beck's analysis in some ways closely resembles those of (the somewhat less widely admired) feminists concerned with reproductive technology in the mid-1980s discussed in chapter 5, who similarly emphasized the lack of sufficient public debate of the introduction of IVF, and who interpreted this lack of deliberation as a measure of the counterdemocratic hegemony of the medical profession, as well as the emergence of conflict in the wake of a more reflexive technological ambivalence. Beck's claim that IVF conveniently establishes a reliable source of human research embryos has also long been a feminist concern, as described, for example, by Gena Corea in her 1985 critique of reproductive technologies as "the application of animal husbandry to human beings" by an elite "power structure" lacking any "conscious policy":

Th[e] language of therapy used in describing IVF obscures the fact that medicine is not just a healing art but is also an institution of social control. IVF gives the power structure potent tools for such control. It makes a certain scenario possible: the application of animal husbandry to human beings in processes that will reduce women to breeders and offer a centralized group of white men control over who is born into the world. This would not necessarily be a conspiracy or even a conscious policy. The efforts of diverse men to create technologies that will increase male control over women and reproduction may be unformalized and intuitive, but nonetheless effective. (1985: 123–124)

Here, then, in reverse composition, is the relation of domestication to technology described earlier, once again on the reproductive frontier, but much less optimistically so. Where both Beck and Corea point to the dehumanizing, antidemocratic, and subjugating legacies of the potent tools made available via human IVF, others, such as Brand, now argue the human condition has not been so different from animal husbandry all along, and that more advanced human husbandry is no longer an optional extra, but must instead be intensified.

And yet! (as Heidegger would say) whether or not its introduction was democratic or consensual, or its risks were sufficiently debated in advance, IVF has become, since the 1980s when its introduction might still have appeared to affect only a tiny minority of citizens, a vast and well-established global industry—indeed one that is not only as regular as air travel over the North Pole, but increasingly reliant on the airline industry to connect consumers with the reproductive products they require. The project of taking biology in hand is now more than ever one that is consciously, politically, publicly, and consensually annexed to an expanding biomedical, biopolitical, and bioeconomic future of cultured biology. To argue that IVF should not exist may be credible for the same reasons organ transplantation is still objected to by some. Or Facebook. But the time has passed for such objections to have any likelihood of abolishing this technology. Ethical and political concerns are not gone, but they have migrated, have been sidelined, or, as in the case of Cardinal Keith O'Brien's objections to embryo research described earlier, have become the object of ridicule. Direct opposition to either IVF or embryo research is now confined to a small minority in global terms. And although calls such as Beck's for a more meaningful public engagement with scientific innovation continue to emphasize the importance of moving it further upstream (a goal that to a degree is manifest in the context of new initiatives such as synthetic biology), the logic of IVF, as discussed in chapter 1 of this book, is now both publicly celebrated and irrevocable. Dissenting concern has moved elsewhere — for example, to humanizing animals, nanotechnology, and the regulation of trade in human tissues, cells, and organs. Far from being banned, or even curtailed (or, for that matter, even meaningfully monitored in most parts of the world), IVF, as Brand notes, has become taken for granted. The "avalanche of problems" anticipated by Beck may indeed be manifest as an ongoing debate over stem cells, embryo research, cloning, and designer babies. But these concerns do not appear to have substantially undermined either continuing public support of research to develop new biological tools such as iPS cells, nor to have diminished popular or philanthropic endorsement of such endeavors. Indeed, as chapter 5 has shown, IVF has become not only normal but normative.

In retrospect, the case of IVF suggests that insofar as people are voting with their feet by queuing up for an ever-widening range of almost entirely privatized reproductive services, this technology is supported by a widespread, diverse — and increasingly global — public consensus. Whether or not IVF was foisted upon an initially naive and unconsenting public, as Beck alleges, and regardless of whether it increases male control of reproduction, as Corea predicted, the progress of IVF since the mid-1980s (as a science, an industry, and a market) can hardly be described as either slow or hesitant. It is no longer even significantly controversial. Five million miracle babies later, IVF looks like other frontiers that are already behind us.

But as chapter 6 has also shown, the rise of IVF has not been unaccompanied by the ambivalence Beck described and the expansion of technological control of reproduction Corea more unambivalently predicted would be subordinating. What the case of IVF thus also foregrounds is the need for more complex models of technological change, and a wider conversation to address the sociological character of these changes. This is one reason I have argued that the feminist debates over reproductive technologies in the 1980s, and in particular the effort to integrate the understanding of IVF technology with the analysis of technologies of gender and kinship, offers a perspective that is of increasing value to understand the evolution of the biosciences more broadly. The fact, for example, that engagement with both the promise and the practice of IVF turns out to be much more complicated than it might initially appear yields a powerful insight not only into the question concerning technology more generally, but the ongoing difficulty of how to analyze the current question concerning biology that this book attempts to explore.

Arguably, what the feminist analysis of IVF reveals with especially significant implications for the future of the biosciences is the absence of adequate attention to reproduction not only in the analysis of technology, but in the effort to theorize social and political structures in general. The difference between Beck's account of new reproductive technologies and those of feminists in the same period lies mainly in the feminist emphasis on the extent to which reproduction was not included within the public political process to begin with. Moreover, what feminist analyses have demonstrated is that if the explicit technologization of reproduction has made this absence in social and political theory more visible, it has not made it more legible or tractable. Had Foucault observed the emergence of a complex worldwide debate over the relationship between IVF and regenerative medicine, or had he followed the debate over designer babies in *Le Monde*, he might have been inspired to revisit the "strangely muddled zone" of reproductive technology and its significance to biopolitics. No doubt Marx would have been a profuse commentator on the rise of biocapital in the context of stem cells and regenerative medicine. And even Lévi-Strauss must have been tempted at times to consider the complex exchange of gametes that is now a routine procedure in the heart of Paris as a new mythic paradigm, or even grammar.

What the absence of such contributions reveals in retrospect is precisely what the feminist analysis of reproductive technology has shown all along, namely that the scope and depth of biopolitics has only just begun to be revealed or charted, but also that from the point of view of gender politics this is hardly novel. In the same way the meaning of "biopower," as Foucault rightly argued, has been hampered by too narrow a definition of politics, so too was his expansion of the term "technology" to encompass the discursive process of subject formation a feminist theory manqué (pace Rubin 1975: 185). Missing from its remit was not only an adequate account of gender but, more surprisingly, of sex, and in particular of the heteronormative apparatus through which sexual reproduction is both organized and channeled. Much as the introduction of IVF may have been imagined as a means of facilitating normative heterosexual, conjugal, and familial ties — and much as it may have been seen as analogous to biological reproduction in vivo — it has turned out, as Strathern predicted, not quite to reproduce these preconditions exactly. Instead, this technology occupies a parallel universe that now supplements an imagined original to which it is never entirely resolved.

That this process of supplementation has itself been replicated in the new traffic connecting biology and technology more widely — in which one is at once synonymous with but exceeds the other, just as the tools of the micromanipulator exceed the frame of cellular reconstruction—only reveals more clearly why IVF was never a simple case of giving nature a helping hand to begin with. Repositioning this technique within the longer history of retooling reproductive substance, and especially the effort to include within this history the recognition that conventional gender and kinship structures are as much part of this retooling as hand-beveled pipettes, opens a new window onto the question of what "biotechnology" actually means.

It turns out to be in the dehyphenated space of this now familiar neologism that biotechnology, like biopolitics, or for that matter biology, still has much to reveal. So far, what the lens of IVF reveals is both that we already have a more contingent understanding of biology, and a more biological model of technology. So much has already been argued throughout this book, and accounts for its title. In turning, then, in the second part of this chapter to a more concrete engagement with the new reproductive frontier opened up by IVF, and to the ongoing effort to domesticate biology as a technology, as well as the new kinship and gender norms this technology relies upon for its own reproduction, it is once again the view up close to the encounter with IVF as both a technology and a way of life that is explored. The aim of this section, which returns to the question of the frontier, is mainly to view this problem from another angle—again from another technology, namely photography. Shifting, then, as in the last chapter, into a different kind of culture medium, we turn to the British artist photographer Gina Glover and *The Art of A.R.T.*

In the following tour of an art installation in an ART clinic, we encounter the reproductive frontier as a highly political space, but one that, for all of the reasons discussed in the first section of this chapter, as yet lacks a very precise political, sociological, or philosophical analysis. In the newly normative space of an IVF waiting room, we also reencounter the ongoing ambivalence toward technological possibility so consistently described in the feminist literature on IVF. Indeed a "strangely muddled zone," to reinvoke Foucault's description somewhat differently, the space of reproductive pioneering is both anxiously and intimately ambivalent—while remaining ripe with possibility and exerting a curious allure. Here, in closest contact with the process of retooling reproductive substance, is also a space of careful thought and extended imaginative reach conjoined with a queer sort of human husbandry. It is to the lessons we can learn from this space of biological relativity, as depicted by an artist in residence, that we now turn to reconsider the open-ended questions of how the futures of new tools and new kinships are conceived by those who are living with them closest to hand.

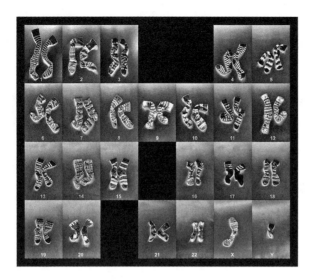

Art in the Age of Reproductive Technology

Having worked with the Guy's and St. Thomas's ACU since the late 1990s, I was already familiar with the award-winning installation the British artist Gina Glover had completed in the Guy's Hospital Genetics Clinic in 2002–2003 before I learned that she had been commissioned to create a second exhibit in the new IVF–stem cell facility, *The Art of A.R.T.*, completed in 2008. From my previous ethnography on preimplantation genetic diagnosis, which was partly based in the Guy's Genetics Clinic (Franklin and Roberts 2006), I was familiar with Gina's most famous hospital installation piece—*Chromosome Socks* (figure 7.2). When I arranged to interview Gina about her new installation, in the autumn of 2009, we thus agreed to meet in the Guy's clinic foyer where her previous work remains a favorite talking point.

As Gina explained to me while standing beside her signature photo light box, *Chromosome Socks* emerged from a year-long residency in the Guy's cytology lab and came to be the centerpiece for the installation not only because it worked visually, but because it was the process of making this piece that enabled Gina to clarify her artistic method: "I mean how it originated was that what I observed when I was working in cytology, where they were looking at chromosomes, was their sensibility to have stripy scarves, stripy socks, stripy this, stripy that. Everywhere I looked there was all this stripiness. People [had them] had on their notice boards, the men were wearing stripy ties. . . . It was extraordinary, the stripiness of everything." This stripiness—the sartorial sign of cytology, based on the banding of chromosomes that is cytology's stock in trade—was both visually and symbolically suggestive. It was also an idiom that was ready to hand both in the lab and at home—indeed it established a connection between these two different parts of the cytologists' lives. In the same way that the cytologists' socks traveled with them from home to work, so too were socks a naturally striped pair of familiar objects used in the translation of genetic diagnosis to patients. For her artwork, Gina sought to exploit these connections by asking the geneticists to donate their socks for her project. "And then I would talk to people and they would talk about socks in a washing machine, or spaghetti, and things like that, and so the idea of socks was originally formulated from remarks they made. And so I collected, and they gave me, [their socks]. This is a geneticist's child's sock [pointing to the smallest pair of socks]. And so all the socks were donated to me, but I didn't have quite enough so I bought a few more at Brixton market, just to top it up a bit."

Knitting together, as it were, the public and the private lives of the geneticists, their own biological relations, as well as the domestic and commercial economies, the socks proved to be an ideal artistic medium. To enhance their "socks appeal," Gina photographed the socks against a bright white background, later Photoshopped to form a halo around each pair. She then mounted the glowing socks on a pearly gray backlit grid, each pair itemized with bright orange numbers to create an oversized glowing montage mimicking, but mutating, the screens used for diagnosing chromosomal disorders. The use of bright color animated the pairs, while the halos enlivened them with light. The effect is not unlike a sock party piece—perhaps a disco. "I kind of wanted them to look a bit psychedelic. I think chromosomes should dance," Gina explained.

This was not the first incarnation of the socks piece, however. For her first shoot Gina had photographed the socks in a domestic garden, in what she describes as a more "documentary" style—a style, as it turned out, the cytologists found hard to follow (figure 7.3). Pinning the socks to a laundry line, Gina had originally imagined the elementary units of cytology crossed with the familial associations of a garden, a home, and housework. This pastoral, Edenic, yet domestic and ordinary location, however, proved too generic an image. The addition of a dog running under the hanging socks only made it more closely resemble a bucolic ad for laundry detergent. "Originally I didn't understand about a karyotype. So I put the socks on a washing line. Which I was very proud of, and it had taken me a whole day to arrange them, and to get a dog to go through, and get the garden looking okay, and to be the right kind of garden to put them in, and of course came back and was told very, very

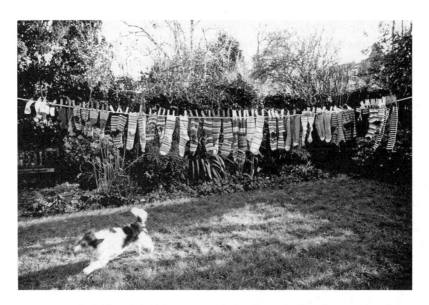

FIGURE 7.3. Gina Glover's initial attempt to depict the work of cytology attempted (unsuccessfully) to deploy a more pastoral setting. Reproduced with permission of the artist, Gina Glover.

firmly that that didn't work, and that wasn't right, and it was totally meaning-less." In retrospect, Gina agreed the garden setting wasn't quite right: "What didn't work with the washing line was that it was in a back garden. It almost needed to be a washing line in Venice." The socks needed to be somehow out of place to show up: the image needed to be incongruous, but with a point to the mismatch between object and place. The bright socks needed to be back-grounded, she felt, against something more rectilinear, more contrasting, and less like where socks might be found ordinarily. But most importantly, she realized, she had not paid adequate attention to the work of the cytologists: the image did not connect with them in part because it was too removed, too superficial, too untranslatable. Estranged from their donated socks by Gina's initial stab at re-presenting them artistically, the cytologists failed to compre-hend her image. There was not enough affinity to pull them in.

What Gina next created drew less on the pastoral image of the domestic garden than on a different home ground for the cytologists: the primal scene of medical genetic screening—their own professional domestic window— the light box. By cutting, pasting, and rearranging the vividly banded pairs of stripy socks into a kind of table (just as a cytologist would), and mounting them in illuminated gridlike squares, Gina reproduced one of the defining visual technologies of cytology, the karyotype, which is used to match pairs of chromosomes and thus to detect genetic abnormality. As in a scientific karyotype, her image is both standardized and individual. Each pair of socks repeats the general pattern, but not consistently, as each chromosome, and pair, is unique. There is variation in the color and shape of each sock, and each pair is shot against a slightly different background—resulting in a series of portraits that make up a population, defined by their similarity, but also by their serial uniqueness.

In both its mode of production and its final form, then, the resulting image is itself an imitation that is defined by both its similarity and uniqueness. It is at once a faithful depiction of a karyotype and a clever masquerade, a pastiche, and a torque of a familiar technics: *Chromosome Socks* is an imitation of a karyotype that is more dramatically dressed up, and in fact not a karyotype at all, but a comment on one. Clearly, it is an artist's representation of a karyotype. It relies on the visual pun of socks that look like chromosomes arranged into a karyotype-like grid, but one that has been enhanced even beyond Kodachrome brightness, as if it is a karyotype on steroids—enlarged, vivid, and theatrical. A translation of technique that doubles back on its makers in the labor of its making, its remade-ness becomes akin to homegrown methods, while introducing a new way of seeing them. At the same time that the image relies upon conventional and familiar mechanisms of scientific display, it re-presents them by putting a mundane domestic object center stage, the humble sock. One need not know that most of these socks were donated by people working in the clinic to recognize that they are ordinary domestic objects that would have belonged to someone. It does not matter whether or not they have been worn, or by whom, for these socks to epitomize everyone's everyday ordinary, as well as the personal and the individual, and the quirky.

Similarly, although they are systematically arranged and displayed in numbered rows, from largest to smallest (as would be a proper karyotype), the overall image is noticeably asymmetrical. Only one row of socks is complete—the rest have gaps. In between the dancing pairs of psychedelic socks are blank empty squares—at once relieving the eye from too much vivid, in-your-face stripy sockiness, but also subtly suggesting the unseen, the unseeable, and the unknown—the incomplete. The way of seeing this piece of artwork thus establishes fuses the professional bioscientific gaze with the daily familiar of the domestic routine: it offers us a picture of clinical genetics as nonthreatening, familiar, and somewhat comical. Adult and child socks share a kinship of technology—literally banded together as a stripy group of individuals and pairs united under the glare of exactly the surveillance Foucault described as a new, disciplining norm of genealogy as technics. Knowingly ironic, and an obvious caricature, the witty image nonetheless retains a mildly pedagogical flavor, recapitulating the ubiquity of domestic analogies used in the context of genetic counseling, where DNA is commonly analogized to such familiar images as beads on a string, an alphabet, a book, or a recipe, and the mixing together of genes is compared to spaghetti, or socks in the washing machine.

In her discussion of "the biological gaze," such as that practiced by clinical geneticists in the lab, Evelyn Fox Keller (1996a) emphasizes its interdependence with touch, as well as its ethos of action, through which sight is allied to the handling of objects to investigate the causes of things. This feature of the biological gaze can also be understood diagnostically, for example, in the use of tracers to identify genes for specific diseases, in order to prevent the establishment of a pregnancy using an affected embryo. Indeed, the agency of the biological gaze — its attachment to the identification of causes through intervention, in order to achieve greater control over outcomes — is arguably the whole point of clinical genetic applications such as preimplantation genetic diagnosis. As in Gell's account of technological reaching, Keller notes that "the history of the biological gaze . . . has become increasingly and seemingly inevitably enmeshed in actual touching, in taking the object in hand, in trespassing on and transforming the very thing we look at" (1996a: 108). The probing, imaginative eye, she argues, requires the probing hand to enquire more fully into the mechanisms that make things work:

> The fact is that scientists have found a way to walk up to the object and touch it; no longer do they peer through the microscope with their hands behind their backs. This in fact was the great contribution the rise of an experimental ethos brought to nineteenth century biology: the desire — and increasingly the skill — to reach in and touch the object under the microscope, and thereby "to make it real." In other words, once the microscope was joined with the manual manipulations of experimental biology — marking, cutting and dissecting under the scope . . . the microscope became a reliable tool for veridical knowledge. By the close of the nineteenth century, hand and eye had begun to converge. (1996a: 112)

It was in experimental embryology, argues Keller, that the union of "representing and intervening," as Ian Hacking describes it (1983: 189–190), became most prominent. Citing the classical experiments performed by Spemann that are discussed in chapter 3, Keller notes:

At first with relatively crude instruments—perhaps a glass rod drawn very finely, or a hair from a baby's head—and later, in the twentieth century, with carefully machined microtomes and micromanipulators—researchers could not only represent but actually intervene in the choreography of the minute primal stages of life. They could isolate the fertilized egg, watch it divide, gently mark one of the cells with a dab of dye and follow it as it continued to divide . . . or they could carefully separate the cells . . . to see if the two halves of the young embryo could independently form whole bodies. (1996a: 112)

It is by these means, she argues, that the biological gaze evolved from a practice not unlike astronomy into a hands-on science seeking to identify the causes of development (or, in Spemann's case, the source of organization) by separating out and testing the very smallest units of life—that is, by manipulating them. In this way, the gaze became a probe searching for the fulcrums of action, and aiming to identify the fundamental units that would, in turn, offer greater biological control. Linked to this change in the gaze was thus also a shift in what was being looked for—no longer mere classification, as Foucault described it, but instead, as Keller notes, "the means to alter—to induce a change in—the course of natural phenomena" (1996a: 115). It was by this means, she claims, that scientists such as H. J. Muller, the classical geneticist trained in T. H. Morgan's lab in New York, were led to envisage a future in which control of genetic mutation would "place the process of evolution in our hands" (Muller cited in Keller 1996a: 116).

As Gina Glover's image demonstrates, by imitating with her artist's hand and eye precisely the touching and probing that motivate the scientists' way of seeing, the biological gaze conveys more than just looking—it is also about touching, selecting, manipulating, and recomposing its objects. A highly skilled practice, acquired only through prolonged training, it is not surprising that the biological gaze, and its contiguous logics of clinical surveillance and therapeutic intervention, as well as of biological causality, are not always legible or obvious to the nonspecialist eye—for example, to patients in the Guy's Genetics Clinic, to whom the glaringly visible signs of a positive or negative diagnosis that are like billboards to the cytologist or clinician may be literally invisible. This same process of translation is the object of Glover's work, only altered by introducing yet another way of seeing, in the form of the artist's handiwork, which retouches the karyoscape, rerendering it through the ordinary idiom of stripy socks. Differently trained, and differently focused, the eye of the photographer-artist is skilled in the process not only of seeing, but of seeing how things are seen, and of revealing new ways of seeing both at once—the sight itself, and how it is composed. Like the experimental embryologist, or cytogeneticist, the photographer is also an adept practitioner of the arts of seeing, as well as the use of technology to probe and manipulate the object under observation or to frame and reframe events (now especially possible in the highly manipulable digital media). For an artist such as Glover, whose work involves both photography and the manipulation of photographic images, often by manually cutting and pasting them into larger compositions (such as *Chromosome Socks*), the language of cytogenetics is, in a sense, already second nature.

The biological gaze that Glover imitates—namely that of the cytogeneticist—is thus powerfully reinhabited by the artist, who has opened this gaze up to the viewer, in part by reconstituting it as identical in form, and labor, but not in content. As a result, the image offers a way of literally seeing through science, and yet also beyond it, as *Chromosome Socks* is not so much a scientific image as an image of science. Glover's art is thus doubly translational: it both complements and decenters the highly technical scientific work of karyotyping by producing an image that resembles genetic counselors' analogies, while inverting their epistemological gravity. At the same time, by supplementing the biological gaze, which is itself a supplement to its objects, Glover introduces once again the relativity that now accompanies spectatorship of the biological—be it as a patient, a clinician, or as a viewer of the evening news, where digitally recorded clips of micromanipulation accompany descriptions of stem cells, cloning, and regenerative medicine.

THE ART OF A.R.T.

Following its award-winning success in the Genetics Clinic, the method Glover devised for *Chromosome Socks* was translated into a different context in order to complete the project in the new ACU at Guy's, opened in the spring of 2009 by Robert Edwards. Overseas at the time, I was unable to attend the opening, and did not view the finished installation until the following autumn. Visiting it for the first time, I immediately recognized some of Glover's familiar themes as soon as I got out of the elevator on the eleventh floor on my first visit to the new lab. Under the title *The Art of A.R.T.*, just opposite the elevator doors was a series of digital images of embryos arranged in a traditional developmental sequence, only now enhanced: Glover had in-filled the cells of a developing blastocyst with pink cherry blossom, using Photoshop.

When I interviewed Glover she explained that the photographs of a blossom had been taken near her London home, and had become a central theme

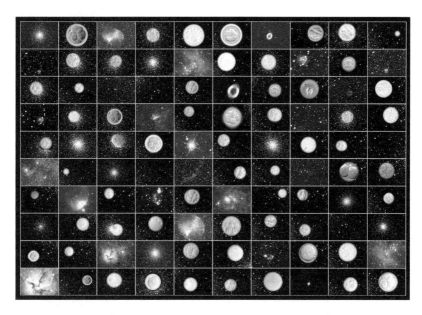

FIGURE 7.4. *Very Small and Far Away.* Reproduced with permission of the artist, Gina Glover.

in the installation as a whole, elsewhere reshaped as giant floating chromosomes, and recurring as a motif across several of the collage images. As well as symbolizing springtime and renewal, the pink blossom set against the blue background was suggestive of the conventional color coding of sex. Significantly, the pink cherry tree blossom also transformed the signature blue of micromanipulation imagery into open sky, while also thus inverting the viewers' gaze upward: whereas an embryo observed through the lens of the micromanipulator is below the viewer, who is looking down, Glover's embryo blossoms appeared to be floating in the sky above, their faint white aureoles like the wispy edges of clouds.

A similarly celestial theme is evident in *Very Small and Far Away* (figure 7.4), also in the central elevator waiting area opposite the clinic's main entrance, where the title of this permanent installation *The Art of A.R.T.* is prominently displayed in large letters, announcing to the viewer that this exhibit is fully part of how this clinic understands its work. This giant galactic Photoshopped collage of cellular and celestial orbs drawn from inner and outer space is backgrounded, like Bennett's frontier thinker, against a starry night sky. While referencing the ancient tradition of comparing embryology to star gazing (Gilbert 1994), these astronomical images also index the artist's playful interpretation of scientific

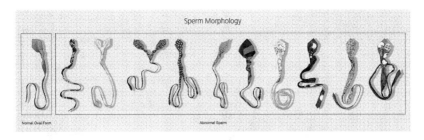

FIGURE 7.5. *Sperm Morphology*. Reproduced with permission of the artist, Gina Glover.

imagery—repeating a signature theme in Glover's work as a whole. Commenting on the overlapping languages of astronomy and embryology—such as the birth and death of stars, and the aureoles and coronas of cells—Glover noted the striking visual similarities between the orbs of inner and outer space, while also revealing, as she put it, the varied ways of being round: "They are all round but they are different kinds of round." It had been important to enhance these effects of similarity and difference, she explained, not only by making the tiny cells bigger, and the giant stars smaller, but by making the entire image very large—upwardly imitating, again, the sky itself—as a galaxy. "I have this on a postcard at home," she said. "It just doesn't work when it is that small."

Just inside the clinic, in a place of suitable prominence, stands the companion piece closest to *Chromosome Socks* in the *Art of A.R.T.* installation, in this case featuring enlarged, Photoshopped ties to represent the diagnosis of sperm morphology (figure 7.5). Once again the ties have been donated and subsequently posed (tied), then shot, cut, reshaped, composed, and further manipulated using Photoshop. Like the socks, the ties are displayed to resemble biological entities as they would be viewed scientifically in the context of clinical analysis. Again, the ties are vibrant and colorful, seeming to squirm against their clinically white graph-paper background. Like *Chromosome Socks* the image is both comical and instructive, scientific and domestic—an imitation of diagnosis and a re-creation of diagnosis as art. Once again, too, in the cutting and pasting of the photographs to create a disciplined montage of selected elements, Gina's labor as an artist reproduces that of the scientists whose work she is depicting.

Directly opposite the ties is *Eggs Donation* (figure 7.6)—a neat, orderly display of eggs donated by female members of the clinical staff, who are named and commemorated in the tiny museum-like labels underneath each individual specimen. The eggs vary slightly in size but greatly in appearance

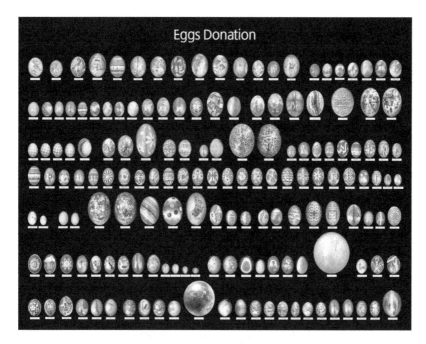

FIGURE 7.6. *Eggs Donation*. Reproduced with permission of the artist, Gina Glover.

and the wide range of materials out of which they have been fashioned—some painted, some made of stone, some that are real (birds') eggs, that are now (Photoshopped) egg specimens on display. At once depicting order and variety, the eggs contrast with the sperm ties opposite in being set against a stately black background, much as they might be in a museum display. Thus, again, while a quasi-scientific idiom is being imitated, it is also being reinhabited by donated personal objects.

A slightly different take on eggs animates *Ex Ovo Omnia* (figure 7.7)—a collection of more than one hundred hens' eggs dressed in colorful knitted cozies. In contrast to the formal curatorial, faintly Victorian, table of donated eggs, this egg population appears ready to go: they are out of the box and on the move. The sense of animation is enhanced by the cartoonish assemblage of characters depicted in a palette reminiscent of children's toys or TV programs. These eggs are interactive and sociable, some appearing to converse in pairs, share a hat, or glance at one another. They are variously positioned standing, sitting, and lying down—together conveying a sense of a community. By their very nature they could be described as culinary, domestic, and companionable. They are also cute and their tone is far from clinical, or even

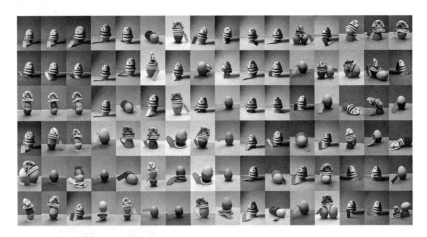

FIGURE 7.7. *Ex Ovo Omnia.* Reproduced with permission of the artist, Gina Glover.

serious. At the same time, the reference to the cozies having been bought on the Internet, and the presence of price tags, carries a less comical implication of a market in eggs—the eggs themselves also commodities purchased by the artist, no doubt in a supermarket. Similarly, one might wonder whether some of the eggs lying down are dead, or duds—perhaps hard-boiled, past their shelf life, or struck down by salmonella.

In describing both of these pieces, Glover comments on her growing obsession with eggs during her residency (figure 7.8). "It is the same thing that happens when you go through IVF treatment," she said. "You become obsessed with eggs. It got so that I was seeing eggs everywhere." We spent a long time in front of a collage titled *Seeing Eggs Everywhere*, made up of several hundred round objects resembling egg cells collected throughout Glover's various travels. For Glover this piece explicitly engages with her sense of entering into a kind of parallel universe to that of the IVF patients and the staff of the clinic in their obsession with eggs (which in humans are, like embryos, round). Echoing her galaxy of orbs is this busy "obsessive" concentration of "shots that have come from everywhere," including a shopping trip with her daughter, also an artist, who lives in New York. "It is as much about what is going on here [she points to her head] as the process [of IVF] I'm describing."

EMBRYOS AS WINDOWS

Gina Glover is not the first artist to investigate IVF as a way of seeing, nor is she the first to envision the embryo as window on new life. These themes have been taken up by other artists, many of whom are included in Suzanne

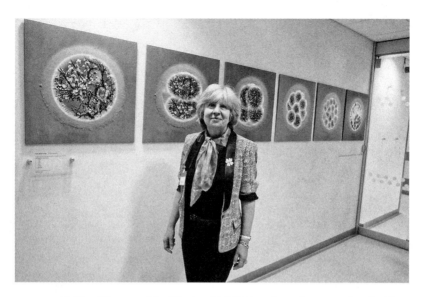

FIGURE 7.8. Gina Glover explains *The Art of A.R.T.* Photo by author, reproduced with permission of the artist, Gina Glover.

Anker and Dorothy Nelkin's (2004) *The Molecular Gaze*, including Anker herself. Among the best-known prior art in this field was produced by the British conceptual artist Helen Chadwick during the 1990s — coincidentally in the lab of one of the embryologists who now works at Guy's, Virginia Bolton (Franklin 1999).

Like Glover, Chadwick immersed herself in the technique of IVF, and became fascinated by the culture of embryo culture. She too used photography as a medium and repeated the seeing-and-touching work of the embryologists' biological gaze to prepare her images, responding with her artists' hands and eyes to the powerful visual aesthetics of embryology and its still-artisanal sense of craft. For her series *Stilled Lives* in 1995, Chadwick created large Plexiglas sculptures of jewelry — a ring, a brooch, a necklace — in which she embedded photographic images of eggs and embryos derived from her work in the lab. Her hands-on training with embryologists had taught Chadwick how to grade embryos for clinical use, much as a jeweler would assess a precious gem. In her artwork, Chadwick built on these associations — not only in terms of the precious value of embryos, but in terms of the delicate manual skills needed to handle and manipulate them (Warner 1996). Chadwick, whose art frequently concerned her own body, became fascinated, for example, by the way lab technicians would use suction pipettes — incorporating their breath into the process of creating new life. Similarly, she was captured by the drama of life's delicacy in the petri dish, where some eggs developed beautifully, but others, inexplicably, failed to thrive. Much of Chadwick's embryo art was focused on the proximity between life and death in the context of IVF, and how this tension was repeated in her own art through photography. Her title *Stilled Lives* captures this ambivalence, since the photograph at once entombs its dead image in emulsion and animates it as a photographic image simulating real life.[14]

Like Glover, Chadwick was struck by the power of the embryological gaze to redefine the world around her. Perhaps affected by the same "eggs are everywhere" obsession described by Glover, Chadwick frequently depicted embryos in the company of seeds, flowers, eyes, hair loops, and air bubbles, suggesting a shared kinship of form, as well as natural history. This kinship of form is extended in Chadwick's work, like Glover's, to stars and the galaxy, as in Chadwick's piece *Nebula*. But whereas Chadwick's experience of IVF was based largely in the lab, Glover's artwork combines the experiences of patients, scientists, and clinicians—attempting to give voice to the world of IVF they together inhabit—in part through transformative ways of seeing that become a shared language in pursuit of a shared goal. Repeatedly she depicts both the strangeness and the ordinariness of the world of IVF in her photographic compositions, which attempt to translate these experiences into a visual vocabulary. Thus, for example, in *Yes!*—Glover's calendric imitation of counting the days of an IVF cycle—she uses rows of pregnancy test wands to translate the experience of waiting for results during the process of IVF into a stylized, repetitive sentence of images ending in victory (figure 7.9). At times she employs the actual voices of both clinicians and patients, collected during her residency, by superimposing their words over composite images she has made to express them visually. Hence in *Nigella* she has incorporated extracts from transcripts from her local interlocutors, much as an ethnographer might (figure 7.10).

This sense of the social fabric of relationality contextualizing everything about the often fraught and inevitably highly charged emotional experience of undergoing IVF is not easily captured visually, and this may be one reason Glover uses the medium of fabrics extensively throughout her work. These fabrics include not only socks and ties, or cozies, but quilts and also Suffolk Puffs, a distinctive fabric construction created by gathering cloth into stylized bunches, shaped like buds, and used in quilting, upholstery, and home decorating. The incorporation of this traditional domestic craft into Glover's artwork draws associations not only with homemaking, but with female labor,

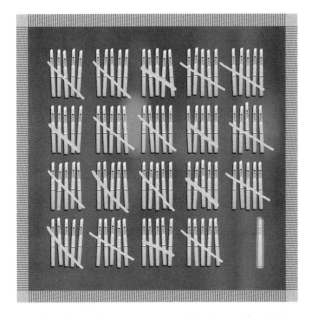

FIGURE 7.9.
Yes! Reproduced with
permission of the
artist, Gina Glover.

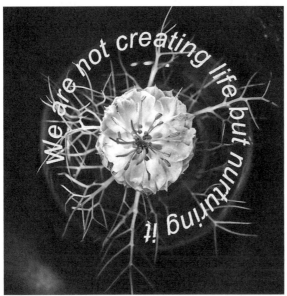

FIGURE 7.10.
Nigella. Reproduced
with permission
of the artist, Gina
Glover.

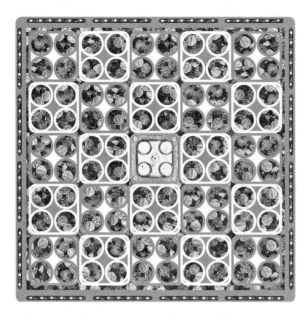

FIGURE 7.11.
Suffolk Puffs.
Reproduced with
permission of the
artist, Gina Glover.

expertise, and manual skill—the domestic arts. Glover's photomontage of a quilt made of Suffolk Puffs in petri dishes captures the social role of fabric in her wider aesthetic vocabulary, suggesting the extent to which people's entire lives are, in a sense, stuffed into a tiny glass world as they make their passage through the ordeal that is IVF (figure 7.11). At the same time, the clustering of so many tiny worlds together as a patchwork quilt evokes the sense of solidarity often forged among couples undergoing IVF, and conveys the collective effort involved in such a project, including the professional IVF team moving things forward. Indeed from this point of view, the quilted quality of so many of Glover's Photoshopped compositions might also be seen to define her role as a residential, translational, frontier artist—knitting together the fabric of the IVF world into photomontages that are at once beautiful patchworks, finely crafted objects, composites of a myriad domestic bits and pieces, and necessary means of keeping out the cold.

THE REPRODUCTIVE FRONTIER

The art of quilting, one of the traditional feminine domestic crafts celebrated by Judy Chicago in her landmark installation piece *The Dinner Party*, is suggestive not only of feminized labor, or art, but also the frontier. In its associations with the economical reuse of leftover fabric, the practicality born of necessity, the provision of much-needed protection against the elements, and the crucial importance of neighborly assistance (the quilting bee being the feminine equivalent of barn raising), the quilt continues to evoke a frontier heritage. In addition to the sexual division of reproductive labor referenced throughout Glover's *Art of A.R.T.* is thus a longer inheritance of the gendered norms of both domestic labor and technology, evident, for example, in the use of Suffolk Puffs. In turn, these legacies evoke the familiar interiority of domestic worlds, be they the delicate china collections of middle-class Victorian dining rooms, or the busy kitchens of suburban housewives in present-day London.

Writing of the American frontier, the literary theorist Annette Kolodny (1975, 1984) describes a gendered space, in which cultivation acquires contradictory meanings of both harmony and destruction. On the one hand a space of promise, hope, and future fulfillment, the expanding westward frontier also left in its wake a trail of environmental pillage that early commentators such as the naturalist and explorer James Audubon described as an abuse of the land. Guiding the westward expansion, Kolodny argues, were familiar gendered archetypes of reproduction, sexuality, and marriage, ultimately manifest as a defining ambivalence toward "the lay of the land."[15] Citing Frederick Jackson Turner's famous 1893 frontier hypothesis, she notes that he "made explicit what had always been the experiential truth of the American continent: the West was a woman, and to it belonged the hope of rebirth and regeneration" (Kolodny 1975: 137). "European men, institutions and ideas," wrote Turner,

> were lodged in the American wilderness, and this great American West took them to her bosom, taught them a new way of looking upon the destiny of the common man, trained them in adaptation to the conditions of the New World, to the creation of new institutions to meet new needs; and ever as society on her eastern border grew to resemble the Old World in its social forms and its industry, as it began to lose faith in the ideal of democracy, she opened new provinces, and dowered new democracies in her most distant domains with her material treasures. (Turner cited in Kolodny 1975: 137)

Such a vividly gendered description, argues Kolodny, cannot be dismissed as merely metaphoric in its language, for the gendered polarities evident in this passage are too ubiquitous to ignore, and too structurally prominent in frontier life to overlook, complex and contradictory though they may be. These gendered images she suggests, are crucial to understanding the postfrontier colonial ethos Turner described as the founding basis of the American character and nation—an ethos that has now been transferred, with equally complex implications, into the pursuit of scientific and technological frontiers, such as reproductive biomedicine:

> Colonization brought with it an inevitable paradox: the success of settlement depended on the ability to master the land, transforming the virgin territories into something else—a farm, a village, a road, a canal, a railway, a mine, a factory, a city, and finally, an urban nation. As a result, those who initially responded to the promise inherent in a feminine landscape were now faced with the consequences of that response: either they recoiled in horror from the meaning of their manipulation of a naturally generous world . . . or they continue[d] pursuing the fantasy in daily life. (1975: 7, references removed)

In labeling this phenomenon the "uniquely American pastoral impulse" (1975: 8), and claiming that it is a defining legacy of ambivalence formed in the context of frontier experience and mythology, Kolodny's analysis raises important questions about the transfer of the American frontier analogy into science.[16] Indeed, nothing about her attention to the formative roles of gender polarity, the sexual division of labor, the imagery of rebirth, or the idiom of conjugality in the making of the American frontier ethos would be unfamiliar to feminist theorists of science more generally, including Evelyn Fox Keller, who points out in her analysis of gender and science:

> Of course, not all scientists have embraced the conception of science as one of "putting nature on the rack and torturing the answers out of her." Nor have all men embraced a conception of masculinity that demands cool detachment and domination. Nor even have all scientists been men. But most have. And however variable the attitudes of individual male scientists toward science and toward masculinity, the metaphor of a marriage between mind and nature necessarily does not look the same to them as it does to women. . . . In a science constructed around the naming of an object (nature) as female and the parallel naming of a subject (mind) as male, any scientist who happens to be a woman is confronted with an a priori contradiction in terms. (1996b: 174)

The implications of both Kolodny's and Keller's arguments in the context of a new scientific frontier that is premised upon ever greater control of the female reproductive system are precisely those mapped out so powerfully in the feminist literature on new reproductive technologies discussed in chapter 5. And it is no wonder that these implications have been the subject of strongly worded and often passionate feminist writing, as well as ongoing feminist debate. If, as also noted earlier, the dominant turn in this literature has been away from a more archetypal or categorical analysis of patriarchy versus women's bodies and instead toward the contradictory, ambivalent, equivocal, and often unresolved worlds of the people who inhabit this new frontier zone, with all its porosity and indeterminacy, the question of how technologies of gender both make and are remade upon the reproductive frontier remains a necessarily prominent one. Arguably, in fact, it is what the lens of gender or sex as technologies reveals about the development of IVF that we have yet fully either to perceive or articulate.[17]

In her description of her monumental feminist artwork, *The Dinner Party*, celebrating the regendering of artistic creativity, Judy Chicago (1996) describes not only her attempt to recover lost and undervalued feminine art forms, such as embroidery and ceramics, but also her effort to reclaim public space for these woman-identified, and often privatized, artisanal arts. Across her immense triangular (vaginal) table, Chicago deploys various media to produce a celebration of female artistic achievement, using the thirty-nine place settings commemorating goddesses and important historic women to showcase forgotten and marginalized feminine domestic arts, such as china painting, lace making, and needlework. Her "organic iconography" of plates derives from her own personal struggle to express herself as a female artist (memorably recorded in her autobiography, *Through the Flower*, 1977), and is intended to inspire women to create images of themselves "as subjects rather than as objects" (1996: 5). Decrying the "absence of public monuments," the "absence of political leaders," and the "absence in our museum of images" (1996: 5), Chicago sought to reclaim public space for female self-expression as well as to inspire women to produce more assertive imagery of themselves.

A significant part of the development of *The Dinner Party* project from its inception was an emphasis on teamwork. Initially with a few friends and supporters, and later with large teams of up to thirty people, Chicago attempted to integrate a sense of group process into the finished work by encouraging dialogue about the piece as it developed. At evening potluck dinners every Thursday, discussions were held to address both technical problems and the broad philosophical and political issues raised by the piece. These conversations, which punctuated the process of completing *The Dinner Party* project, are described by Chicago (1996: 8) as "sometimes confrontational" and "often emotionally draining," but above all as crucial to the work, and to the ability to integrate dialogue and process into the finished piece.

Indeed, *The Dinner Party* project has continued to generate debate — it remains a talking point; it continues to stimulate conversation; and it continues to inspire criticism as well as praise. Like the contemporaneous feminist debates about reproductive technologies, it continues to evoke a sense of collectivity, as well as division. In its material form the project remains didactically curatorial—reminding viewers of the narrow definition of high art and who has been excluded from this tradition. Overall it succeeds in its original aims—of publicly exhibiting the world of female art, of putting women's experience on display, and thus creating an artistic soil out of which other similar projects can grow in the future.

Sitting in the waiting room of the Guy's ACU, surrounded by Gina Glover's artwork, it is clear she has accomplished a similar task. By reflecting the experiences of IVF patients back to them through her Art of A.R.T., she too has used artistic form to stimulate dialogue and to uncover the emotional realities of assisted reproduction. By visualizing women's (and men's) experience of IVF, and hanging it on the wall, she has transformed the often uncomfortably public experience of this technique into a new form of kinship. By incorporating her own autobiography as a woman, a mother, an artist, a traveler, a tourist, a photographer, a shopper, a collector, and a Londoner into her work, she has infused her images with the ordinary business of living a life—thus integrating herself into the sociality she is depicting as an invitation for others to do the same. As I have often observed myself while visiting the clinic, the images become interactive windows for the assembled members of the waiting room—not all of them patients, some being children or relatives of individuals or couples having treatment. Similarly, the staff members in the clinic and the lab take considerable pride in the presence of Gina's work, which they describe as both an inclusive aesthetic and a constructive visual presence that assists them in the work they do.

The atmosphere of the clinic is noticeably different because of the presence of the installation as a whole, fused as it is with the clinic's architecture, thus signifying not only an interest in patients' lives, emotions, and labor, but the desire to recognize and include these nonclinical aspects of patients' lives in the daily working life of the clinic. The prominence of artwork in the elevator exit area, before visitors have even entered the clinic, sends a powerful message about what kind of clinic it sees itself to be: it is not a clinic that shies away from the struggles that living IVF involves, the questions it poses, the hurdles it presents, or the doubts it may raise. It is a clinic that hangs on its walls questions that do not have easy answers.

This is another reason why The Art of A.R.T. is a distinctive window onto the culture of embryo culture and the world of IVF. The work of bioartists such as Helen Chadwick and Gina Glover, along with many others, such as Suzanne Anker, enable us not only to contemplate, but to reinhabit the biological, molecular, and embryological ways of seeing that define the remaking of human reproductivity in the context of contemporary bioscience. They effect an artistic translation of translational sciences such as IVF and stem cell research, providing the basis for reflection, conversation, and dialogue. On display in the Guy's ACU is an installation that highlights the constitutive ambivalence of IVF—its "curiouser and curiouser" character posed as a series of re-presentations of its artifice, and as a series of questions about living the remaking of life. Skillful bioartists are making these questions, reflections, and ambivalences more prominently visible as works of art, and thus as windows onto the question concerning technology as this question becomes ever more intimately biological. By exploring not only the biological gaze of the scientist but the biographical ways of seeing of those who live in closest proximity to biotechniques, artists such as Gina Glover have imaginatively transformed the scientific lens into a window through which to observe and contemplate the looking-glass world of IVF. From this vantage point, it becomes possible to reconsider what kind of frontier territory is being inhabited, or domesticated, in the context of new reproductive technologies on both sides of the hole in the wall, or open door, connecting them.

Although her work does not explicitly concern human embryonic stem cell derivation, Glover's art is nonetheless helpful as a means of exploring the IVF–stem cell interface, as throughout her installation are reminders of the work that is involved in handling life as well as the emotional and physical demands of treatment. Inside the lab, biologists are making human cellular models in order to see into the workings of human biology: these new human tools, including IVF itself, comprise a way of seeing that is based on replicating the object being investigated—imitating it with a purpose, we might say. This is, at the most obvious level, the whole point, for example, of a dish model of disease: it has advantages over animal models not only because it is human, and accessible, but because experimentally it can be manipulated and observed more directly—it is "the best tool you can get." This way of seeing through the synthetic and the bespoke is how IVF was first developed—as a handmade model of human conception in glass.

Outside the lab are the IVF patients who are engaging with the retooling of reproductive substance in the most intimate and personal way—by attempting to achieve a successful pregnancy. And yet, like the experimentalism of science, this attempt to move forward often fails, and even when it succeeds may lead in unexpected directions. At once guided by the biological gaze, this way of seeing is also blind in many of the most important respects. What it can see is dependent on what becomes its background, but even the very best visual tools of science are often deceptive in what they show—as both patients and clinicians are well aware. And there is of course a whole world that is never the object of the scientific gaze to begin with. Following the path of scientific progress requires becoming literate in these gaps and ambivalences, as well as learning how to read a karyotype.

As Anker and Nelkin (2004) note in their important analysis of bioart, artists have to a certain extent turned the logic of the instrumental biological gaze on its head—or inside out. The handmade synthetics that artists see through are their own creations and are dedicated to human artifice in, of, and for itself—often using their own bodies, biologies, and autobiographies as resources for what Beatriz da Costa and Kavita Philip (2008) describe as "tactical biopolitics." As Anker and Nelkin point out, the tools, materials, and techniques used by scientists and bioartists increasingly overlap—indeed they are frequently identical.[18] But as Anker and Nelkin also note, "ultimately the images generated by scientists and those provided by artists are based on quite different epistemologies. . . . They represent quite distinct ways of knowing the world" (2004: 189).

For anthropologists of science too, this conceptual difference holds an important methodological lesson, particularly perhaps for ethnography, which also relies on imitation as a learning tool, and writing as a technology, or art, of creative revealing. As it turns out, the anthropology of the life sciences is also a lens for seeing the remaking of biological life, using well-worn techniques for depicting social relationships—such as collecting observations and writing about them. Similarly, in Gina Glover's artwork is evident the importance not only of new biological tools, but of living with them—ambivalently, emotionally, and physiologically. Her artwork demonstrates how these biological and biographical relations to technology are knitted together on the frontier of reproductive pioneering—a frontier defined by the coupling of substance and tool. As well as revealing the art of ART, Gina Glover's artwork depicts a new frontier of biological relativity in which the social, the biological, and the technical are lived ambivalently together.

In this way, Glover's artistic insights are similar to those produced by Rayna Rapp (1999) in her ethnographic description of the moral pioneering engaged in by women in the context of new reproductive technologies. As Rapp notes, the advent of new reproductive technology also creates "moral pioneers" situated on "a research frontier," where women being offered difficult and unprecedented decisions and choices are also "making concrete and embodied decisions about the standard for entry into the human community" (1999: 3). Contesting the privatization and invisibility of this context of moral pioneering, she argues, "A classic feminist analysis might begin by noting that women have long been relegated to the sociocultural domain of the family, intimacy and the private; thus important cultural and political tensions concerning the limits of individualism, privacy and bodily integrity have been played out by our potentially reproductive bodies. . . . Multiple iterations of our sex/gender system index our medico-legal system. . . . Women are thus culturally positioned to think about their reproductive capacities, desires, and decisions as a private dimension of public life" (306). Rapp, like Strathern, describes the emergence of new reproductive technologies such as amniocentesis as "an impromptu and large-scale social experiment" (309), adding that the work of moral pioneering is one of reshaping "a more social terrain" in which these technologies can be more consciously and ethically inhabited. The exclusion of reproduction from the public sphere, and its relegation to the privatized and feminized world of personal reproductive decision making, deprive the larger society of a crucial resource, she argues.

Arguably this privatization of reproduction, reproductive ethics, and reproductive politics is one of the conditions that is changing after IVF. One of the consequences of the rapid expansion of IVF over the past thirty years, and its expansion into stem cell research, in labs such as the one at Guy's, has been to make more publicly visible the political importance of a highly feminized and privatized reproductive frontier. Indeed, Rapp's use of the terms "pioneering" and "frontier" encourage such a change, invoking as they do idioms more traditionally associated, as Kolodny argues, with a masculine realm of exploration and discovery. Somewhat unexpectedly, perhaps, the hole in the wall puncturing the border between IVF and stem cell research is thus also a window connecting one definition of the political in the past with another that is already taking shape in the present—under a very different definition of biopolitics that has more in common with reproductive politics. In the same way we may be cautious about adopting the idiom of the frontier at all, given its militaristic and colonial origins, so too we would rightly be wary of overestimating the influence of the way of seeing introduced by the newly porous and hybrid relationship between bioscience and reproductive biomedicine. To pursue this effort further, it will be necessary to understand and depict with greater clarity the extent to which experimental science is never separate from the experiment of being social at all.

EIGHT After IVF

The future of kinship that is explored in this book through the lens of IVF inevitably raises the question of how kinship has been thought in the past—especially since the kinship concept is itself a tool, in both quotidian and academic life. The history of kinship theory is itself relational in the sense that kinship models are proposed and reproposed analytically and comparatively over time (Carsten 2004; Strathern 2005), and so too is it an evolving technology. While I have been writing this book, for example, I have been teaching kinship theory to students by examining how the very earliest debates about marriage, family, parenthood, and kinship out of which anthropology and sociology emerged in the late nineteenth century are related to current public consultation exercises occurring in the midst of the vast dissemination of shared reproductive substance in the present. Such debates not only belong to academic dialogue, they are active in social life—arguably in no small part due to the rise of new reproductive technologies over the past thirty years (Franklin and McKinnon 2001). Hence, while writing this conclusion I also prepared a short presentation for the Nuffield Council of Bioethics in London to assist them in their inquiry concerning mitochondrial donation—a new species of technological transfer of reproductive substance engendering debate about children with three genetic parents. Such an inquiry is a typically recursive exercise—a reiteration of kinship substance as sign, to model a problem, in this case addressing an ethical question about a code of conduct. Pronuclear and maternal spindle transfer techniques (PNT and MST), the council explains on the background information sheet prepared for their inquiry, raise new ethical questions, which they phrase in terms of kin ties, such as, "What might the use of these techniques signify for the relationships of the resulting child to the three adults with whom it shares a genetic condition?" How, the members of the council's working group would like to know from expert witnesses from the social sciences, social psychology, and other disciplines, "might mitochondrial DNA be associated with a person's identity?" The scope of such kinship dilemmas is not narrowing as reproductive and genetic biomedical interventions become more precise: to the contrary (and handily for anthropology teaching), the kinship dilemmas engendered by these applications have now become analogies for one another in the increasingly complex field of technologically assisted reproductive possibilities. Hence, the council asks, "could the relationships . . . between the mitochondrial donor and a person born with their donated mitochondria be seen as similar to those involved in: a) organ or tissue transplantation? b) gamete donation? c) donation of other bodily material?" Or, the members of the working group would like to know, "should [they] be seen as unique?" (Nuffield 2012).

Politically, it is now the established norm in the United Kingdom, where many innovative biomedical technologies affecting reproduction in both humans and nonhumans have been developed and introduced, for the implementation of translational science to be accompanied by a formal process of public consultation and dialogue. Often these translational biomedical efforts originate in formal and semiformal consultation and dialogue between patient groups and clinicians, leading to the involvement of scientists and clinicians to see if new solutions can be found, as is the case with PNT and MST, which are intended to alleviate the burden of severe inherited mitochondrial (genetic) disease. Without overstating the role of dialogue (or rehearsing its shortcomings), it is not inaccurate to point out that modern health measures responding to rare, often obscure, genetic diseases typically include a dialogic component at both ends of, and often throughout, the process of their development. This component is indeed perceived as critical to translational success. Ensuring that a consultation process, or talk, is built into a proposed application is now considered to be a crucial component in the introduction of new technologies (Burchell et al. 2009; Davies 2008).

If, in other words, the proposed clinical introduction of mitochondrial transfer rehearses a familiar process of seeking public consent to rewrite heredity in the name of improved human health, so too we might suggest that both this technical process of genetic reinscription and the larger hybrid genre of biomedical translation to which it belongs, are multiply authored, combining not only numerous voices, or forms of dialogue, but different kinds of technological comparison. As the Nuffield Council notes, the situation of a child being born who has genetic relationships to three people is in some ways novel: "the genetic link between a mitochondrial donor and the individual created using this donation has a relatively ambiguous social framework by which to contextualise it" (Nuffield 2012: 2). At the same time, they add, such possibilities already have analogies in the form of other kindred procedures: "The possible ambiguity in the perception of the social relationship between the resulting child and the donating woman that would be brought about after the use of maternal spindle and pronuclear transfer is also seen in the range of language used to describe the parentage of people born after the use of these procedures" (2).

As well as belonging to an increasingly familiar genre of technologically assisted biology, the novel transfer of reproductive substance in the context of PNT and MST thus already inherits "the range of language used to describe the parentage of people born after the use of these procedures." In addition, the council notes, "there is an online market for information about mitochondrial heritage [although] not a great deal is known about perceptions of any social meaning within this genetic relationship" (Nuffield 2012: 2). As they have already suggested, analogies can be drawn to other forms of tissue and cell donation, as well as assisted conception technologies such as IVF. And these analogies are part of the translational process by which reproductive substance has become more publicly acknowledged through media such as the Internet.

Here, as in the history of kinship theory, a relation is established between past and future models of parenthood in the formation of the body politic. The Nuffield consultation replicates this process of serial modeling by introducing a range of comparative contexts and examples in its call for dialogue about the future of kinship. The future of new kinship technologies is thus contextualized through comparisons to those forms of biomedical assistance that already have human histories, such as IVF. We might call this process "conditional comparison" in the way the histories of recent technological innovations condition the prospect of their expansion in the future. And this is a conventional form of consultation, characterized by the weighing up of unknown and ambivalent future technological possibilities against what can be known from the past: many, if not most, public dialogues about the future of technology now take this form.

The following account of conditional comparison illustrates more precisely how this process functions, and also why it is important to understanding the relation of being after that is so significant to the history of technology, and to being after IVF. Using a much older example, from one of Plato's dialogues about technology, it is possible to see how dialogue functions as a kind of contact zone in which it is not only interaction with technology that is at stake, but the question of being after, in several senses of this term—after in time, after as in pursuit, after as descent or succession, and after as style. As Haraway notes, these are the many forms of being after that are united in the contact zone: "Contact zones are where the action is, and interactions change interactions that follow. Probabilities alter; topologies morph; development is canalized by the fruits of reciprocal induction. Contact zones change the subject—all of the subjects—in surprising ways" (2008: 451). As the following example suggests, the contact zone is thus itself a reproductive frontier—a space of ambivalent possibility that is shaped, often unpredictably, by multiple interactions. At stake on the frontier is precisely what will come after, and how this can be controlled (or not). And at stake in the question concerning technology is precisely the same set of contingencies. At stake in the future of reproductive technology is therefore not only the question of what kind of kinship will come after MST, but who will be part of the interaction, or dialogue, that shapes and guides this process.

The fear of technological futures that the following example illustrates is thus one to which, as we shall see, the politics of reproduction is both central and primary. For it is the anxiety engendered by the specter of technology racing ahead and spiraling out of control that haunts the threshold of new techniques such as IVF with the "monstrous" possibility of a degenerative "after." The ambivalence that attaches to reproductive technologies such as IVF has many dimensions, but the question of which "after" will ensue from the next technological step forward is one of the most familiar of its forms. It is the fear of degeneration in the wake of technological change, set against the more confident expectation of an improved, more fruitful, future, that has long characterized technological ambivalence. But equally evident, and somewhat more curious, is the strikingly repetitive and overdetermined form of the question concerning technology as one in which it is the future of kinship—and the question of what kind of kinship it will be—that is seen to be at stake, even in some of the very oldest dialogues about changing technological inheritance.

Hothouse

In the Platonic dialogue titled *Phaedrus*, after the young literary impressario whose peripatetic conversation with Socrates is its subject, the technology at issue is the written word. In the closing section of the dialogue, Socrates reflects on the relation of writing to speech, denigrating writing as a degenerate copy of living words. Using the analogy of horticulture, he contrasts the forced hothouse growing of plants for a party with their "sensible" agricultural production in order to castigate written speeches, and the damage they do to men who mistake the mere possession of information conveyed through "alien marks" for the active, vital integrity of spoken rhetoric (Plato 2005: 62–64). The proper pursuit of truth through speaking, argues Socrates, produces wisdom as knowledge of its absence. Writing, by contrast, produces absence of memory in place of truth. "Socrates: So tell me this: the sensible farmer who had some seeds he cared about and wanted to bear fruit—would he sow them in some Garden of Adonis [forced pots] and delight in watching the garden become beautiful in eight days . . . for the sake of amusement on a feast day [or] would he make use of the science of farming and sow them in appropriate soil, being content if they reached maturity in eight months?" (2005: 64). Only "the man who thinks he has left behind a science in writing" and is thus "full of simplicity," Socrates advises his young companion, would confuse "written words" with "the man who knows the subjects to which the written things relate" and can speak of them unassisted by technical devices (63). So too does Socrates warn that writing is but "black water sown through a pen" producing sterile "words that are incapable of speaking in their own support, and incapable of adequately teaching what is true." The "garden of letters" is not only "without fruit" but is a sterile caricature of speech. It is incapable of generating "a seed from which others grow in other soils" or of "rendering the seed forever immortal," and thus lacks the virtue of "making the one who has it as happy as a man can be" (65).

Writing, Socrates continues, is but a "phantom" with the "strange feature . . . like painting" of standing "as if alive" and yet remaining mute, defenseless, and passive. It lacks a proper origin to give it any character of its own because it is a mere copy. Letters, he claims, give but "the appearance of wisdom":

The offspring of painting stand there as if alive, but if you ask them something, they preserve a quite solemn silence. Similarly with written words: you might think that they spoke as if they had some thought in their heads, but if you ever ask them about any of the things they say out of a desire to learn, they point to just one thing, the same each time. And when once it is written, every composition trundles about everywhere in the same way, in the presence both of those who know about the subject and those who have nothing at all to do with it, and it does not know how to address those it should address, and not those it should not. When it is ill treated and unjustly abused, it always needs its father to help it; for it is incapable of either defending or helping itself. (Plato 2005: 63)

Suffused with the language of reproduction and fertility, as well as generation and paternity, these passages from Plato's dialogue depict technology in one of its formative dehumanizing moments in the history of philosophy—one that equates written words with deceit, illegitimacy, and death. A temptation, or even magical elixir, the artifice of written inscription is equated with a loss of humanity, a loss of truth, and a loss of self. This emphasis on loss and degeneration is the same theme that later animates the work of both Husserl and Heidegger in their discussions of technology, and motivates Derrida's lifelong effort to reclaim a place for the "garden of letters" in the horticultural aspirations of the "sensible farmer." The "crisis of the European sciences" depicted by Husserl as one of "mathematization" finds its echo in the fear of loss that Habermas (2010), arguing in this same tradition, later denigrates as technological automatism.

But what is of particular note in this passage from one of the foundational inherited texts of classical philosophy concerning the degenerative effects of technological reproduction is the dense intertwining of the issue of technological futurity with the reproduction of parenthood and the conventional structures of kinship. The relation of being after is entirely at stake in this dialogue, in which the misapplication of technology is equated not only to a loss of humanity but to a warping of kinship relations. Being after writing, in the sense of modeling oneself upon its artifice, is compared to being an abject orphan unrelated by kinship: "it does not know how to address those it should address, and not those it should not." The relation of "after" suggested by Plato's comparison of writing to misspent horticulture, to barrenness, and to wilful ignorance is one that equates technological reproduction not only with diminished individual capacity and exclusion from kinship, but terminal failure of the elementary reproductivity kinship organizes.

Plato's depiction of the dehumanizing effects of being after a technology that caricatures an original is a powerful strand in the history of philosophy, and one that is centrally animated by the specter of degeneration. Hannah Arendt similarly described the "banality" of "artificial life" and the "forgetting" of "normal expression in speech and thought" that accompany "new scientific and technical knowledge" in the opening pages of *The Human Condition*, published in 1958, in response to the development and use of atomic weapons. A German Jewish refugee, she was understandably cautious about the seemingly inverse relationship of "the modern scientific worldview" and "science's great triumphs" to the role of "thinking and speaking"—especially since, she warned, "speech is what makes man a political being" (Arendt 1958: 3). Technology is what makes us human, she admitted, but we should never let even the greatest glories of human artifice to allow us to forget that "life itself is outside this artificial world" (2). Like Socrates (Plato), she uses a form of potted life to illustrate her point—the test-tube baby. "The human artifice of the world separates human existence from all mere animal environment, but life itself is outside this artificial world, and through life man remains related to all other living organisms. For some time now, a great many scientific endeavours have been directed toward making life also 'artificial,' [such as those] manifest in the attempt to create life in the test-tube" (2).

Such ambitious artifice, Arendt warns, presumes for future man "an exchange" of the "free gift" of human life "for something he has made himself" (1958: 2–3)—in sum, for an artificial human condition, and thus for a relation of being after that is defined by loss. Such an exchange, she cautions, would create a potentially "final" forgetting that "would be as though our brain . . . were unable to follow what we do, so that from now on we would indeed need artificial machines to do our thinking and speaking." The conditions that define human existence after the test-tube baby would no longer be those of the earth, birth, nature, or "life itself" but instead a "desire to escape" that would require a "turning-away" from these elementary human conditions, by a "cutting of the last tie" to them in a "fateful repudiation" (2). "If it should turn out to be true that knowledge (in the modern sense of know-how) and thought have parted company for good, then we would indeed become the helpless slaves, not so much of our machines as of our know-how, thoughtless creatures at the mercy of every gadget which is technically possible, no matter how murderous it is" (3). But how is it that knowledge and know-how part company for good through artifice? Is this "cutting of the last tie" between technology and thought equivalent to the Platonic denunciation of writing as a diminution of humanity?

Only a year after publication of *The Human Condition*, in 1959, Jacques Derrida gave his first lecture on the work of Husserl, "'Genesis and Structure' and Phenomenology"—in which he publicly launched his critique of the philosophical tradition of logos, or logocentrism, as the basis of transcendental humanism precisely by offering an alternative account of kinship and technology. Turning to the anthropological materialism of both Marx and the French paleontologist André Leroi-Gourhan, Derrida introduced an account of *techne* as the invention of the human—the ground on which human thought invents itself—only ever in an artificial world, and indeed only ever as the artifice that is "man." Following Leroi-Gourhan, who argues that the human body—its upright skeletal posture, the molding of the human hand, the flattening of the human face—coevolves with the apparatus humans invent, from flints and pots to language and signs, Derrida (1974) reads the history of "originary technics" as one of regeneration.

Like Marx, many of Derrida's analogies for technology are biological. Thus he understands writing as a living system comparable to an organism, with a kinship to other technologies, for which one of his many analogies is grafting. In order even to begin to read a written text, one must become enjoined with its physiology, he claims, just as the text itself is the live offspring of previous couplings. In his critique of Plato's *Phaedrus*, aptly titled *Dissemination*, Derrida's (1981) vocabulary borrows and mutates Plato's terminology to reconstitute technics as both growth and life. From the outset Derrida describes writing as a "tissue," morphing Plato's depiction of logos as a *zoon*, "an animal that is born, grows, belongs to the *phusis*" (Derrida 1981: 79). Through this metaphor, Derrida grafts his own reading of Plato's text into its body, making it live according to different "rules of the game." He reconstitutes the reader's living relationship to the written text "as an organism, indefinitely regenerating its own tissue behind the cutting trace, the decision of each reading" (1981: 63). For Derrida, writing is not dead or barren because it is a copy of an original, but instead more lively because it is recombinant.

To further his point, Derrida morphically engages Plato's analogy between technological and reproductive futurity. In contrast to the open-ended possibilities of living technics figured by the hybrid, regenerative graft, Derrida critiques Plato's idealized image of logos as a "household . . . from which one does not escape" (1981: 81), a place of ordered co-habitation, governed by the proper laws of kinship as a (patri)lineage. Writing, as Derrida notes, has been accorded the status of an orphan in Plato's kinship system, "deformed by its very birth" (148). In Plato's view, writing is "not well born" both because it is "not entirely viable" and because it is "outside of the law" (Derrida 1981: 148). The relation of proper speech to this household ought to be properly filial— the offspring should know their names "by heart." This is the position Plato advocates through his analogy to the serious farmer, who does not waste his seed, thus giving rise to the title of Derrida's response as *Dissemination*. As Derrida summarizes Plato's (Socrates's) logic in his account (above) of proper planting by the serious farmer, it is a parable of propriety—of proper seeds: "Here is the analogy: simulacrum-writing is to what it represents . . . as weak, easily exhausted, superfluous seeds giving rise to ephemeral produce (floriferous seeds) are to strong, fertile seeds engendering necessary, lasting, nourishing produce (fructiferous seeds). On the one hand, we have the patient, sensible farmer; on the other, the Sunday gardener, hasty, dabbling, and frivolous. On the one hand, the serious; on the other the game and the holiday. On the one hand cultivation, agriculture, knowledge, economy; on the other, art, enjoyment and unreserved spending" (1981: 150, original Greek terms removed). In Derrida's summation of Plato's agricultural parable, he emphasizes not only the pattern of opposing natural truth to moribund artifice that lies at the heart of Platonism, and at the root of logocentrism, but also their relationship to technological futurity—imagined through the idioms of kinship and procreation, as well as horticulture. Thus, we can interpret the analogy to include the proper relation of offspring who answer when their names are called, and take root in the correct soil to become well cultivated. However, Derrida's point is that these very distinctions constantly dissolve into themselves, relying upon the very terms they imagine as other to them, in the process of espousing an imagined transcendence. After all, Plato's critique of writing was delivered in writing: "while condemning writing as a lost or parricidal son, Plato behaves like a son *writing* this condemnation," writes Derrida (1981: 153).

Derrida pointedly compares his own analytical process of dissolving boundaries ("deconstruction") to another horticultural practice—to grafting (a form of cloning)—in a footnote in *Dissemination* addressed to the comparison of writing and agriculture in *Phaedrus*:

> Within the problematic space that brings together, by opposing them, writing and agriculture, it could easily be shown that the paradoxes of the supplement . . . are the same as those of the graft, of the operation of grafting . . . of the grafter, of the grafting knife and of the scion. It could also be shown that all the most modern dimensions (biological, psychical, ethical) of the problem of graft, even when they concern parts believed to be . . . perfectly "proper," . . . are caught up and constrained within the graphics of the supplement. (1981: 184–185)

In other words, to write about the dangers of writing is to perform an act that undoes its own propriety, because the means by which this end is achieved exceed and contradict the logic of its purpose. This is what Derrida refers to as "the graphics of the supplement"—a recursive process he compares to grafting in the way a handheld tool connects an "alien" part to the original stem. Each part—scion (root), plant (stem), tool (knife), and hand (grafter)—exists within a larger whole at once "dissolvable" and integral—and regenerative. The graft is not dissimilar to the analogy used by Strathern (1992a) to describe merographic thinking—through which a partial connection "from another angle" can displace one meaning for another—a process she describes as substitution in her critique of the metaphysics of nature and culture. The horticultural analogy of the graft is also familiar from the context of embryology, where Strathern's analogy, like Derrida's, reverberates (indeed, revertebrates).

Both models take on suggestive connotations in the context of Spemann's famous tied embryo—and grafted blastomeres—where a different sort of metaphysical principle, of organization, exists in a complex relation to both technics and the pursuit of truth. Here, the logic of the supplement is empirically replicated in the role of artifacts—those scientific results which may be the consequence of the experimental apparatus rather than the vital processes under investigation. The relevance of this way of "stem thinking" for understanding IVF becomes clearer when we recall its origins as a model system, used in model organisms, to model biological effects. At once an imitation and a substitute for the in vivo process it models in vitro, IVF graphically supplements what is already known about early development by replicating it in glass in a manner that both reveals how it works and changes this process into something else — by making of it a living supplement to demonstrate the laws of life (and indeed to produce new offspring). In a complicated kind of grafting, or more accurately transplantation, or forcing, induced pluripotent stem (iPS) cells are similarly used to model biological processes such as cellular differentiation—while at the same time rendering them more opaque, since the iPS cell is not exactly the same as its unforced equivalent. As in the history of much experimental embryology and IVF, the recombinant path opened by technological innovation does not necessarily lead directly to applications, or even to precise questions. The success of the iPS cell could even be said to have raised more questions than it answers by dissolving the very concepts it reveals.

In vitro fertilization can similarly be described as emerging out of an openended relationship between technical success and scientific progress, or, as Plato might have it, the pursuit of the greatest happiness.[1] In vitro fertilization was born out of the free play of experimental embryology, and the effort to replicate biological mechanisms and pathways, in order both to understand and to alter them, using technology to rewrite substance. The evolution of IVF technology, while narratable in retrospect as cumulative and even linear, was much more haphazard "going forward" toward what remains in many ways a barely charted biological frontier. Consistent with Derrida's textual model of the reinvention of the human via the reinvention of technique, IVF could be described as a site of *transférance*, mutating the Derridean idiom (surely the greatest mark of respect) to describe the ambiguity and supplementarity of the transfer of this technology "into man."

Tellingly, it is this tradition of transférance that leads to human embryonic stem cell propagation—the forcing of lineages of human cells into new forms in the aid of both increasing human knowledge and improving the quality of human lives. Conceived as a process of translation, this field of scientific work recapitulates precisely the pattern Derrida describes as a revivification of historical inheritance at the level of reinscription. Reprogramming a cell to differentiate to order occurs against the backdrop of a constant disorder that is carefully managed in a clean room facility such as the one described in chapter 2. The passaging of stem cells is thus literally and technically described as the translation of lineages of cells into new kinds of biological life. This dense recapitulation, whether it is read as an analogy or not, repeats a distinctive pattern of technological recursion, and one that can be traced through embryology, kinship theory, and philosophy alike.

In attempting to reflect on the genealogy of this novel work of transférance, this book has sought to widen the models of both biology and technology through which we might characterize the condition of being after IVF. Beginning with the question of how we might understand being five million miracle babies later, I have argued that this process of remaking life requires us to engage with what is more unusual about this technique than its rapid routinization into something regular might suggest. In asking what the view of biology or technology, or their evolving kinship with each other, looks like from the perspective offered by the IVF window, I have suggested that the looking-glass world of IVF has become curiouser and curiouser as well as more normal, regular, and comfortable. This double aspect of the view from IVF can be seen not only from close up, in the experiences of those who undergo this procedure or provide IVF services, but from a distance, as the IVF window is interfaced to a wider, watching world, for whom the manipulation of human embryos is now a generic form of imagery.

In addressing the question of how IVF works, and by investigating its mechanisms, the role of other technologies has been foregrounded, in order that we can appreciate IVF, in Raymond Williams's terms, as a cultural form, and "in terms of its place in an existing social formation" (1990: 12). From this perspective, IVF emerges as a complex of a specific kind, but also as a placeholder for a larger set of questions I have approached from the point of view of technological ambivalence, or ambivalent progress. These observations contribute to the effort to characterize the condition of biological relativity IVF both makes explicit and reproduces—a curiouser and curiouser condition IVF substantializes as both a scientific frontier and a lived experience. Here, in the complex effort to navigate the topsy-turvy world of IVF, is the moral pioneering described by Rayna Rapp (1999) as well as the unfolding question of what new biological relations are being forged in the interface between IVF and regenerative medicine. On the other side of the hole in the wall is an ongoing process of remaking life that requires more complex description and analysis, fulfilling Hannah Landecker's (2007) description of how biotechnology changes biology, while also demonstrating how technology is becoming more biological. At the same time, and like the idiom of the frontier itself (and much as Derrida would have predicted), the very distinctions these terms rely upon are being dissolved in the context of the retooling of reproductive substance. The ambivalent condition this produces is hardly new: as Peletz (2001) argues, it characterizes the anthropological description of kinship as lived relations perhaps more than any other feature. The legacy of this ambivalence is captured in the many meanings of "after," from "behind in place or order," "next to," "in quest of," "because of," "regardless of," "in imitation of," "in the style of," "in honor of," "with the same name or close to the same name as," "in conformity to," or "according to the nature or desires of" (*American Heritage Dictionary*). The meaning of being after IVF is similar—it describes an ambivalent position that is constantly being reworked, rewritten, and recomposed. We can understand the relationship between biological relativity and technological ambivalence better by tracing them through the lens of IVF, which offers a revealing case study of their coproduction. The fact that the technological means employed in the pursuit of an imagined objective may themselves engender changes in how that objective is defined, or even reveal new and different objectives, demonstrates that one way technology reveals itself is as an evolving relationality. Not only objects but also subjects are remade along the critical path of technological change, inevitably altering a sense of the past as well as the future. To understand technology in this way also offers us a different perspective on reproduction; for example, one in which there is no such thing as biological reproduction on its own. The crucial object lesson offered by the case of IVF, in sum, is a new model of reproductivity in which the birth of viable offspring both depends upon and changes the social conditions that activate reproductive substance. Ironically, in other words, what being after IVF reveals is both the before that an imagined biological naturalism has for so long obscured, and the empty space of technological autonomism that remains to be filled. From this point of view, of course, IVF is not so much a vehicle to channel viable gametes into fruition. The petri dish is not merely a container in which it is now possible to force a new form of biological fertilization into existence. Instead, IVF provides a new model of viable reproduction for which relationality must remain both the smallest and the largest unit of analysis in order to understand how technologies make people, how people make technology, and why neither process is, in any simple sense, ever only a before or after at all.

By pursuing the question of what it means for the human embryo to have become a tool, I have set a thought experiment in motion that grafts together a
mosaic of perspectives in order to offer what might be called, following Gina
Glover, a "plural resolution" on the problem of how to interpret the changing relationship of biology and technology. The history of IVF, I have argued,
provides a powerful hermeneutic device for interpreting the question of retooling reproductive substance in particular, and the future of kinship more
generally. At the interface of IVF and stem cell technology, a unique window
has been opened up onto both the future of human regenerative medicine
and the history of the effort to technologize biological reproduction. By trans-
porting this looking glass to a range of other sites and locations, I have offered
snapshots onto the landscape of being after IVF. By adding the models of technology and sex from Marx and Foucault to a discussion of IVF, I have argued
that they offer important resources for charting the bumpy path of this technique's emergence, but that they lack adequate capacity to explain what IVF
is reproducing, exactly, or how it changes the very same biological processes
it is imagined to imitate. The resources needed to address gender, technology,
and sex, as well as power and inequality, developed within feminist theory are
all the more important in the context of addressing reproductive technology,
which is also why feminist debates on these topics have occupied a major part
of this book. The complex ambivalence toward IVF first documented by feminist researchers in the 1980s has been extended through an ongoing effort,
largely within the social sciences, to chart this frontier. This literature now
constitutes one of the most extended, empirically based, analytical engage-
ments with the question of living the remaking of life that is available today.
To the extent that, for all of the reasons explored in this book, an enduring
ambivalence toward this technology would appear to be one of its defining

sociological, philosophical, anthropological, and historical characteristics, it will repay future analysts of this field to explore it further. The ambivalent progress that characterizes IVF is a feature of biological relativity more generally, and is as legible in the frontier analogy of scientific exploration as it is in Gina Glover's *Art of A.R.T.* or in the induced pluripotent stem cell.

A different future for speech than the one depicted in *Phaedrus* is the one in which dialogue is not opposed to technics but is instead built into it—making technics dialogic, as it were. This is the vital sense of dialogue as it is espoused by Hannah Arendt (1958) through her concern about IVF and "artificial life," and her reminder of the dangers of remaining silent in the face of the "banality" of technology. Pertinent though it may be to point out that we have not become helpless slaves to our gadgets half a century later (although there is certainly ongoing concern about this possibility), and metaphysical though her appeal to life itself may have been at the time, it is nonetheless such a model of dialogue this book shares. To the extent that the conversation outlined in this book offers a different set of starting points from which to view the remaking of life, that sees in it neither apocalyptic doom nor transhumanist evangelism, but instead an ongoing process of navigating the same ambivalent relationship to technology that characterizes identity or society itself, *Biological Relatives* has contributed to the kind of dialogue Arendt imagined. If this book has introduced useful tools for analyzing biological relativity, technological ambivalence, and the condition of being after IVF, so much the better for a dialogic future of technics. And if the value of attending closely to the experiences of people who inhabit the evolving reproductive frontier has been instructive, this too is a contribution to wiser speech and thought. The grafting of careful thought into our regenerative relationship to biology as technology, to the retooling of reproductive substance, to the hole in the wall, and to the open door to the petri dish, is the best contribution to the future of kinship we can make, in speech or in writing or in both. It is the best tool available for the curious work of culturing biology both in and out of glass.

NOTES

1. The manufacture of "artificial cells" is described, among other things, as a "frontier science," referring to the moving boundaries between life and nonlife, artifact and tool, or nature and artifice. Shinya Yamanaka received the BBVA Foundation "Frontiers of Knowledge" award in 2010 for his pioneering work on the manipulation of cellular differentiation pathways.

2. The proposed use of IVF, which was originally designed as an experimental research technique used in basic scientific research on reproduction and development, for human clinical applications generated enormous debate and media coverage as early as the 1940s, and throughout the 1960s and 1970s (see, e.g., Edwards 1989). However, as Robin Marantz Henig (2004: 173–176) chronicles in one of the few histories of this technique available, the story of IVF in the two decades following its success in 1978 is one of "radical transformation" from distrust to acceptance to not noticing at all.

3. Like other social analysts of science and technology, I place a high importance on hands-on experiences in the lab, where learning what is involved in various techniques and procedures greatly increases the ability to "see through" such methods, as is discussed further in chapter 2.

4. For a discussion of the methods used to fuse mammalian embryos, see Rafferty (1970: 54–55), and for the classic account of the importance of these tools to developmental biology, see McLaren (1976).

5. Clarke (1998: 276) attributes the neglect of attention to the reproductive sciences—in both the academic and popular literature—in part to the amount of energy and attention directed toward the Human Genome Project.

6. The new kinds of biological relatives produced by IVF include, for example, a multiplication of maternities, divided into genetic and gestational branches, as well as new types of siblings, such as twins born years apart or donor siblings connected via the Internet. These new types of biological relatives have led to changes in the law, and newly explicit definitions of parenthood, as well as complex models of biological relatedness in various contexts of bioscience and biomedicine.

7. Although there is some debate about whether iPS cells would eliminate the need

for human embryos, donated fresh embryos from IVF programs remain the gold standard in human embryonic stem cell research (see further in Franklin 2006a, 2006b, 2007b, 2008).

8. I use the term "matrix" to describe IVF both to emphasize its importance as a place of technological intersection and because "matrix" refers to "a situation or surrounding substance within which something else originates, develops or is contained." The dictionary definition of "matrix" also refers to "formative cells or tissue" and to "the womb." A matrix is further defined as "ground substance," a "binding substance" (such as concrete), and also as a "mold or dye." The term derives from Latin to refer to "breeding animal" or "mother" (*American Heritage Dictionary*). I sometimes also refer to IVF as a "platform technology" to describe its use as a base for staging various kinds of technological deployment. This is somewhat different from, although not incompatible with, the concept of "biomedical platforms" developed by Peter Keating and Alfred Cambrosio to describe a distinctive series of biotechnical "steps" in a procedure (Keating and Cambrosio 2003: 3).

9. Foucault published *La Volonte de Savoir*, Volume 1 of his series on the history of sexuality, in 1976.

10. "When we compare these discourses on human sexuality with what was known at the time about the physiology of animal and plant reproduction," Foucault observes, "we are struck by the incongruity. Their feeble content from the standpoint of elementary rationality, not to mention scientificity, earns them a place apart in the history of knowledge. They form a strangely muddled zone" (1990: 54).

ONE Miracle Babies

1. The etymological stem of the use of "mere" to mean "alone" — as in "mere biology" — is the Old French *mier*, or pure, from the Latin stem *merus*. The use of "-mere" as a suffix, as in "blastomere," derives from the related Latin stem *meros*, meaning part. In a sense, biological relativity occurs when "mere" in the sense of "only" (merely biological) is transformed to mean "-mere" in the sense of "part of."

2. A crucial distinction between Carlson's and Brand's versions of the "biology is technology" argument or analogy, and those that are used to describe sex or gender as technologies, is that the former are seeking to naturalize, in the sense of normalize, this conjunction, whereas the latter seek to achieve the reverse effect, of denaturalizing these same norms.

3. In his discussion of the ambivalence of mimicry in the context of colonization, Homi Bhabha uses the expression "almost the same, but not quite" to point to the double articulation of imitation, and the extent to which it troubles normalized powers and disciplinary knowledges. In his model of ambivalence, imitation produces a "partial presence" that is at one level strategic, but also menacing, by introducing a "strategic confusion of the metaphoric and metonymic axes of the cultural production of meaning" (Bhabha 1984: 129–130). In the context of IVF, the ambivalence of mimicry is deepened by the extent to which it "strategically confuses" the biological reproduction of persons as well.

4. Foucault's genealogical method offers a means of tracing the emergence of the invisible norms that constitute both individualized subjects and general knowledge practices (a process that is described as technological). His methodology has been particularly useful in the effort to provide a history for elements of human life that are often imagined as ahistorical, such as sexuality or biology. Reproduction, of course, fits into this model very naturally. I have expanded on the Foucauldian method by splicing it with an anthropological one, namely Clifford Geertz's (1973) concept of "thick description"—a term he used to resist the call for anthropology to become a normal science, arguing it should remain an interpretive one. *Biological Relatives*, like *Dolly Mixtures* (Franklin 2007b), attempts to provide a thick genealogy for the emergence of modern technologies of reproductive substance.

5. Robert Edwards's declining health prevented his attendance at the Nobel Laureate Award Ceremony in Stockholm, where he was represented by his wife, family, and colleagues. See Nobelprize.org, "The Nobel Prize Award Ceremony 2010," http://www.nobelprize.org/nobel_prizes/medicine/laureates/2010/award-video.html.

6. For useful histories of IVF, see Biggers (1984), Challoner (1999), Edwards (2001), Fishel and Symonds (1986), or Henig (2004).

7. Watt's contribution to the history of energy production is somewhat circuitously memorialized as wattage, for example, through the lightbulb (which he did not invent), on which his name, eponymously electrified, appears as a unit of energy. He thus belongs to a unique patrilineage of energy units named for famous scientists including the farad, after Michael Faraday; the joule, after James P. Joule; the newton, after Isaac Newton; and the volt, after Alessandro Volta.

8. Other theorists of technology, such as both the ethnopaleontologist André Leroi-Gourhan (1993) and Karl Marx (see below), have argued this watershed was much earlier, and have emphasized the crucial influence of human coevolution with technology dating back to the Paleolithic era. Marx and Leroi-Gourhan's models are the basis for Derrida's (1974, 1981) conception of "originary technics" (Noland 2009) and the recent reinvention of Derrida as a theorist of technology (Stiegler 1998).

9. References to Marx throughout this book refer to Marx/Engels Collected Works (MECW) available online at Marxists Internet Archive, http://www.marxists.org/archive/marx/works/cw/index.htm. *The Economic Manuscripts of 1861–3*, comprising the twenty-three notebooks that form the basis for several of his works, contain as a lengthy addition to Part 3, on "Relative Surplus Value," his notes titled "Division of Labor and Mechanical Workshop. Tool and Machinery." This and several other chapters are to be found in Volume 33 of MECW and are cited accordingly. Despite the fact that more polished versions of some of the direct quotations from these notebooks used in this book can be found, for example, in Volumes 1 and 3 of *Capital*, I have chosen to use the original notebook versions, which are often richer in technical detail and reveal Marx's extensive knowledge of machines, as well as his somewhat surprising fondness for Darwin.

10. "Man possessed living automata from the beginning, in the shape of animals, and the employment of animal power for the pulling and carrying of burdens, for riding, driving, etc., is older than most handicraft instruments. Hence if one wished to char-

acterise this as the decisive feature, machinery would be further developed among the Scythians than the Greeks; at least, the former employed these living locomotives to a greater extent" (MECW, Vol. 33: 391).

11. This description contains Marx's answer to the question of what distinguishes a machine from a tool—a question he pursues in debate with Charles Babbage. "Once the tool is itself driven by a mechanism, once the tool of the worker, his implement, of which the efficiency depends on his own skill, and which needs his labour as an intermediary in the working process, is converted into the tool of a mechanism, the machine has replaced the tool. In this case the mechanism must already have attained a degree of development which makes it capable of receiving its motive power from a mechanically driven prime motor, instead of receiving it as before from a human being or an animal, in short from prime motors which possess voluntary movement" (MECW, Vol. 33: 432).

12. For a review of various attempts to theorize "biocapital," see Helmreich (2008).

13. As I argued in the chapter on "Capital" in *Dolly Mixtures* (2007b: 46–72) as well as in previous publications on stem cells (2001b, 2003a, 2006a, 2006b), theorizing biocapital is different from theorizing biocapitalism, which arguably does not yet exist. Moreover, theorizing biocapital requires returning to the basic meanings of capital, including both livestock and tools. Significantly, the word "capitalism" rarely occurs in Marx's work. He is principally a theorist of the forms of capital that exist before capitalism, and the nature of the forces that transform these pre- or protocapitalist forms of stock in the context of what he frequently referred to as "bourgeois economic interest."

14. Darwin relied heavily on the reported observations of his largely male colleagues for his meandering account of sexual selection, which is based in no small part on the behavior of domesticated livestock, imported birds such as pheasants, and household pets. A more intriguing ethological interpretation of "sex work" among animals is the more complex (and less predictably Victorian) model of sexual selection offered by Bruce Bagemihl (1999) as part of his account of sex not as a biological division but as a field of diverse performances and interactions maximizing the adaptive potential of sexual reproduction by preserving its diversity—a perspective with a significant precedent in Julian Huxley's ([1914] 1968) remarkable work on the complex tactical signaling performed by pairs of grebes.

15. See further on the "traffic in nature" and the digital quality of naturalization to switch back and forth as a cultural technics in Franklin et al. (2000). This digital function also characterizes the relationship between the natural, or biological, and the artificial in the context of experimental science, as is explored further in chapter 3.

16. One way to interpret Foucault's concept of genealogy is that it relies in a similarly magical manner upon the ability to realign partial and contingent histories in retrospect as singular paths stemming from known origins—arguably a core logic of kinship and descent systems as well as narratives of technological evolution.

17. In contrast to the incest taboo that is the foundational law engendering the "deployment of alliance," the modern family is "the most active site of sexuality" where "incest . . . is constantly being solicited and refused," making the family "a hotbed of constant sexual incitement" (Foucault 1990: 109).

18. For an account of the rise of mammalian developmental biology in the United Kingdom, see Graham (2000), and more broadly in Alexandre (2001). See also R. G. Edwards (2004, 2005) and Johnson (2011).

19. For histories of embryo transfer, see Betteridge (1981, 2003) and Biggers (1984). See further in chapter 3.

20. The modern use of high-speed transportation combined with culture and cryopreservation methods to enable a complex worldwide trade in human and animal germplasm, reproductive substance, and other biological materials extends the long history of livestock egg and embryo transfers, some of which as early as the 1950s, were cosponsored by commercial airlines such as TWA (Chang and Marden 1954). The airline industry also features prominently in the online video promoting the American Embryo Transfer Association and its goal of "Global Genetic Improvement through Embryo Technology" (www.aeta.org).

21. Elsewhere I have used the term "transbiology" to describe this importance of transfer to translation (Franklin 2006a, 2010b).

22. This addition, or supplement, of technological assistance neither removes nature from the process of conception nor replaces it by technology: it combines both. What Strathern (1992a, 1992b) articulated so clearly was how IVF establishes new roles for biology and technology based on their interchangeability. This substitutability, discussed further in chapter 4, is what, in Strathern's view (1992a, 1992b), displaces an understanding of technology as a set of tools that can be applied to biology or nature. In vitro, the distinction between embryo, tool, and experiment disappears. This process can also be described as part of the strategic ambivalence that characterizes imitative biotechnologies.

23. For a comparison of stem cell debates internationally, see Geesink et al. (2008), and Prainsack et al. (2008). Even in the United States, it should be noted, a majority of the population supports stem cell research.

TWO Living Tools

1. Haraway's first book, on the history of embryology, was published in 1976. Her influential articles on primatology in *Signs* (1978a, 1978b), enormously unusual when they were first published, and the first to begin to chart the technologies of sex and gender at work in the narration of human emergence, were published the same year Louise Brown was born. All of the essays in her now-classic volume *Simians, Cyborgs, and Women*, exploring "modern biology as a system of production and reproduction," were written in the late 1970s and 1980s (Haraway 1991: 2).

2. The aim is also to make of human reproductive substance more effective shareware: it is estimated that a single human embryonic cell line could produce treatments for several million patients.

3. The earlier version of "A Cyborg Manifesto" was titled "The Ironic Dream of a Common Language for Women in the Integrated Circuit: Science, Technology, and Socialist Feminism in the 1980s or a Socialist Feminist Manifesto for Cyborgs." This version contains all of the hallmarks of the later one, but includes several pages of discussion of new reproductive technologies including IVF.

4. In Firestone's view, as she explains at length, sexual politics would always restrict even the seemingly unstoppable Baconian drive for scientific discovery for the very simple reason that the drive itself was sexed.

5. This is what the terms "performance" and "performativity" have come to mean in science studies or science and technology studies more generally through the work of scholars such as Susan Leigh Star (1989, 1995), Mike Lynch (1985), and Andrew Pickering (1995), among others.

6. In his definition of labor, Marx is famously insistent on the difference between human and animal labor, commenting, for example, "A spider conducts operations that resemble those of a weaver, and a bee puts to shame many an architect in the construction of her cells. But what distinguishes the worst architect from the best of bees is this, that the architect raises his structure in imagination before he erects it in reality" (MECW, Vol. 35, *Capital*, Vol. 1, Book 1, C 7, section 1). My purpose in this section, however, is not to debate Marx's anthropocentrism, but instead to point to his attention to the liveliness of his account of human-tool relations.

7. "Relics of bygone instruments of labour possess the same importance for the investigation of extinct economic forms of society, as do fossil bones for the determination of extinct species of animals" (MECW, Vol. 35, *Capital*, Vol. 1, Book 1, C 7, section 1).

8. Conversely, the capitalist's ability to turn "dead substance" and "dead labor" into capital is described as monstrous reproduction: "By turning his money into commodities that serve as the material elements of a new product, and as factors in the labour-process, by incorporating living labour with their dead substance, the capitalist at the same time converts value, *i.e.*, past, materialised, and dead labour into capital, into value big with value, a live monster that is fruitful and multiplies" (MECW, Vol. 35, *Capital*, Vol. 1, Book 1, C 7, section 1).

9. Suction pipettes, although preferred by many embryologists, are no longer viable tools in a clean room environment due to rigid anticontamination protocols. What Emma is explaining here is that even though her lab has in the past hand-manufactured "perfect" pipette templates for stem cell propagation and sent them to a company to be manufactured under accredited (sterile) conditions, so they could be marketed as a medicinal product in compliance with GMP requirements, not enough consumer demand exists at present to sustain the market. Here, as elsewhere, the issue of scale is thus a critical factor in the enterprising up of human embryonic stem cell production.

THREE **Embryo Pioneers**

1. For a fuller description of the origins of Roosevelt's request and the origins of the "Endless Frontier" report, see Kevles (1977). On the basis of extensive archival research, Kevles argues FDR did not himself write the letter, but that it was penned by members of his office in "the President's style" (Kevles 1977: 17), having as its centerpiece a vision of "a new and humane industrial frontier" (19) upheld by a "magna carta of science" (11) intended to protect the urge of "free men everywhere and at all times" (13) to pursue knowledge for its own sake.

2. That the report and subsequent bill to establish the Office of Scientific Research and Development later disappointed its author and his staff in some respects is also an important legacy of the "Bush Doctrine" and its aftermath, as documented by historian Larry Owens (1994).

3. The origins of the use of the term "frontiers of knowledge" are obscure and date back at least to the mid-nineteenth century. William Herschel (1830: 6) refers, for example, to "the very frontier of knowledge . . . where no human thought has penetrated." The extent to which this is a specifically American use of "frontier" is thus debatable. The idiomatic use of "frontier" (which comes from French, meaning front) in reference to knowledge does not appear in the *Oxford English Dictionary* (1985 ed.), nor in the *Concise Oxford Dictionary*, although it is the third of its three definitions in the *American Heritage Dictionary*. "The critical path" refers both to the frontier sense of pathfinding and the effort to find critical biological pathways in the causation of illness and disease.

4. The older sense of the frontier as a place is not absent from the list of books appearing on the first page of a search of Amazon.com for the single word "frontier," where there are still frontier explorers, frontier history, and frontier artifacts to be found. These, however, are interspersed among frontiers of baking, kayaking, health, and personal therapy—as well as knowledge.

5. See Clarke (1998: 40–46) and Rossiter (1979) for histories of agriculture and animal science in the United States. See Marx (1964) for an account of the American pastoral ideal and see Gardner (2002) for an overview of American agricultural history in the twentieth century.

6. These universities figure prominently in Bush's report. See Clarke (2007) and Dziuk (1993) for more detailed historical studies of the Society for the Study of Reproduction. "Champaign" refers to the large fields (prairies) used for farming in the central Illinois region.

7. The use of artificial insemination techniques in livestock to improve breeding soundness had become a well-established practice in American agriculture before World War II, but was not the focus of concentrated scientific research in the U.S. until the postwar period (Clarke 1998: 159). Agricultural research on artificial insemination in livestock played a crucial role in the development of IVF. Robert Edwards, for example, used bovine embryos from the Animal Research Station at Cambridge for his early research into fertilization. Reproductive biologist Ian Gordon describes John Hammond's research on embryo transfer in cattle as "a natural follow-on to his pioneering efforts with AI" (2003: 4).

8. Both Adele Clarke and Philip Pauly similarly emphasize the importance of hands-on exploratory experimentalism to the history of the reproductive sciences, Clarke (1998: 18) referring to the "dense situations" that link "the practical value of 'golden hands'" to the formation of disciplinary concerns and Pauly to the importance of the history of the breeding arts as comprising a "form of *techne*, and not a science on the academic model" that emphasizes "traditions of skill" and "artisanal goals" over "basic principles" (2007: 264).

9. For accounts of how technology influenced scientific understandings of infertility and its treatment, see Orland (2001), Marsh and Ronner (1996), and Pfeffer (1993).

10. As Jane Maienschein (1986: 84) notes, the debates over Roux's experiments were compared by Herbert Spencer Jennings in 1926 to "a Gilbertian comic opera" because of their theoretical inconclusiveness.

11. Needham, a biochemist and later historian of biology, borrows the phrase "limiting factors" from physiology. He describes embryology prior to the nineteenth century as "a medley of *ad hoc* hypotheses" (Needham 1935: 17), arguing that even in the twentieth century it lacked a clear conceptual basis. As a result, he claimed, "Experimental embryology, Morphological embryology, Physiological embryology and Chemical embryology form today a vast range of factual knowledge, without one single unifying hypothesis" (18).

12. This is also the pattern that characterizes the development of the iPS cell discussed earlier.

13. This is why the idiom of the frontier remains problematic, invoking as it does military origins, the legacies of colonial imperialism, and more recent associations with the military-industrial science of nationalist economic and political agendas. The goal of progress, and today especially scientific progress, thus remains historically linked to the kinds of movement, agency, and activity the frontier analogy presupposes — epitomized by pioneers exploring uncharted territory, and the forward march of settlement, and thus also the tensions and ambivalences these histories engender. As Jasanoff (2007) argues, it has become one of the dominant axioms of "the biosociety" that public discomfort concerning "the frontiers of science" becomes particularly acute when the territory being domesticated is biological interiority. I return to these themes in chapters 6 and 7.

14. The American frontier idiom was famously forged in opposition to the Old World traditions of Europe. See further discussion in Franklin (2007b: 131–135).

15. The term "manifest destiny" describes a mid-nineteenth-century American ethos justifying territorial expansion in the name of progress, and legitimating progress in the name of the already existing evidence of its benefits. Hence, in terms of both American political values (the emphasis on liberty) and economic aspirations (the benefits of land and resource acquisition through settlement), manifest destiny, like the ethos of the frontier, worked as rhetorical devices to align a version of the past (as evidence of improvement) with a moral mission for the future (as an imperative to improve) — even when this effort required military force (initially against native peoples and later toward other nations).

16. Sir Ian Lloyd (1921–2006) was a conservative MP who came of age himself during the era of the scientific frontier manifesto and its expansion. A South African by birth, he was also a leading parliamentary spokesperson on science and technology, as well as an enthusiast of mechanical engineering, having authored a series of books on the history of the Rolls-Royce motor company in the 1970s.

17. The continuities that link nineteenth-century embryology to today's stem cell science are neatly encapsulated by Hopwood, who suggests, "In nineteenth century universities and medical schools embryology was a key to the science of life; around 1900 modern biology was forged within it; and as developmental biology it buzzes with excitement today" (2009: 285).

18. Far better and more informed genealogies of embryological technique have been

written by more skilled and qualified authors, and hence this chapter should be primarily considered as part of a series of reflections on how technologies work in order to better analyze how they intersect and work in and through one another.

19. Monica Casper (1998) usefully develops the concept of "work object" in the context of reproduction, and this term is originally used in the context of Mead's (1934) concept of "social objects." As Casper shows, work objects, in her case the unborn fetus, are constituted in the context of working communities, whose objects thus recapitulate existing norms and values (see further in Ehrich et al. [2008] re the human embryo as a "moral work object"). My use of the term here extends these arguments by suggesting that reproductivity in general becomes one of the work objects of embryology, and furthermore that it is in the context of these workings that a distinctive fusion of technology and reproductive substance is forged.

20. These events are discussed in much more substantial detail by historians of science, who continue to debate the role of technology in the development of embryology. See in particular Hopwood (1999, 2000, 2009), Horder et al. (1985), Gilbert (1994), Maienschein (2003), Needham (1959), Oppenheimer (1967), and Nyhart (1995).

21. The distinction between mere description and experimentation has been challenged, not least since experimentation requires careful observation. Roux used a hot pin to destroy half of a two-cell embryo in order to test his theory of mosaic development.

22. It is also conventional to distinguish between the pre-Darwinian emphasis on histogenesis and growth and the late nineteenth-century embryological emphasis on morphogenesis, also described as "the origin of form" (cf. Hamburger 1962).

23. It is the transparency of certain organisms (e.g., zebra fish and sea urchins) and parts of organisms (e.g., most embryos and egg cells) that increases their utility for experimentation, which is similarly diminished by opacity, as in the case of canine ova (hence the difficulty of dog cloning).

24. Large marine organisms, such as sea urchins, are conveniently possessed of transparent bodies, accessible gametes, and rapid reproductive cycles. They are ideal organisms for observing and manipulating fertilization in vitro, and their ready availability has long ensured they remain among the handiest of model organisms for embryologists. They also have historic importance to the field. Oscar Hertwig, Ernst Haeckel, Hans Driesch, and Theodor Boveri, among others, all undertook influential embryological studies of sea urchins that are now considered foundational to developmental biology. While they are the object of study, such model organisms thus also perform many other functions, serving, for example, as textbook organisms and tools of the trade as well as comprising legacy objects on which certain kinds of classical experiments are performed as part of routine embryological training.

25. Like most scientists, Spemann was part of a team, and much of the work with which he is associated was undertaken by his less celebrated coworkers, most notably his graduate student Hilde Mangold. This same pattern characterizes the invention of technique more generally, which is commonly far less individual than the eponymous naming of Bunsens or petris would suggest.

26. See Sander and Faessler (2001: 3).

27. Heape is responsible for the student laboratory manual on rabbit embryo re-

covery published as an appendix to the second edition of Foster and Balfour's *Elements of Embryology* in 1883.

28. Heape was elected to the Royal Society in part for his embryo transfer work, and Biggers's (1991) detailed reconstruction of his experiments was written to commemorate the technique's centenary.

29. Ultimately it would require further experimentation to disprove telegony in the form of the Penicuik experiments, conducted in Scotland by James Ewert in 1899.

30. Heape coauthored the second edition of Balfour's influential embryology manual (Foster and Balfour 1874).

31. Heape's work was primarily in vivo: his transfer was in vivo A to in vivo B, and it established their parity. This is one of many ways embryo transfer can be used as an exploratory tool, while also serving as a technique of moving material between model systems.

32. Gordon, in his comprehensive overview of embryo transfer in cattle, refers to "embryo *in vitro* production technology," or "IVP," a term that emphasizes the development over time of an increasing number of productive uses for IVF and embryo transfer. I use the terms "platform technology" and "stem technology" to similarly emphasize the expansion over time of different uses of IVF.

33. Following completion of his PhD at Harvard in 1927, Pincus received a National Research Council Fellowship allowing him to conduct research in Cambridge under the reproductive physiologist John Hammond and at the Kaiser Wilhelm Institute in Berlin with the geneticist R. Goldschmidt. He published his "Observations on the Living Eggs of the Rabbit" (1930) on the basis of his Cambridge work, marking his first major move in the direction of the study of oogenesis, a field of research he would pursue for the rest of his career.

34. Loeb had studied under the Austrian plant physiologist and agriculturalist Julius Sachs and had been inspired by the physicist and social reformer Josef Popper-Lynkeus (an early advocate of converting the mechanical energy of waterfalls into electricity). He was equally influenced by Ernst Mach, the physicist-philosopher for whom scientific concepts were seen as tools for social reform (see further in Maienschein 2009).

35. Indeed it is a truism today that biology is not only a technology, but simply is technology, full stop. Such is the raison d'être, for example, of synthetic biology, which is based on the premise that we cannot fully understand biological systems, living systems, until we can build them from scratch (see Keller 2009). This definition of biology is discussed further in chapter 8.

36. As Chang (1968: 16) points out, technically Pincus did not claim to have definitively achieved fertilization in these experiments.

37. As he states in his preface, "I am possessed by the belief that accurate quantitative observations afford the means for elucidating the nature of biological processes" (Pincus 1930: vii–viii).

38. Increasingly, this genealogy is defined not only by certain privileged objects of study, such as favored model organisms, or even the techniques used to investigate them, but by the relationship between the two — indeed the coevolution of stem techniques and organisms, as well as the core questions and concepts to which they come to be attached through repeated application.

39. The technical evolution, and recapitulation, of techniques such as in vitro culture for the study of biological development takes on additional interest from the point of view of what might be described as the feedback loop, or recursion, between the evolving tools of technogenesis (e.g., the adaptation of a technique for a new use) and their objects (e.g., the mechanics of development, aka developmental biology). We see here again the complex archaeology of the means by which technologies are reproduced (e.g., embryo transfer) in order to synthesize reproduction (e.g., artificial parthenogenesis). This, again, is why the union IVF confirms is not only that of sperm and egg, but more broadly the coupling of the reproduction of technique to the technicization of reproduction—which is one reason why reproductive technology is such an intriguing, and dense, area of study.

40. If any single sentence recapitulates the union of the premodern natural history of observation and description with the postexperimental turn toward intervention as understanding, I have not found it yet.

41. Tellingly in this sentence, "its life history" could refer as accurately to "the experimental investigation" as to "the growth and development of the mammalian ovum."

FOUR Reproductive Technologies

1. One of the reasons I began my first book on IVF (Franklin 1997) with an extensive discussion of the so-called virgin birth debate in anthropology is because of the extent to which this debate endlessly rehearses the obviousness of the very facts whose nonobviousness the debate reveals. While it is obviously true that it takes a sperm and an egg to make a baby, this explanation only works in retrospect, when there is a baby, and does not explain why reproduction sometimes works and sometimes fails. As Annette Weiner wrote in the 1970s, once biological reproduction is no longer "the axis on which all else turns," it becomes clear that "the issues are . . . more complex" (1978: 238).

2. The argument that kinship systems reproduce themselves for themselves— repetitively and in perpetuity—is the condition of reproductivity (culture) that Lévi-Strauss argues is made possible, and viable, through the law of exogamy. As we shall see in this chapter, the argument that this reproductivity is essentially for itself does not require that it be given an arbitrary biological basis in the natural value of women's reproductive capacity. In fact, such a naturalistic claim only obscures and limits the most powerful implication of structuralist anthropology, which, as Derrida points out, is its persuasive emphasis on the excessive generativity of the technical systems through which human sociality reproduces itself (Kirby 2011).

3. Or, more radically, is there a strictly biological sense of the term "reproduction" at all?

4. It should be noted that Strathern's reference to the meroblast is primarily to distinguish merographic thinking from mereographic thought, although as it turns out the fortuitous inclusion of the meroblast is highly apt.

5. It is precisely the technical nature of merographic thinking that underscores the similarity between Mol's (2002) and Strathern's (1992a) accounts of biomedical objects.

6. That all of the work involved in making IVF work can then be retrospectively (or

even prospectively) naturalized as something that would have happened anyway by itself is another example of the utility of merographic logic.

7. These various (old and new) kinds of relatives would include those that are biological before they are cultural, cultural because they are biological, born because they are biologically formed, formed because they are biologically cultured, born because they are made, made because they will be born, failed because they were not biologically viable (or unhappily cultured), etc., etc. The merographic move is as useful for imagining progress as it is for recomposing failure (it works as an after as well as a before). The more of the merographic is, simply, endless. As Strathern notes, "there is endless fractal potential for the replication of combinatory phenomena across different scales" (2005: 168n).

8. The term "convention" is derived from the Latin *conventionalis*, meaning agreement, assembly, or covenant. Although according to the *Oxford English Dictionary* the use of the term "social convention" was not taken up in English usage until the eighteenth century, and the use of convention to refer to tradition developed even later, these senses of the term are original to it in Latin, so that the term "social convention," for example, is a tautology, or more precisely pleonasm, because it repeats the same idea twice. A convention can only be social, and *conventionalis* originally referred in Latin to social activities. In the human sciences, the use of the idea of "convention" as a binding or shaping set of rules was taken up particularly widely within psychology and sexology in the 1970s. The early use of "gender identity," for instance, is a classic example of the idea of convention being used to describe the powerful molding mechanisms of socialization (to Durkheim, a convention was a contract). Throughout her essay, Rubin's interest is both in how these conventions direct human subjects to become certain kinds of persons (e.g., men or women), and how they require repression: "The division of the sexes has the effect of repressing some of the personality characteristics of virtually everyone, men and women" (1975: 180). The mechanics of convention, in other words its work, is to shape persons — or force them into molds.

9. Lévi-Strauss refers to women's reproductive capacity variously throughout his work, and the references are usually hybrids of the idea of property as a distinctive physical characteristic — as in the biological properties of the placenta — and as a valuable good in the sense of something that is desirable to others. He refers variously to "the quality intrinsic to these women" (Lévi-Strauss 1969: 481), and the "biological considerations" as to "the properties of these individuals" (482).

10. This would be the "is female to nurture as male is to culture" counterargument.

11. After all, this was a logic that even Lévi-Strauss himself questioned in his famously confused and disingenuous parting comment that (*mais bien sur!*) "woman could never become just a sign and nothing more, since even in a man's world she is still a person, and since in so far as she is defined as a sign she must be recognised as a generator of signs" (1969: 496). We might add that since the first and second halves of this sentence contradict each other, they only compound the error of the conflation he appears to want to qualify by admitting women are still persons. He is in effect saying that "woman" is valuable (a) because she is not "just" a sign, but (b) because she will generate more signs like her.

12. Wittig's term for the unexamined and primitive heterosexism of Lévi-Strauss's

account of the exchange of women, "the straight mind" (1992), is a parody of the title of his later book *The Savage Mind*. As Rubin points out, much of Wittig's (1969) surrealist lesbian novella *Les guérillères* is clearly written as a critique of Lévi-Strauss (and Lacan). Jacques Derrida, also a fierce critic of Lévi-Strauss, claimed that his entire argument was not only tautological, but symptomatic of the defining logocentrism of Western philosophy: "It could perhaps be said that the whole of philosophical conceptualization, systematically relating itself to the nature/culture opposition, is designed to leave in the domain of the unthinkable the very thing that makes this conceptualization possible: the origin of the prohibition of incest" (Derrida 1978: 283–284). Foucault offers yet another view in *La Volonté de Savoir*, published in nearly the same year as Rubin's essay, 1976, where he argues that it is the positioning of the threat of incest at the center of a hyperaffectively charged nuclear family life in the second half of the nineteenth century that produces the crucial incitements necessary to the birth of modern sexuality (an analysis that remained famously silent on the sex/gender system).

13. Rubin cites the 1972 republication in Macksey and Donato's anthology *The Structuralist Controversy* (reprinted in a fortieth anniversary edition in 2007 by Johns Hopkins University Press) of "Structure, Sign, and Play," Derrida's lengthy critique of Lévi-Strauss, first published in 1966. Notably, Derrida's critique of Lévi-Strauss in this essay, one of his earliest, describes the nature-culture dichotomy as "congenital to philosophy" and claims that Lévi-Strauss is using old tools to expose the weaknesses of the "old machinery" of which he remains a part. He contrasts the "sterility" of this approach to monstrous gestation in his conclusion (Derrida 1978: 278–294).

14. By his own admission, Lévi-Strauss was primarily a theorist of myth and mythmaking, and acknowledged not only that his own method was highly speculative but that it might itself be mythical. By this he also implies that he himself did not think the nature-culture opposition was so much a true ontological fact as a valuable sociological method, or decoding device. This is where he parts company with many social anthropologists, many of whom prefer to consume their facts empirically raw rather than hermeneutically cooked.

15. These are the very same values, it might be added, that had just begun to be implemented as human IVF at Bourn Hall in Cambridge as *Nature, Culture and Gender* went to press.

16. Readers familiar with *Embodied Progress* (Franklin 1997) will be aware that some of the material rehearsed in this chapter partially resembles the account in that earlier book of this debate, where indeed similar arguments are made about employing IVF as a "defamiliarizing lens" on technologies of kinship. Since the argument presented here both leads in a slightly different direction and is set in the midst of a rather different overall structure, I have included this material again despite the risk of appearing to repeat myself.

17. Notably, the question of biology was crucial to the women's health movement throughout the 1970s (*Our Bodies, Ourselves* had begun as the We and Our Biology group in Boston in the 1970s), and had been explored in many popular 1970s feminist texts, including those of Firestone and Greer (which in turn had been anticipated as early as the 1940s by both Ruth Herschberger and Simone de Beauvoir).

18. The rapidly expanding corpus of Melanesian ethnography was, like feminist an-

thropology, one of the important contexts in which these categories had already been substantially challenged and retheorized as part of a shift toward a more reflexive post-structuralist anthropology (see for example Wagner 1975).

19. "Dual organizations" were central to the binary precepts of structuralist anthropology, which, following the structure of Hegelian dialectics, released cultural creativity through a process of opposition and resolution. They were also crucial to the models of structural functionalism, which relied on the structure of descent groups as a basic principle of social reproduction.

20. The analysis of gender and sex as cultural accomplishments introduced by ethnomethodologists such as Harold Garfinkel (1967), like the account of gender as a performance by Erving Goffman (1976), are sometimes compared to Butler's critique of gender identity in the context of feminist post-structuralism. Although such accounts, and others in the tradition of sociology, social psychology, and phenomenology that approach gender and sex as situated interaction, ritual display, performance, and role theory, etc., overlap with both Butler's account and those derived from feminist anthropology, they are very differently oriented, and do not seek to explain either the persistence of a natural or biological base for gender and sex, nor the intractability of gender inequality. Importantly, it is the role of biological explanations within the human sciences, and the critique of identity, that most strongly motivates Butler, while it is the role of reproduction in particular that concerns feminist anthropology. The word "biology" does not appear in Goffman's (1976) account of "the moral career" of individuals, for example, and neither Garfinkle nor Goffman concerned themselves with biological determinism.

21. The point that has been made not only by Strathern (1992a, 1992b) but by many other analysts of the digital switching back and forth that characterizes the hybrid logic of kinship thinking (both in its Anglophone guise, and more widely) is that this kinship model was never reliant on nature per se, but on techniques of naturalization that are themselves a cultural technology. This is the meaning of kinship technics as they are analyzed, for example, in the "new kinship studies," to which questions of technology have been central (see, e.g., Edwards 2000; Edwards et al. 1993; Edwards and Strathern 2000; Edwards and Salazar 2009; Franklin and McKinnon 2001; Franklin et al. 2000; Haraway 1997, 2008; and Thompson 2005; as well as Strathern 1999, 2005).

FIVE Living IVF

1. This phrasing deliberately echoes Georges Canguilhem's insistence upon the indivisibility between knowing or analyzing life or living things and the actual living of a concrete life: "The universal relation of human knowledge to living organization reveals itself through the relation of knowledge to human life" (2008: xix). A kindred anthropological axiom would be that to understand technologies of kinship or gender it is necessary to understand how they are lived in real life.

2. One of the reasons that feminist debates concerning NRTs have only recently begun to receive more attention is because of the extent to which they were initially seen merely to concern white, Western, middle-class women's infertility in developed

nations—an assumption that overlooks the very extensive use of IVF worldwide and the initial trials of clinical IVF in a largely working-class patient cohort in Lancashire.

3. For reviews of the feminist debate over NRTs in the 1980s, see Burfoot (1999), Donchin (1986, 1989), Farquhar (1996), Lublin (1998), Overall (1987), and Thompson (2005). For a Foucauldian analysis, see Sawicki (1991).

4. For example, the entire corpus of Western philosophy could be described as divisive, if we understand this term according to its original meaning as "analytic" or "making or perceiving distinctions."

5. If the high regard in which the British parliamentary system is held serves as any guide, the ability to maintain highly divisive and acrimonious debate is nothing short of a political ideal.

6. The feminist debate over NRTs can be read, for example, as anticipating, confirming, and extending what Zygmunt Bauman (1993: 10), writing in the 1990s, describes as "the ambivalence of man-made design" or Ulrich Beck (1992) characterizes as "reflexive modernity." As we see in chapter 7, Beck's critique of IVF overlapped with those of many feminists opposing IVF in this period (and see more pointedly Beck-Gernsheim 1989). Like many bioethicists, Beck was more concerned with how IVF would affect humanity than women, leading him, like Habermas (2003) and Fukuyama (2002), to focus on the eugenic potential of IVF.

7. These volumes emerged out of the June 1979 conference held at Hampshire College in Amherst, Massachusetts, titled "Ethical Issues in Human Reproduction Technology: Analysis by Women," organized by Helen B. Holmes, a feminist biologist with expertise in population genetics, human biology, and bioethics.

8. Hence, Rothman (1984) suggests, the possibility of having much more information about the fetus can have the paradoxical effect of making users of amniocentesis more conscious of the right not to have certain information, such as ambiguous test results or genetic information that could adversely affect their relationships to other family members. Choice in this context can also become prescriptive: to the extent she can be held liable for a preventable outcome, the choice to undertake amniocentesis can become a means of women's subordination, rather than empowerment.

9. Dworkin's model of the reproductive brothel is developed in her 1983 book on right-wing women.

10. The Feminist International Network of Resistance to Reproductive and Genetic Engineering, founded in 1985, is discussed further below. It began as the Feminist International Network on the New Reproductive Technology (FINNRET) at the Second Interdisciplinary Congress on Women in Groningen, Netherlands, in April 1984. In July 1985 an "emergency" conference was held in Vallinge, Sweden, where a more explicitly oppositional form of the network was accompanied by a name change.

11. Lublin, for example, suggests, "Not only do FINRRAGE feminists claim that the use and development of technology is male dominated, but they allege that men conspire to control this arena" (1998: 66), although she later adds that "there is a diversity of views within the group" (67).

12. UBINIG is a policy and action research organization formed in 1984 by activists seeking alternatives to mainstream development programs based in Dhaka. See further at www.ubinig.org.

13. In this case, the three scientists were coauthors, not coeditors.

14. Crowe's research was not included in Klein's anthology for the likely reason that it was published in a very similar Australian anthology edited by Jocelynne Scutt in 1990, *The Baby Machine*.

15. The question of the extent to which being on the "fertility road" or the IVF quest can function as a mechanism to repair lost or threatened conjugal or familial identities is taken up further in this and later chapters.

16. This finding also points to the question of how IVF can become a duty: precisely because you know your chances of actually becoming pregnant through IVF are slim, it is crucial to be seen to be pursuing this goal, to which the alternative is "just giving up," and thus being seen not to value the pursuit of children highly enough.

SIX IVF Live

1. In addition to the early work on IVF in the 1980s discussed in chapter 5, major monographs on IVF beginning in the 1990s include Becker (2000), Franklin (1997), Inhorn (1994), Kahn (2000), Thompson (2005), and Throsby (2004) as well as Sandelowski (1993).

2. Early attention to the importance of achieved parenthood is evident in a range of studies from the 1990s onward including, for example, Lewin's analysis of lesbian motherhood in which she describes the "crafting" of kin ties as a form of "natural achievement" (1993: 184). Similarly, Ginsburg (1998: 110) describes a transformation from ascribed gender identities to achieved identities in the context of struggles over reproduction and nurture in her 1989 study of abortion activists. A different kind of achieved identity is described in the literature on adoption, particularly by Judith Modell (2002: 182, and see also 1994), who refers to "the achievement of identity" and to "made" identities, later described by Thompson (as "strategic naturalization" [2005; and see also Cussins 1996]). To the extent that this model of achieved identity has become one of the major themes in the literature on IVF, it underscores the point made earlier that IVF can enable its users to achieve certain identities by aligning themselves with its means even if the end they are intended to enable does not materialize.

3. Given the long association between pilgrimages of various kinds and the quest for a child in the context of infertility, it is in some ways surprising that a more systematic comparison between these two phenomena has not been undertaken, all the more so as such a comparison is frequently either explicitly referred to, or an implicit structural analogy, in many ethnographic studies of new reproductive technologies, including my own (1997) as well as those of Inhorn (1994), Paxson (2003), and Clarke (2010).

4. The emphasis in the literature on achieved parenthood includes in some of its earliest forms, such as the work of Lewin (1993: 164), an almost artisanal view of kinship as the subject, in Lewin's words, of "curiously crafted strategies." This emphasis on craft, and "recrafting," is also found in Thompson (2005: 256) alongside the dominant emphasis in her work on making parenthood.

5. Sadly, it is so much the better if the narrative is especially tragic, if the aim is to demonstrate devotion and sacrifice.

6. The steps or stages of IVF are themselves hybrid constructs. Ovulation and fertilization, for example, refer to natural processes that in the context of IVF are technologically assisted—as evident in other steps of IVF, namely ovarian stimulation, egg aspiration, embryo transfer, etc. A result is that IVF elongates the process of conception, transforming what is biologically a relatively brief period of time (about twenty-four hours) into a lengthy procedure normally lasting several weeks (not including the period of planning the procedure and arranging it). As noted above, it is not uncommon for the IVF process in total to take place over several years, or even as much as a decade.

7. The sociality of the clinic often reproduces the conventional gender division of labor common to medical settings of male consultant aided by largely female staff, which also exaggerates these gender differences.

8. Although it is increasingly possible for nonnormative kinship and gender identities to be accommodated within the world of IVF (indeed, some clinics specialize in offering fertility services to lesbian and gay consumers), the strain of inhabiting this "hypergender-appropriate" world may be severe, as Laura Mamo (2007) shows in her important study of lesbians' exhausting experiences of fertility treatment.

9. The experience of one's own biology on an IVF program is also, again paradoxically, most similar, if you are a woman, to the experiences of male patients undergoing gender transition by submitting to a hormonal regime that replaces their original and familiar one.

10. This form of modern double consciousness associated with technology can be closely related to the ambivalence this technology also produces—again, a recursion of identity technics in the context of a similarly doubled reproductivity.

11. My thanks to Sara Ahmed for the reference to feminist phenomenology.

12. Another term for this, after Thompson (2005), might be "strategic biologization" (also after Spivak's [1985] "strategic essentialism")—both in terms of whether something is biologized or not (e.g., the drive to reproduce) and how it is biologized (e.g., in relation to the start of pregnancy). That the amount of strategic adjustment occurring during any ART procedure is part of its workload is not in question. However, the forms of biological consciousness, biological knowledge, or biological identity operating here are less well characterized, especially insofar as they are, in effect, novel forms of technological consciousness, technical knowledge, and tactical identity in the context of IVF.

13. In addition to making it possible to be partially pregnant, IVF has also made it more difficult to be, as it were, just or simply pregnant. Various new forms of pregnancy have arisen in the wake of IVF. The existence of assisted and achieved pregnancy have left in their wake, for example, new categories for previously unmarked forms of pregnancy including unassisted, natural, and spontaneous pregnancies. A pregnancy that is established by a test result two weeks after embryo transfer may reveal a positive pregnancy indicator that is later revealed to have been an artifact of treatment known as a chemical pregnancy—which is such a particularly undesirable form of pregnancy that patients are often repeatedly warned in advance to be wary of the test result until they have had it confirmed two weeks later (advice it may be easier to

follow rationally than emotionally). In vitro fertilization also increases the chances of ectopic, or tubal, pregnancies, as well as multiple pregnancy. A pregnancy can also be more than one of these types, for example a spontaneous multiple pregnancy.

14. One of the primary meanings of "heroic" is "exaggerated characterization" (*American Heritage Dictionary*). In the *Oxford English Dictionary* "heroic" is defined as "having recourse to bold, daring or extreme measures; boldly experimental, attempting great things" (1971: Volume 1, 246). A female hero is of course a heroine—a woman of great fortitude who undertakes acts of greatness.

15. A number of excellent studies have documented the globalization of IVF not only as a means of family formation but a form of consumer culture. As Marcia Inhorn (2003) documents in her study of globalizing reproductive technologies, these means bring with them the effects of economic stratification, which can exacerbate, rather than relieve, the distress of infertility.

16. Paxson (2004: 214) makes explicit reference to the arguments of Teresa de Lauretis's (1987) model of gender as a technology and points out that Foucault's version of technologies of sex draws on ancient Greek philosophy.

17. It might be said that IVF combines an effect of origin with a means of effecting an origin.

18. This was the logic of the right-to-life effort to implicate women in the guilt of abortion both by facilitating bonding through ultrasound, and by revulsion at the sight of dismembered fetal remains (Petchesky 1987).

19. As both Lisa Cartwright (1995) and Hannah Landecker (2007) have documented, the history of the cinema has its origins in the effort to explore the mechanics of cell biology.

20. The contrast is particularly evident in relation to Nilsson's photos, the work of preparation for which is noticeably absent, as it is only the finished object in the form of a photograph he sought to produce.

21. The reliance on microinjection in the context of assisted conception is exemplified by the increasingly routine use of ICSI in IVF in order to avoid contamination of the egg's environment during fertilization. Also, ICSI is used to avoid sperm cell contamination when performing polar body removal or blastomere biopsy.

SEVEN Frontier Culture

1. See Ahmed for an insightful account of "facing" as an orientation that becomes "the point from which 'we' emerge" (2006: 15).

2. To my knowledge, this is the first publication ever to use this phrase as its title, although the expression appears to have been in routine use since at least the mid-nineteenth century.

3. Robert Edwin Peary (1856–1920) claimed to have reached the North Pole in 1909, the first explorer to do so. An American explorer, a graduate of Bowdoin College, and a civil engineer by training, he employed indigenous Inuit techniques to conduct Arctic expeditions. The ship he captained for his most famous expeditions was named *Roosevelt*.

4. In both the United States and Australia, where the frontier narrative plays a cru-

cial role in the national imaginary, the "no-man's-land" (*terra nullius*) occupied by white settler colonists was already occupied by highly civilized people, whose displacement was often brought about by violent and illegal acts of occupation.

5. For an insightful account of this question, see Amy E. Wendling's (2009) discussion of Marx's analysis of technology, in which she argues Marx's model of technology changes significantly in the wake of his "energeticist turn," a view that accords with this book's emphasis on Marx's technological biologism.

6. As Habermas notes: "Today, in the industrially most advanced systems, an energetic attempt must be made consciously to take in hand the mediation between technical progress and the conduct of life in the major industrial societies, a mediation that has previously taken place without direction, as a mere continuation of natural history" (2010: 87).

7. "Envisaging the possibility of a technology that would constitute a theory of the evolution of technics, Marx [and Engels] outlined a new perspective," claims Stiegler (1998: 2). He cites Marx: "Technology reveals the active relation of man to nature, the direct process of the production of his life, and thereby it also lays bare the process of the production of the social relations of his life, and of the mental conceptions that flow from these relations" (Marx cited in Stiegler 1998: 16). In sum, he argues, Marx and Engels offered a technical version of biological evolution, as well as an evolution of technics.

8. Theorists in this tradition would include not only Leroi-Gourhan, who is discussed earlier, and who is closely followed by Lemonnier as well as other anthropologists and ethnologists of technique, but more recently Tim Ingold. A version of this project continues to be advanced under the rubric of anthropological materialism.

9. Bryan Pfaffenberger describes the progressive evolutionary model of need-driven, adaptation-oriented, strategic technological advance as the "Standard View," referring in part to its commonsense appeal. Lewis Binford (1965) argues, for example, that the primary meaning of technology is always instrumental and pragmatic, after which it may acquire a secondary social or cultural meaning. The opposite view, that social and cultural meanings are more primary than technology, has been put forward by Sahlins (1972, 1976), among others, as well as Lemonnier (1993).

10. The term "contact zone" is also closely associated with the work of Mary Louise Pratt (1992: 2) to describe interactions on the colonial frontier. Her use of the term "contact" derives from the use of "contact languages," such as pidgin, to describe hybrid or mixed strategies of interaction.

11. Perhaps not surprisingly, the literature which emphasizes that technology is an essential, but not determining, variable in the causal histories of social change has developed in close partnership with arguments from science studies, such as those of Madeleine Akrich (1992) concerning technology transfer, and Bruno Latour (1987, 1993) emphasizing the dependency of how techniques work not only on factors unrelated to their efficiency, but on the viability of social relations and cultural constructs that support their coming into being as hybrid entities. This argument is similarly prominent in anthropology, as illustrated earlier by Gell (1988) and more recently by Lucy Suchman (2007).

12. Such an argument has been made by an increasing number of social theorists,

including Stefan Helmreich (2008), Vicky Kirby (2011), and Myra Hird (2009). In such arguments humans are already a kind of in vitro life contained by the culture medium of the technologically saturated milieu. The concept of the "Anthropocene" similarly resembles the model of the petri dish, by implying a kind of contamination of the evolutionary process that is "manmade."

13. Less than twenty years after the publication of Roosevelt's endless frontier doctrine for science, Dwight D. Eisenhower was to publicly express his fears that the so-called military-industrial-science complex would alienate the American public from the "insidious penetration" of a technoscientific elite. In 1961, in his farewell speech, Eisenhower called on Americans to hold science in respect but to beware the "danger that public policy could itself become the captive of a scientific-technological elite" (Eisenhower 1961).

14. Made from the rendered remains of domesticated livestock, emulsion is itself a technological substance derived both from the "culture of nature" and denatured biology, manifest as media. See further in Shukin (2009: 104–114).

15. This ambivalence is differently evoked in Leo Marx's (2000) account of the paradoxes of American pastoralism, an argument that revolves centrally around the contradictory figure of the machine in the garden.

16. The need to colonize people as well as land in the context of frontier expansion also has implications for the question of whose biological substance becomes domesticated as a tool—an ongoing question that has been widely debated within anthropology in the context of the Human Genome Project (Goodman et al. 2003).

17. The effort to analyze the highly stratified post-IVF world of reproductive tourism, or "cross-border reproductive care," which has only recently begun to be pursued in a more systematic manner (Inhorn and Gurtin 2011), strongly reinforces the argument of this book that IVF makes explicit the intersection of what Derrida describes as "originary technics," meaning identity, thought, and language, with the methods more commonly associated with technology, including direct manual intervention of the use of tools. The models of intersectionality proposed from within feminist theory, including Haraway's (1983, 1985) early work on technology and cyborg politics, make clear that the gendering of reproductive substance, or even sex, cannot be separated from the technics of race, nationality, or class.

18. Increasingly, bioartists such as Oron Cotts, of the Tissue Culture and Art project, have been formally trained in leading scientific labs to learn the techniques they now use for bioart. Science is itself a technical art, and the history of experimental science is highly reliant upon aesthetic criteria, visual culture, and the skilled handling of tools.

EIGHT After IVF

1. As Sara Ahmed notes, "the very possibility of being pointed toward happiness suggests that objects are associated with affects before they are even encountered" (2010: 27). Happiness, as she notes, is "end orientated" (26).

REFERENCES

Ahmed, Sara. 2006. *Queer Phenomenology: Orientations, Objects, Others*. Durham, NC: Duke University Press.

Ahmed, Sara. 2010. *The Promise of Happiness*. Durham, NC: Duke University Press.

Akrich, Madeline. 1992. "The De-Scription of Technical Objects." In Wiebe Bijker and John Law, eds., *Shaping Technology, Building Society: Studies in Sociotechnical Change*, 205–224. Cambridge, MA: MIT Press.

Alexandre, H. A. 2001. "History of Mammalian Embryological Research." *International Journal of Developmental Biology* 45: 457–467.

Anker, Suzanne, and Sarah Franklin. 2011. "Specimens as Spectacles: Reframing Fetal Remains." *Social Text* 29(1): 103–125.

Anker, Suzanne, and Dorothy Nelkin. 2004. *The Molecular Gaze: Art in the Genetic Age*. Cold Spring Harbour, NY: Cold Spring Harbour Laboratory Press.

Anzaldúa, Gloria. 1987. *Borderlands/La Frontera*. San Francisco: Spinster's Ink.

Ardener, Edwin. 1972. "Belief and the Problem of Women." In J. La Fontaine, ed., *The Interpretation of Ritual: Essays in Honour of A. I. Richards*, 135–158. London: Routledge.

Arditti, Rita, Renate Duelli Klein, and Shelley Minden, eds. 1984. *Test-Tube Women: What Future for Motherhood?* London: Pandora.

Arendt, Hannah. 1958. *The Human Condition*. Chicago: University of Chicago Press.

Austin, C. R. 1961. *The Mammalian Egg*. Oxford: Blackwell.

Austin, C. R., and R. V. Short, eds. 1972. *Reproduction in Mammals*, vol. 5: *Artificial Control of Reproduction*. Cambridge: Cambridge University Press.

Bagemihl, Bruce. 1999. *Biological Exuberance: Animal Homosexuality and Natural Diversity*. New York: St. Martin's.

Bartky, Sandra. 1993. *Gender and Domination*. London: Routledge.

Bauman, Zygmunt. 1993. "Postmodernity, or Living with Ambivalence." In J. P. Natoli and L. Hutcheon, eds., *A Postmodern Reader*, 9–24. Albany: State University of New York Press.

Bavister, Barry D. 2002. "Early History of *In Vitro* Fertilization." *Reproduction* 124: 181–196.

Beck, Ulrich. 1992. *Risk Society: Towards a New Modernity*. London: Sage.

Becker, Gay. 2000. *The Elusive Embryo: How Women and Men Approach New Reproductive Technologies.* Berkeley: University of California Press.

Becker, Howard S. 1963. *Outsiders: Studies in the Sociology of Deviance.* New York: Free Press.

Beck-Gernscheim, Elisabeth. 1989. "From the Pill to Test-Tube Babies: New Options, New Pressures in Reproductive Behaviour." In K. S. Ratcliff, ed., *Healing Technology: Feminist Perspectives,* 23–40. Ann Arbor: University of Michigan Press.

Beer, Gillian. 1983. *Darwin's Plots: Evolutionary Narrative in Darwin, George Elliot and Nineteenth-Century Fiction.* London: Ark.

Bennett, Jesse Lee. 1925. *Frontiers of Knowledge.* Chicago: American Library Association.

Berer, Marge. 1985. "Breeding Conspiracies: Feminism and the New Reproductive Technologies." *Trouble and Strife* 6 (summer): 29–35.

Berlant, Lauren. 2006. "Cruel Optimism." *differences* 17(3): 20–36.

Betteridge, Keith J. 1981. "An Historical Look at Embryo Transfer." *Reproduction and Fertility* 62: 1–13.

Betteridge, Keith. 2003. "A History of Farm Animal Embryo Transfer and Some Associated Techniques. *Animal Production Science* 79(3): 203–244.

Bhabha, Homi. 1984. "Of Mimicry and Man: The Ambivalence of Colonial Discourse." *October* 28: 125–133.

Biggers, J. D. 1984. "*In Vitro* Fertilization and Embryo Transfer in Historical Perspective." In Alan Trounson and Carl Wood, eds., *In Vitro Fertilization and Embryo Transfer,* 3–15. London: Churchill Livingstone.

Biggers, J. D. 1991. "Walter Heape, FRS: A Pioneer in Reproductive Biology." *Journal of Reproduction and Fertility* 93: 173–186.

Binford, Lewis. 1965. "Archeological Systematics and the Study of Culture Process." *American Antiquity* 31(2): 203–210.

Birke, Lynda. 1986. *Women, Feminism and Biology: The Feminist Challenge.* London: Wheatsheaf.

Birke, Lynda, Sue Himmelweit, and Gail Vines. 1990. *Tomorrow's Child: Reproductive Technologies in the 90s.* London: Virago.

Bowker, Geoffrey, and Sandra Leigh Star. 1999. *Sorting Things Out: Classification and Its Consequences.* Cambridge, MA: MIT Press.

Brand, Stewart. 2010. *Whole Earth Discipline.* London: Atlantic Books.

Breeze, Nancy. 1984. "Who Is Going to Rock the Petri Dish? For Feminists Who Have Considered Parthenogenesis When the Movement Is Not Enough." In Arditti et al. 1984, 397–401.

Bullard, Linda. 1987. "Killing Us Softly: Toward a Feminist Analysis of Genetic Engineering." In Spallone and Steinberg 1987, 110–119.

Bunch, Charlotte. 1982. "Copenhagen and Beyond: Prospects for Global Feminism." *Quest: A Feminist Quarterly* 5(4): 25–35.

Burchell, Kevin, Sarah Franklin, and Kerry Holden. 2009. *Public Culture as Professional Science.* London: London School of Economics.

Burfoot, Annette, ed. 1999. *Encyclopedia of Reproductive Technologies.* Boulder, CO: Westview.

Bush, Vannevar. 1945. "Science: The Endless Frontier." *Transactions of the Kansas Academy of Science* 48(3): 231–264.

Butler, Judith. 1990. *Gender Trouble: Feminism and the Subversion of Identity*. New York: Routledge.

Canguilhem, Georges. 2008. *Knowledge of Life*. New York: Fordham University Press.

Carby, Hazel. 1987. *Reconstructing Womanhood: The Emergence of the Afro-American Novelist*. New York: Oxford University Press.

Carlson, Robert H. 2010. *Biology Is Technology: The Promise, Peril, and New Business of Engineering Life*. Cambridge, MA: Harvard University Press.

Carsten, Janet. 2001. "Substantivism, Antisubstantivism, and Anti-antisubstantivism." In Franklin and McKinnon 2001, 29–53.

Carsten, Janet. 2004. *After Kinship*. Cambridge: Cambridge University Press.

Cartwright, Lisa. 1995. *Screening the Body: Tracing Medicine's Visual Culture*. Minneapolis: University of Minnesota Press.

Casper, Monica. 1998. *The Making of the Unborn Patient: A Social Anatomy of Fetal Surgery*. New Brunswick, NJ: Rutgers University Press.

Cassidy, Rebecca. 2007. "Introduction: Domestication Reconsidered." *Where the Wild Things Are: Domestication Reconsidered*. Oxford: Berg.

Cavalli-Sforza, Luigi Luca. 1984. "Isolation by Distance." In Aravinda Chakravarti, ed., *Human Population Genetics: The Pittsburgh Symposium*, 229–248. New York: Van Nostrand Reinhold.

Chadwick, Helen. 1995. *Stilled Lives*. Edinburgh: Portfolio Gallery.

Challoner, Jack. 1999. *The Baby Makers: The History of Artificial Conception*. London: Macmillan.

Chang, M. C. 1958. "Capacitation of Rabbit Spermatozoa in the Uterus with Special Reference to the Reproductive Phases of the Female." *Endocrinology* 65: 619–628.

Chang, M. C. 1968. "In Vitro Fertilization of Mammalian Eggs." *Journal of Animal Science* 27: 15–21.

Chang, M. C., and W. G. R. Marden. 1954. "The Aerial Transport of Fertilized Mammalian Ova." *Journal of Heredity* 45(2): 75–78.

Chicago, Judy. 1977. *Through the Flower: Autobiography of a Feminist Artist*. New York: Anchor.

Chicago, Judy. 1996. *The Dinner Party*. New York: Penguin.

Childe, V. Gordon. 1952. "The Birth of Civilization." *Past and Present* 2: 1–10.

Clarke, Adele. 1995. "Research Materials and Reproductive Science in the United States, 1910–1940." In Susan Leigh Star, ed., *Ecologies of Knowledge: Work and Politics in Science and Technology*. Albany: State University of New York Press.

Clarke, Adele. 1998. *Disciplining Reproduction: Modernity, American Life Sciences and "The Problem of Sex."* Berkeley: University of California Press.

Clarke, Adele, and Joan H. Fujimura, eds. 1992. *The Right Tools for the Right Job: At Work in Twentieth-Century Life Sciences*. Princeton, NJ: Princeton University Press.

Clarke, John. 2007. "The History of Three Scientific Societies." *Studies in History and Philosophy of Science* 38(2): 340–357.

Clarke, Morgan. 2009. *Islam and New Kinship: Reproductive Technology and the Shariah in Lebanon*. Oxford: Berghahn Books.

Clifford, James. 1983. "On Ethnographic Authority." *Representations* 1(2): 118–146.

Clifford, James, and George Marcus, eds. 1986. *Writing Culture*. Berkeley: University of California Press.

Collier, Jane, and Sylvia Yanagisako, eds. 1987a. *Gender and Kinship: Essays toward a Unified Analysis*. Stanford, CA: Stanford University Press.

Collier, Jane, and Sylvia Yanagisako. 1987b. "Introduction." In Collier and Yanagisako 1987a, 1–13.

Corea, Gena. 1985. *The Mother Machine: From Artificial Insemination to Artificial Wombs*. New York: Harper and Row.

Corea, Gena, Jalna Hanmer, Renate D. Klein, Janice G. Raymond, and Robyn Rowland. 1987. "Prologue." In Spallone and Steinberg 1987, 1–12.

Corea, Genoveffa. 1984. "Egg Snatchers." In Arditti et al. 1984, 37–51.

Crowe, Christine. 1985. "Women Want It: In Vitro Fertilization and Women's Motivations for Participation." *Women's Studies International Forum* 8: 547–552.

Crowe, Christine. 1987. "'Women Want It': *In Vitro* Fertilization and Women's Motivations for Participation." In Spallone and Steinberg 1987: 84–93.

Crowe, Christine. 1990. "Bearing the Consequences: Women Experiencing IVF." In Scutt 1990, 58–66.

Cussins, Charis. 1996. "Ontological Choreography: Agency through Objectification in Infertility Clinics." *Social Studies of Science* 26(3): 575–610.

da Costa, Beatriz, and Kavita Philip, eds. 2008. *Tactical Biopolitics: Art, Activism, and Technoscience*. Cambridge, MA: MIT Press.

Darwin, Charles. 1874. *The Descent of Man, and Selection in Relation to Sex*. 2nd ed. London: John Murray.

Davies, Sarah R. 2008. "Constructing Communication: Talking to Scientists about Talking to the Public." *Science Communication* 29(4): 413–34.

De Chadarevian, Soraya, and Nick Hopwood, eds. 2004. *Models: The Third Dimension of Science*. Stanford, CA: Stanford University Press.

Deech, Ruth, and Anna Smajdor. 2007. *From IVF to Immortality: Controversy in the Era of Reproductive Technology*. Oxford: Oxford University Press.

de Lauretis, Teresa. 1984. *Alice Doesn't: Feminism, Semiotics, Cinema*. Bloomington: Indiana University Press.

de Lauretis, Teresa. 1987. *Technologies of Gender: Essays on Theory, Film, and Fiction*. Bloomington: Indiana University Press.

Department of Health. 2011. *Taking Stock of Regenerative Medicine in the United Kingdom*. London: HMSO.

Derrida, Jacques. 1974. *Of Grammatology*. Trans. Gayatri Spivak. Baltimore, MD: Johns Hopkins University Press.

Derrida, Jacques. 1978. *Writing and Difference*. Trans. Alan Bass. London: Routledge.

Derrida, Jacques. 1981. *Dissemination*. Trans. Barbara Johnson. Chicago: University of Chicago Press.

Donchin, Anne. 1986. "The Future of Mothering: Reproductive Technology and Feminist Theory." *Hypatia* 1(2): 121–138.

Donchin, Anne. 1989. "The Growing Feminist Debate over the New Reproductive Technologies." *Hypatia* 4(3): 136–149.

Douglas, Mary. 1970. *Natural Symbols*. London: Barrie and Cresset.

Duden, Barbara. 1993. *Disembodying Women: Perspectives on Pregnancy and the Unborn*. Cambridge, MA: Harvard University Press.

Dworkin, Andrea. 1983. *Right-Wing Women*. New York: Perigee Books.

Dyson, Anthony. 1995. *The Ethics of IVF*. London: Mowbray.

Dziuk, Philip. 1993. "The Society for Reproduction: 25 Years in Retrospect." *Biology of Reproduction* 48: 28–32.

Edwards, Jeanette. 2000. *Born and Bred Oxford: Idioms of Kinship and New Reproductive Technologies in England*. Oxford: Oxford University Press.

Edwards, Jeanette, Sarah Franklin, Eric Hirsch, Francis Price, and Marilyn Strathern. 1993. *Technologies of Procreation: Kinship in the Age of Assisted Conception*. Manchester: Manchester University Press.

Edwards, Jeanette, and Charles Salazar, eds. 2009. *European Kinship in the Age of Biotechnology*. Oxford: Berghahn.

Edwards, Jeanette, and Marilyn Strathern. 2000. "Including Our Own." In J. Carsten, ed., *Cultures of Relatedness: New Approaches to the Study of Kinship*, 149–166. Cambridge: Cambridge University Press.

Edwards, R. G. 2001. "The Bumpy Road to Human In Vitro Fertilization." *Nature Medicine* 7(10): 1091–1094.

Edwards, R. G. 2004. "Stem Cells Today: Origin and Potential of Embryo Stem Cells." *RBMOnline* 8(3): 275–306.

Edwards, R. G. 2005. "Introduction: The Beginnings of In-Vitro Fertilization and Its Derivatives." In Robert Edwards and Francisco Risquez, eds., *Modern Assisted Conception*, 1–7. Cambridge: Reproductive Healthcare Ltd.

Edwards, R. G., B. D. Bavister, and P. C. Steptoe. 1969. "Early Stages of Fertilization In Vitro of Human Oocytes Matured In Vitro." *Nature* 221: 632–635.

Edwards, Robert. 1989. *Life before Birth: Reflections on the Embryo Debate*. London: Hutchinson.

Edwards, Robert, and Patrick Steptoe. 1980. *A Matter of Life: The Story of a Medical Breakthrough*. New York: William Morrow.

Ehrich, Kathryn, Clare Williams, and Bobby Farsides. 2008. "The Embryo as Moral Work Object: PGD/IVF Staff Views and Experiences." *Sociology of Health and Illness* 30(5): 772–787.

Eisenhower, Dwight D. 1961. "Farewell Address." American Rhetoric: Top 100 Speeches. Accessed November 5, 2011. http://www.americanrhetoric.com/speeches /dwightdeisenhowerfarewell.html.

Eldredge, Niles. 2009. "Experimenting with Transmutation: Darwin, the Beagle and Evolution." *Evolution: Education and Outreach* 2(1): 35–54.

Engels, Frederick. 1962. "The Part Played by Labour in the Transition from Ape to Man." In *Selected Works, Karl Marx and Frederick Engels*, vol. 2. Moscow: Foreign Language Publishing House.

Engels, Frederick. (1884) 2010. *The Origin of the Family, Private Property and the State*. London: Penguin.

Fabian, Johannes. 1983. *Time and the Other: How Anthropology Makes Its Object*. New York: Columbia University Press.

Farquhar, Dion. 1996. *The Other Machine: Discourse and Reproductive Technologies*. New York: Routledge.

Fausto-Sterling, Anne. 1985. *Myths of Gender: Biological Theories about Women and Men*. New York: Basic Books.

Firestone, Shulamith. 1972. *The Dialectic of Sex: The Case for Feminist Revolution*, rev. ed. New York: Bantam.

Fishel, Simon, and Malcolm Symonds. 1986. *In Vitro Fertilisation: Past, Present, Future*. Oxford: Blackwell.

Fitzgerald, Deborah. 1990. *The Business of Breeding: Hybrid Corn in Illinois, 1890–1940*. Ithaca, NY: Cornell University Press.

Foster, Michael, and Francis Maitland Balfour. 1874. *The Elements of Embryology*. London: Macmillan.

Foucault, Michel. 1973. *The Order of Things: An Archaeology of the Human Sciences*. New York: Vintage (translation of *Les mots et les choses*, Editions Gallimard, 1966).

Foucault, Michel. 1990. *The History of Sexuality*, vol. 1: *An Introduction*. Trans. Robert Hurley. New York.: Vintage.

Franklin, Sarah. 1991. "Fetal Fascinations: New Dimensions to the Medical Scientific Construction of Fetal Personhood." In Sarah Franklin, Jackie Stacey, and Celia Lury, eds., *Off-Centre: Feminism and Cultural Studies*, 190–205. London: HarperCollins.

Franklin, Sarah. 1995. "Science as Culture, Cultures of Science." *Annual Review of Anthropology* 24: 163–184.

Franklin, Sarah, ed. 1996. *The Sociology of Gender*. Cheltenham, U.K.: Edward Elgar.

Franklin, Sarah. 1997. *Embodied Progress: A Cultural Account of Reproduction*. London: Routledge.

Franklin, Sarah. 1999. "Dead Embryos: Feminism in Suspension." In Lynn M. Morgan and Meredith W. Michaels, eds., *Fetal Subjects, Feminist Positions*, 61–82. Philadelphia: University of Pennsylvania Press.

Franklin, Sarah. 2001a. "Biologization Revisited: Kinship Theory in the Context of the New Biologies." In Franklin and McKinnon 2001, 302–322.

Franklin, Sarah. 2001b. "Culturing Biology: Cell Lines for the Second Millennium." *Health* 5(3): 355–354.

Franklin, Sarah. 2003a. "Ethical Biocapital: New Strategies of Cell Culture." In Franklin and Lock 2003b, 97–128.

Franklin, Sarah. 2003b. "Re-thinking Nature-Culture: Anthropology and the New Genetics." *Anthropological Theory* 3(1): 65–85.

Franklin, Sarah. 2006a. "The Cyborg Embryo: Our Path to Transbiology." *Theory, Culture and Society* 23(7–8): 167–188.

Franklin, Sarah. 2006b. "Embryonic Economies: The Double Reproductive Value of Stem Cells." *Biosocieties* 1(1): 71–90.

Franklin, Sarah. 2006c. "The IVF–Stem Cell Interface." *International Journal of Surgery* 4(2): 86–90.

Franklin, Sarah. 2007a. "Crook Pipettes: Embryonic Emigrations from Agriculture to Reproductive Biomedicine." *Studies in the History and Philosophy of Science* 38(2): 358–373.

Franklin, Sarah. 2007b. *Dolly Mixtures: The Remaking of Genealogy*. Durham, NC: Duke University Press.

Franklin, Sarah. 2008. "Embryo Transfer: A View from the UK." In Francesca Molfino and Flavia Zucco, eds., *Women in Biotechnology: Creating Interfaces*. Berlin: Springer.

Franklin, Sarah. 2010a. "Revisiting Reprotech: Shulamith Firestone and the Question of Technology." In Mandy Merck and Stella Sandford, eds., *The Further Adventures of the Dialectic of Sex*, 29–60. London: Palgrave Macmillan.

Franklin, Sarah. 2010b. "Transbiology: A Feminist Cultural Account." *Scholar Feminist Online* 9(1–2).

Franklin, Sarah. 2013. "In Vitro Anthropos: New Conception Models for a Recursive Anthropology?" *Cambridge Anthropology* 31(1).

Franklin, Sarah, Charles Hunt, Glenda Cornwell, Valerie Peddie, Paul Desousa, Morag Livie, Emma L. Stephenson, and Peter R. Braude. 2008. "HESCCO: Development of Good Practice Models for hES Derivation." *Regenerative Medicine* 3(1): 105–116.

Franklin, Sarah, and Lamprini Kaftantzi. 2008. "Industry in the Middle: Interview with Intercytex Founder and CSO, Dr Paul Kemp." *Science as Culture* 17(4): 449–462.

Franklin, Sarah, and Sharon Kaufman. 2009. "Ethical and Consent Issues in the Reproductive Setting: The Case of Egg, Embryo and Sperm Donation." In Ruth Warwick, Deirdre Fehily, Ted Eastlund, and Scott A. Brubaker, eds., *Tissue and Cell Donation: An Essential Guide*, 222–243. Oxford: Wiley-Blackwell.

Franklin, Sarah, and Margaret Lock. 2003a. "Animation and Cessation: The Remaking of Life and Death." In Franklin and Lock 2003b, 3–22.

Franklin, Sarah, and Margaret Lock, eds. 2003b. *Remaking Life and Death: Towards an Anthropology of Biomedicine*. Santa Fe, NM: School of American Research Press.

Franklin, Sarah, Celia Lury, and Jackie Stacey. 2000. *Global Nature, Global Culture*. London: Sage.

Franklin, Sarah, and Susan McKinnon, eds. 2001. *Relative Values: Reconfiguring Kinship Studies*. Durham, NC: Duke University Press.

Franklin, Sarah, and Maureen McNeil. 1988. "Reproductive Futures: Recent Literature and Current Debates on Reproductive Technologies." *Feminist Studies* 14(3): 545–561.

Franklin, Sarah, and Helena Ragoné, eds. 1998. *Reproducing Reproduction: Kinship, Power and Technological Innovation*. Philadelphia: University of Pennsylvania Press.

Franklin, Sarah, and Celia Roberts. 2006. *Born and Made: An Ethnography of Preimplantation Genetic Diagnosis*. Princeton, NJ: Princeton University Press.

Friese, Carrie. 2013. *Cloning Wild Life: Making Nature in the Zoo*. New York: New York University Press.

Fujimura, Joan. 1996. *Crafting Science: A Sociohistory of the Quest for the Genetics of Cancer*. Cambridge, MA: Harvard University Press.

Fukuyama, Francis. 2002. *Our Posthuman Future: Consequences of the Biotechnology Revolution*. New York: Farrar, Straus and Giroux.

Gardner, Bruce L. 2002. *American Agriculture in the Twentieth Century: How It Flourished and What It Cost*. Cambridge, MA: Harvard University Press.

Garfinkel, Harold. 1967. *Studies in Ethnomethodology*. Englewood Cliffs, NJ: Prentice-Hall.

Geertz, Clifford. 1966. "Religion as a Cultural System." In Michael Banton, ed., *Anthropological Approaches to the Study of Religion*, 1–66. London: Routledge.

Geertz, Clifford. 1973. *The Interpretation of Cultures: Selected Essays*. New York: Basic Books.

Geesink, Ingrid, Barbara Prainsack, and Sarah Franklin. 2008. "Stem Cell Stories: 1998–2008." *Science as Culture* 17(1): 1–11.

Gell, Alfred. 1988. "Technology and Magic." *Anthropology Today* 4(2): 6–9.

Genetic Interest Group. 2008. "Background Briefing on Stem Cell Research for Second Reading of the Human Fertilisation and Embryology Bill." Accessed April 11, 2011. http://www.geneticalliance.org.uk/docs/BriefingStemCellResearch.pdf.

Gilbert, Scott F. 1994. *A Conceptual History of Modern Embryology*. Baltimore, MD: Johns Hopkins University Press.

Ginsburg, Faye. 1998. *Contested Lives: The Abortion Debate in an American Community*. Berkeley: University of California Press.

Goffman, Erving. 1976. *Stigma: Notes on the Management of Spoiled Identity*. New York: Penguin.

Gonzalez-Santos, Sandra. 2010. "The Sociological Aspects of Assisted Reproduction in Mexico." PhD Dissertation, University of Sussex.

Goodman, Alan H., Deborah Heath, and M. Susan Lindee. 2003. *Genetic Nature/Culture: Anthropology and Science beyond the Two-Culture Divide*. Berkeley: University of California Press.

Gordon, Ian R. 2003. *Laboratory Production of Cattle Embryos*, 2nd ed. Wallingford, U.K.: CABI.

Graham, Chris. 2000. "Mammalian Development in the UK (1950–1995)." *International Journal of Developmental Biology* 44: 51–55.

Habermas, Jürgen. 1971. *Toward a Rational Society: Student Protest, Science, and Politics*. Boston: Beacon.

Habermas, Jürgen. 2003. *The Future of Human Nature*. Cambridge: Polity.

Habermas, Jürgen. 2010. "Technical Progress and the Social Life-World." In Craig Hanks, ed., *Technology and Values: Essential Readings*, 169–175. Oxford: Blackwell.

Hacking, Ian. 1983. *Representing and Intervening: Introductory Topics in the Philosophy of Natural Science*. Cambridge University Press.

Haldane, J. B. S. 1924. *Daedalus; or, Science and the Future*. New York: E. P. Dutton and Company.

Hamburger, Viktor. 1962. *A Manual of Experimental Embryology*, rev. ed. Chicago: University of Chicago Press.

Hamburger, Viktor. 1988. *The Heritage of Experimental Embryology: Hans Spemann and the Organizer*. New York: Oxford University Press.

Haraway, Donna J. 1976. *Crystals, Fabrics and Fields: Metaphors of Organicism in Twentieth-Century Developmental Biology*. New Haven, CT: Yale University Press.

Haraway, Donna. 1978a. "Animal Sociology and a Natural Economy of the Body Politic, Part I: A Political Physiology of Dominance." *Signs* 4(1): 21–36.

Haraway, Donna. 1978b. "Animal Sociology and a Natural Economy of the Body Politic, Part II: The Past Is the Contested Zone: Human Nature and Theories of Production and Reproduction in Primate Behaviour Studies." *Signs* 4(1): 37–60.

Haraway, Donna. 1979. "The Biological Enterprise: Sex, Mind, and Profit from Human Engineering to Sociobiology." *Radical History Review* 20: 206–237.

Haraway, Donna. 1981. "In the Beginning Was the Word: The Genesis of Biological Theory." *Signs* 6(3): 469–481.

Haraway, Donna. 1983. "The Ironic Dream of a Common Language for Women in the Integrated Circuit: Science, Technology, and Socialist Feminism in the 1980s or a Socialist Manifesto for Cyborgs." Accessed March 21, 2011. http://www.molodiez .org/net/harraway.pdf.

Haraway, Donna. 1984. "Teddy Bear Patriarchy: Taxidermy in the Garden of Eden, New York City, 1908–1936." *Social Text* 11: 20–64.

Haraway, Donna. 1985. "A Manifesto for Cyborgs: Science, Technology, and Socialist-Feminism in the Late Twentieth Century." *Socialist Review* 80: 65–108.

Haraway, Donna. 1989. *Primate Visions: Gender, Race and Nature in the World of Modern Science.* New York: Routledge.

Haraway, Donna. 1991. *Simians, Cyborgs, and Women: The Reinvention of Nature.* London: Free Association Books.

Haraway, Donna J. 1997. *Modest_Witness@Second_Millennium.FemaleMan©_Meets _Oncomouse™.* New York: Routledge.

Haraway, Donna. 2004a. "Ecce Homo, Ain't (Ar'n't) I a Woman, and Inappropriate/d Others: The Human in a Post-humanist Landscape." In *The Haraway Reader*, 47–62. New York: Routledge.

Haraway, Donna. 2004b. "Introduction: A Kinship of Feminist Figurations." In *The Haraway Reader*, 1–6. New York: Routledge.

Haraway, Donna. 2006. "When We Have Never Been Human, What Is to Be Done: Interview with Donna Haraway" [interviewer Nickolas Gane]. *Theory, Culture and Society* 23(7–8): 135–158.

Haraway, Donna. 2008. *When Species Meet.* Minneapolis: University of Minnesota Press.

Heidegger, Martin. 1968. *What Is Called Thinking?* New York: Harper and Row.

Heidegger, Martin. 1982. "Kein Tier hat eine Hand." In *Paramenides.* Frankfurt am Main: Vittorio Klostermann.

Heidegger, Martin. 1993. *Basic Writings: From Being and Time (1927) to The Task of Thinking (1964).* Ed. David Farrell Krell. London: Routledge.

Heidegger, Martin. 1995. *The Fundamental Concepts of Metaphysics: World, Finitude, Solitude.* Bloomington: Indiana University Press.

Helmreich, Stefan. 2008. "Species of Biocapital." *Science as Culture* 17(4): 463–478.

Henig, Robin Marantz. 2004. *Pandora's Baby: How the First Test Tube Babies Sparked the Reproductive Revolution.* New York: Houghton Mifflin.

Herschel, John Frederick William. 1830. *Preliminary Discourse on the Study of Natural Philosophy.* London.

Hird, Myra J. 2009. *The Origins of Sociable Life: Evolution after Science Studies.* London: Palgrave Macmillan.

Holmes, Helen B., Betty B. Hoskins, and Michael Gross, eds. 1980. *Birth Control and Controlling Birth: Women-Centered Perspectives.* Clifton, NJ: Humana.

Holmes, Helen B., Betty B. Hoskins, and Michael Gross, eds. 1981. *The Custom-Made Child? Women-Centered Perspectives.* Clifton, NJ: Humana.

Honigman, David. 2010. "Lunch with the FT: Stewart Brand." *Financial Times*, January 8, 2010.

hooks, bell. 1981. *Ain't I a Woman: Black Women and Feminism*. Boston: South End.

Hopwood, Nick. 1999. "'Giving Body' to Embryos: Modeling, Mechanism and the Microtome in Late Nineteenth-Century Anatomy." *Isis* 90(3): 462–496.

Hopwood, Nick. 2000. "Producing Development: The Anatomy of Human Embryos and the Norms of Wilhelm His." *Bulletin of the History of Medicine* 74(1): 29–79.

Hopwood, Nick. 2009. "Embryology." In Peter J. Bowler and John V. Pickstone, eds., *The Cambridge History of Science*, vol. 6: *The Modern Biological and Earth Sciences*, 285–315. Cambridge: Cambridge University Press.

Horder, T. J., J. A. Witkoski, and C. C. Wylie, eds. 1985. *A History of Embryology*. Cambridge: Cambridge University Press.

Hubbard, Ruth. 1990. *The Politics of Women's Biology*. New Brunswick, NJ: Rutgers University Press.

Hull Fertility Services. 2011. "IVF Step 1: Downregulation." Accessed April 12. http://www.hullivf.org.uk/treatment/ivf/step1.html.

Hurtado, Aida. 1989. "Relating to Privilege: Seduction and Rejection in the Subordination of White Women and Women of Colour." *Signs* 14(4): 833–855.

Huxley, Julian. (1914) 1968. *The Courtship Habits of the Great Crested Grebe: With an Addition to the Theory of Sexual Selection*. London: Jonathan Cape.

Hynes, H. Patricia. 1987. "A Paradigm for Regulation of the Biomedical Industry: Environmental Protection in the United States." In Spallone and Steinberg 1987, 190–205.

IETS (International Embryo Transfer Society). 1993. "Robert Geoffrey Edwards, CBE, FRCOG, FRS: Recipient of the 1993 Embryo Transfer Pioneer Award." *Theriogenology* 39(1): 1–4.

Inhorn, Marcia. 1994. *Quest for Conception: Gender, Infertility, and Egyptian Medical Traditions*. Philadelphia: University of Pennsylvania Press.

Inhorn, Marcia. 1996. *Infertility and Patriarchy: The Cultural Politics of Gender and Family Life in Egypt*. Philadelphia: University of Pennsylvania Press.

Inhorn, Marcia C. 2003. *Local Babies, Global Science: Gender, Religion and In Vitro Fertilization in Egypt*. New York: Routledge.

Inhorn, Marcia C. 2011. "Diasporic Dreaming: Return Reproductive Tourism to the Middle-East." *Reproductive Biomedicine Online* 23(5): 582–591.

Inhorn, Marcia C., and Zeynep B. Gurtin. 2011. "Cross-Border Reproductive Care: A Future Research Agenda." *Reproductive Biomedicine Online* 23(5): 665–676.

Jasanoff, Sheila. 2007. *Designs on Nature: Science and Democracy in Europe and the United States*. Princeton, NJ: Princeton University Press.

Jenkinson, John Wilfred. 1909. *Experimental Embryology*. Oxford: Clarendon.

Johnson, Martin H. 2010. "Robert Edwards: Nobel Laureate in Physiology or Medicine." Lecture given at the Nobel Prize Symposium in Honour of Robert G. Edwards, December 7, 2010, Karolinska Institutet, Stockholm.

Johnson, Martin H. 2011. "Robert Edwards: The Path to IVF." *Reproductive Biomedicine Online* 23: 245–262.

Johnson, M. H., S. B. Franklin, M. Cottingham, and N. Hopwood. 2010. "Why the MRC

Refused Robert Edwards and Patrick Steptoe Support for Research on Human Conception in 1971." *Human Reproduction* 25: 2157–2174.

Jordanova, Ludmilla. 1980. "Natural Facts: A Historical Perspective on Science and Sexuality." In MacCormack and Strathern 1980, 42–69.

Kahn, Susan Martha. 2000. *Reproducing Jews: A Cultural Account of Assisted Conception in Israel.* Durham, NC: Duke University Press.

Keating, Peter, and Alberto Cambrosio. 2003. *Biomedical Platforms: Realigning the Normal and the Pathological in Late-Twentieth-Century Medicine.* Cambridge, MA: MIT Press.

Keller, Evelyn Fox. 1982. "Feminism and Science." *Signs* 7(3): 589–602.

Keller, Evelyn Fox. 1983. *A Feeling for the Organism: The Life and Work of Barbara McClintock.* Oxford: Blackwell.

Keller, Evelyn Fox. 1992. *Secrets of Life, Secrets of Death: Essays on Language, Gender and Science.* New York: Routledge.

Keller, Evelyn Fox. 1996a. "The Biological Gaze." In George Robertson, Melinda Mash, Lisa Tickner, Jon Bird, Barry Curtis, and Tim Putnam, eds., *FutureNatural: Nature, Science and Culture,* 107–121. London: Routledge.

Keller, Evelyn Fox. 1996b. *Reflections on Gender and Science.* New Haven, CT: Yale University Press.

Keller, Evelyn Fox. 2002. *The Century of the Gene.* Cambridge, MA: Harvard University Press.

Keller, Evelyn Fox. 2003. *Making Sense of Life: Explaining Biological Development with Models, Metaphors and Machines.* Cambridge, MA: Harvard University Press.

Keller, Evelyn Fox. 2009. "What Does Synthetic Biology Have to Do with Biology?" *BioSocieties* 4: 291–302.

Kevles, Daniel. 1977. "The National Science Foundation and the Debate over Postwar Research Policy, 1942–1945: A Political Interpretation of Science — the Endless Frontier." *Isis* 68(1): 4–26.

Kirby, Vicki. 2011. *Quantum Anthropologies: Life at Large.* Durham, NC: Duke University Press.

Klein, Renate, ed. 1989. *Infertility: Women Speak Out about Their Experiences of Reproductive Medicine.* London: Pandora.

Koch, Lene. 1990. "IVF — an Irrational Choice?" *Reproductive and Genetic Engineering* 3: 225–232.

Kolodny, Annette. 1975. *The Lay of the Land: Metaphor as Experience and History in American Life and Letters.* Chapel Hill: University of North Carolina Press.

Kolodny, Annette. 1984. *The Land Before Her: Fantasy and Experience of the American Frontiers, 1630–1860.* Chapel Hill: University of North Carolina Press.

Landecker, Hannah. 2007. *Culturing Life: How Cells Became Technologies.* Cambridge, MA: Harvard University Press.

Latour, Bruno. 1987. *Science in Action: How to Follow Scientists and Engineers through Society.* Cambridge, MA: Harvard University Press.

Latour, Bruno. 1993. *We Have Never Been Modern.* Cambridge, MA: Harvard University Press.

Latour, Bruno, and Steve Woolgar. 1979. *Laboratory Life: The Construction of Scientific Facts*. London: Sage.

Leach, Edmund. 1970. *Claude Lévi-Strauss*. London: Fontana.

Lemonnier, Pierre. 1993. *Technological Choices: Transformation in Material Cultures since the Neolithic*. London: Routledge.

Leroi-Gourhan, André. 1993. *Gesture and Speech*. Cambridge, MA: MIT Press.

Lesnik-Oberstein, Karin. 2008. *On Having an Own Child: Reproductive Technologies and the Cultural Construction of Childhood*. London: Karnac.

Lévi-Strauss, Claude. 1969. *The Elementary Structures of Kinship*. Boston: Beacon.

Lewin, Ellen. 1993. *Lesbian Mothers: Accounts of Gender in American Culture*. Ithaca, NY: Cornell University Press.

Lorber, Judith. 1989. "Choice, Gift or Patriarchal Bargain? Women's Consent to In Vitro Fertilization in Male Infertility." *Hypatia* 4(3): 23–36.

Lorde, Audre. 1984. *Sister Outsider: Essays and Speeches*. New York: Crossing Press.

Lovelock, James E., and Lynn Margulis. 1974. "Atmospheric Homeostasis by and for the Biosphere: The Gaia Hypothesis." *Tellus* 26(1–2): 2–10.

Lublin, Nancy. 1998. *Pandora's Box: Feminism Confronts Reproductive Technology*. Lanham, MD: Rowman and Littlefield.

Lynch, Michael. 1985. *Art and Artifact in Laboratory Science: A Study of Shop Work and Shop Talk in a Research Laboratory*. London: Routledge and Kegan Paul.

MacCormack, Carol. 1980. "Nature, Culture and Gender: A Critique." In MacCormack and Strathern 1980, 1–24.

MacCormack, Carol, and Marilyn Strathern, eds. 1980. *Nature, Culture and Gender*. Cambridge: Cambridge University Press.

Macksey, Richard, and Eugenio Donato, eds. 1972. *The Structuralist Controversy: The Languages of Criticism and the Sciences of Man*. Baltimore, MD: Johns Hopkins University Press.

Maienschein, Jane. 1986. *Defining Biology: Lectures from the 1890s*. Cambridge, MA: Harvard University Press.

Maienschein, Jane. 2003. *Whose View of Life? Embryos, Cloning and Stem Cells*. Cambridge, MA: Harvard University Press.

Mamo, Laura. 2007. *Queering Reproduction: Achieving Pregnancy in the Age of Technoscience*. Durham, NC: Duke University Press.

Marden, W. G., and M. C. Chang. 1952. "The Aerial Transport of Mammalian Ova for Transplantation." *Science* 115: 705–706.

Margulis, Lynn, and James Lovelock. 1974. "Biological Modulation of the Earth's Atmosphere." *Icarus* 21(4): 471–489.

Marsh, Margaret S., and Wanda Ronner. 1996. *The Empty Cradle: Infertility in America from Colonial Times to the Present*. Baltimore, MD: Johns Hopkins University Press.

Martin, Emily. 1987. *The Woman in the Body: A Cultural Analysis of Reproduction*. Boston: Beacon.

Martin, Emily. 1991. "The Egg and the Sperm: How Science Has Constructed a Romance Based on Stereotypical Male and Female Roles." *Signs* 16(3): 485–501.

Marx, Karl. 1990. *Capital: A Critique of Political Economy*. London: Penguin.

Marx, Leo. 2000. *The Machine in the Garden: Technology and the Pastoral Ideal in America*. Oxford: Oxford University Press.

Mathieu, Nicole-Claude. 1973. "Homme-Culture et Femme-Nature." *L'Homme* 13(3): 101–113.

McKibben, Bill. 2004. *Enough: Staying Human in an Engineered Age*. New York: St. Martin's.

McLaren, Anne. 1976. *Mammalian Chimaeras*. Cambridge: Cambridge University Press.

Mead, George Herbert. 1934. *Mind, Self and Society*. Chicago, IL: University of Chicago Press.

MECW. "Marx/Engels Collected Works." Marxists Internet Archive. http://www.marxists.org/archive/marx/works/cw/index.htm.

Mies, Maria. 1985. "'Why Do We Need All This?': A Call against Genetic Engineering and Reproductive Technology." *Women's Studies International Forum* 8(6): 553–560.

Minh-ha, Trinh. 1989. *Woman, Native, Other: Writing Postcoloniality and Feminism*. Bloomington: Indiana University Press.

Modell, Judith. 1994. *Kinship with Strangers: Adoption and Interpretations of Kinship in American Culture*. Berkeley, CA: University of California Press.

Modell, Judith. 2002. *A Sealed and Secret Kinship: A Culture of Policies and Practices in American Adoption*. Oxford: Berghahn.

Mol, Annemarie. 2002. *The Body Multiple: Ontology in Medical Practice*. Durham, NC: Duke University Press.

Moraga, Cherríe, and Gloria Anzaldúa, eds. 1981. *This Bridge Called My Back: Writings by Radical Women of Color*. Watertown, MA: Persephone.

Morgan, Lewis Henry. 1877. *Ancient Society; or, Researches in the Lines of Human Progress from Savagery through Barbarism to Civilization*. New York: Henry Holt.

Mundy, Liza. 2007. *Everything Conceivable: How Assisted Reproduction Is Changing Our World*. New York: Anchor.

Needham, Joseph. 1935. "Limiting Factors in the Advancement of Science as Observed in the History of Embryology." *Yale Journal of Biological Medicine* 8(1): 1–18.

Needham, Joseph. 1959. *A History of Embryology*. New York: Arno.

Noland, Carrie. 2009. *Agency and Embodiment: Performing Gestures — Producing Culture*. Cambridge, MA: Harvard University Press.

Nuffield Council on Bioethics. 2012. *Novel Techniques for the Prevention of Mitochondrial DNA Disorders: An Ethical Review*. June. Accessed May 13, 2012. http://www.nuffieldbioethics.org/mitochondrial-dna-disorders.

Nyhart, Lynn K. 1995. *Biology Takes Form: Animal Morphology and the German Universities, 1800–1900*. Chicago: University of Chicago Press.

Oakley, Ann. 1987. "From Walking Wombs to Test-Tube Babies." In Stanworth 1987, 36–56.

O'Brien, Keith. 2008. "Easter Sunday Homily." BBC News, March 21. Accessed October 5, 2010. http://news.bbc.co.uk/1/hi/scotland/7308883.stm.

O'Brien, Mary. 1981. *The Politics of Reproduction*. London: Routledge and Kegan Paul.

Oppenheimer, Jane M. 1967. *Essays in the History of Embryology and Biology*. Cambridge, MA: MIT Press.

Orland, Barbara. 2001. "Spuren Einer Entdeckung. (Re-)Konstructionen der Unfrucht-barkeit im Zeitalter der Fortplanzungsmedizin." *Gesnerus* 58: 5–29.

Ortner, Sherry. 1972. "Is Female to Male as Nature Is to Culture?" *Feminist Studies* 1(2): 5–31.

Ortner, Sherry. 1974. "Is Female to Male as Nature Is to Culture?" In Michelle Zimbal-ist Rosaldo and Louise Lamphere, eds., *Woman, Culture and Society*, 67–88. Stanford, CA: Stanford University Press.

Overall, Christine. 1987. *Ethics and Human Reproduction: A Feminist Analysis.* Boston, MA: Allen and Unwin.

Owens, Larry. 1994. "The Counterproductive Management of Science in the Second World War: Vannevar Bush and the Office of Scientific Research and Development." *Business History Review* 68(4): 515–576.

Parkes, Alan S. 1966. *Sex, Science and Society: Addresses, Lectures and Articles.* London: Oriel.

Parkes, Alan S. 1985. *Off-Beat Biologist: The Autobiography of Alan S. Parkes.* Cambridge: Galton Foundation.

Pauly, Philip J. 1987. *Controlling Life: Jacques Loeb and the Engineering Ideal in Biology.* Oxford: Oxford University Press.

Pauly, Philip. 2007. *Fruits and Plains: The Horticultural Transformation of America.* Cambridge, MA: Harvard University Press.

Paxson, Heather. 2004. *Making Modern Mothers: Ethics and Family Planning in Urban Greece.* Berkeley: University of California Press.

Peletz, Michael. 2001. "Ambivalence in Kinship since the 1940s." In Franklin and McKinnon 2001, 413–444.

Petchesky, Rosalind Pollack. 1984. *Abortion and Women's Choice: The State, Sexuality, and Reproductive Freedom.* Boston, MA: Northeastern University Press.

Petchesky, Rosalind Pollack. 1987. "Foetal Images: The Power of Visual Culture in the Politics of Reproduction." In Stanworth 1987, 57–80.

Pfeffer, Naomi. 1985. "Not So New Technologies." *Trouble and Strife* 5 (spring): 46–50.

Pfeffer, Naomi. 1993. *The Stork and the Syringe: A Political History of Reproductive Medi-cine.* Cambridge: Polity.

Pfeffer, Naomi, and Anne Woollett. 1983. *The Experience of Infertility.* London: Virago.

Pickering, Andrew. 1995. *The Mangle of Practice: Time, Agency and Science.* Chicago: University of Chicago Press.

Pincus, G. 1930. "Observations on the Living Eggs of the Rabbit." *Proceedings of the Royal Society of London* 107(749): 132–167.

Pincus, G. 1936. *The Eggs of Mammals.* New York: Macmillan.

Pincus, G. 1939a. "The Breeding of Some Rabbits Produced by Recipients of Artificially Activated Ova." *Proceedings of the National Academy of Science* 25: 557–559.

Pincus, G. 1939b. "Ovum Culture." *Science* 89: 509.

Pincus, G., and E. Enzmann. 1934. "Can Mammalian Eggs Undergo Normal Develop-ment In Vitro?" *Proceedings of the National Academy of Science* 20: 121–122.

Plato. 2005. *Phaedrus.* Trans. Christopher Rowe. London: Penguin.

Prainsack, Barbara, Ingrid Geesink, and Sarah Franklin. 2008. "Stem Cell Technolo-gies 1998–2008: Controversies and Silences." *Science as Culture* 17(4): 351–362.

Pratt, Mary Louise. 1992. *Imperial Eyes: Travel Writing and Transculturation*. New York: Routledge.

Rabinow, Paul. 1992. "Artificiality and Enlightenment." In J. Crary and S. Kwinter, eds., *Incorporations*, 234–252. New York: Zone Books.

Rafferty, Keen A. 1970. *Methods in Experimental Embryology of the Mouse*. Baltimore, MD: Johns Hopkins University Press.

Rapp, Rayna. 1999. *Testing Women, Testing the Fetus: The Social Impact of Amniocentesis in America*. New York: Routledge.

Raymond, Janice. 1984. "Feminist Ethics, Ecology and Vision." In Arditti et al. 1984, 427–437.

Raymond, Janice. 1993. *Women as Wombs: Reproductive Technologies and the Battle over Women's Freedom*. New York: Harper San Francisco.

Ritvo, Harriet. 1987. *The Animal Estate: The English and Other Creatures in the Victorian Age*. Cambridge, MA: Harvard University Press.

Robertson, John. 1994. *Children of Choice: Freedom and the New Reproductive Technologies*. Princeton, NJ: Princeton University Press.

Rolt, L. T. C. 1967. *The Mechanicals: Progress of a Profession*. London: Heinemann.

Roosevelt, Franklin D. 1944. "President Roosevelt's Letter." National Science Foundation. Accessed February 2, 2012. http://www.nsf.gov/od/lpa/nsf50/vbush1945.htm#letter.

Rosaldo, Michelle, and Louise Lamphere, eds. 1974. *Woman, Culture and Society*. Stanford, CA: Stanford University Press.

Rossiter, Margaret. 1979. "The Organization of the Agricultural Sciences." In A. Oleson and J. Voss, eds., *The Organization of Knowledge in Modern America, 1860–1920*, 211–248. Baltimore, MD: Johns Hopkins University Press.

Rothman, Barbara Katz. 1984. "The Meanings of Choice in Reproductive Technology." In Arditti et al. 1984., 23–34.

Rothman, Barbara Katz. 1986. *The Tentative Pregnancy: How Amniocentesis Changes the Experience of Motherhood*. New York: Norton.

Rowland, Robyn. 1992. *Living Laboratories: Women and Reproductive Technology*. London: Octopus.

Rubin, Gayle. 1975. "The Traffic in Women: Notes on the 'Political Economy' of Sex." In Rayna Reiter, ed., *Towards an Anthropology of Women*, 157–210. New York: Monthly Review Press.

Rubin, Gayle. 1992. "Thinking Sex: Notes for a Radical Theory of the Politics of Sexuality." In C. S. Vance, ed., *Pleasure and Danger: Exploring Female Sexuality*. New York: Pandora.

Russell, Diane E. H., and Nicole Van de Ven. 1976. *Crimes against Women: Proceedings of the International Tribunal*. Milbrae, CA: Les Femmes.

Sahlins, Marshall David. 1972. *Stone Age Economics*. Chicago, IL: Aldine.

Sahlins, Marshall David. 1976. The Use and Abuse of Biology: An Anthropological Critique of Sociobiology. Ann Arbor: University of Michigan Press.

Sandelowski, Margarete. 1990. "Fault Lines: Infertility and Imperiled Sisterhood." *Feminist Studies* 16(1): 33–51.

Sandelowski, Margarete. 1991. "Compelled to Try: The Never-Enough Quality of Reproductive Technology." *Medical Anthropology Quarterly* 5(1): 29–47.

Sandelowski, Margarete. 1993. *With Child in Mind: Studies of the Personal Encounter with Infertility*. Philadelphia: University of Pennsylvania Press.

Sander, Klaus, and Peter E. Faessler. 2001. "Introducing the Spemann-Mangold Organizer: Experiments and Insights That Generated a Key Concept in Developmental Biology." *International Journal of Developmental Biology* 45: 1–11.

Sawicki, Jana. 1991. *Disciplining Foucault: Feminism, Power and the Body*. New York: Routledge.

Schneider, David M. 1968. *American Kinship: A Cultural Account*. Englewood Cliffs, NJ: Prentice-Hall.

Schneider, David. 1984. *A Critique of the Study of Kinship*. Ann Arbor: University of Michigan Press.

Scutt, Jocelyn, ed. 1990. *The Baby Machine: Reproductive Technology and the Commercialisation of Motherhood*. London: Merlin.

Sedgwick, Eve Kosofsky. 1990. *Epistemology of the Closet*. Berkeley: University of California Press.

Seller, Mary. 2008. "Slipping on the Slippery Slope of Progress." *Tablet*, April 5, 2008. Accessed October 9, 2010. http://www.thetablet.co.uk/article/11258.

Sennett, Richard. 2008. *The Craftsman*. London: Penguin.

Shukin, Nicole. 2009. *Animal Capital: Rendering Life in Biopolitical Times*. Minneapolis: University of Minnesota Press.

Smith, Austin G. 2008. "Embryo-Derived Stem Cells: Of Mice and Men." *Annual Review of Cell and Developmental Biology* 17: 435–462.

Smith, Neil, and Phil O'Keefe. 1980. "Geography, Marx and the Concept of Nature." *Antipode* 12(2): 30–39.

Soames, Gemma. 2009. *Sunday Times* (London), February 1, 2009. Accessed April 18, 2011. http://women.timesonline.co.uk/tol/life_and_style/women/families/article5599066.ece.

Solomon, Alison. 1989. "Infertility as Crisis: Coping, Surviving—and Thriving." In Klein 1989, 169–187.

Spallone, Patricia. 1989. *Beyond Conception: The New Politics of Reproduction*. London: Macmillan.

Spallone, Patricia, and Deborah Lynn Steinberg, eds. 1987. *Made to Order: The Myth of Reproductive and Genetic Progress*. London: Pergamon.

Spar, Debora. 2006. *The Baby Business: How Money, Science, and Politics Drive the Commerce of Conception*. Cambridge, MA: Harvard Business School Press.

Speroff, Leon. 2009. *A Good Man: Gregory Goodwin Pincus*. Portland, OR: Arnica.

Spillers, Hortense. 1987. "Mama's Baby, Papa's Maybe: An American Grammar Book." *Diacritics* 17(2): 65–81.

Spivak, Gayatri. 1985. "Criticism, Feminism and the Institution." *Thesis Eleven* 10/11: 175–187.

Spivak, Gayatri. 1987. *In the Other Worlds: Essays in Cultural Politics*. New York: Methuen.

Squier, Susan Merrill. 1994. *Babies in Bottles: Twentieth-Century Visions of Reproductive Technology*. New Brunswick, NJ: Rutgers University Press.

Stanworth, Michelle, ed. 1987. *Reproductive Technologies: Gender, Motherhood and Medicine*. Cambridge: Polity.

Star, Susan Leigh. 1989. *Regions of the Mind: Brain Research and the Quest for Scientific Certainty*. Palo Alto, CA: Stanford University Press.

Star, Susan Leigh. 1995. *Ecologies of Knowledge: Work and Politics in Science and Technology*. Albany: State University of New York Press.

Stephenson, Emma, Caroline Mackie Ogilvie, Heema Patel, Glenda Cornwell, Laureen Jacquet, Neli Kadeva, Peter Braude, and Dusko Ilic. 2010. "Safety Paradigm: Genetic Evaluation of Therapeutic Grade Human Embryonic Stem Cells." *Interface* 7 (Suppl. 6): s677–688.

Stiegler, Bernard. 1998. *Technics and Time, I: The Fault of Epimetheus*. Trans. Richard Beardsworth and George Collins. Stanford, CA: Stanford University Press.

Strathern, Marilyn. 1980. "No Nature, No Culture: The Hagen Case." In MacCormack and Strathern 1980, 174–222.

Strathern, Marilyn. 1984. "Marriage Exchanges: A Melanesian Comment." *Annual Review of Anthropology* 13: 41–73.

Strathern, Marilyn. 1987. "Producing Difference: Connections and Disconnections in Two New Guinea Highland Kinship Systems." In Collier and Yanagisako 1987a, 271–300.

Strathern, Marilyn. 1988. *The Gender of the Gift: Problems with Women and Problems with Society in Melanesia*. Berkeley: University of California Press.

Strathern, Marilyn. 1992a. *After Nature: English Kinship in the Late Twentieth Century*. Cambridge: Cambridge University Press.

Strathern, Marilyn. 1992b. *Reproducing the Future: Anthropology, Kinship and the New Reproductive Technologies*. New York: Routledge.

Strathern, Marilyn. 1999. *Property, Substance and Effect: Anthropological Essays on Persons and Things*. London: Athlone.

Strathern, Marilyn. 2005. *Kinship, Law and the Unexpected: Relatives Are Always a Surprise*. Cambridge: Cambridge University Press.

Suchman, Lucy. 1987. *Plans and Situated Actions: The Problem of Human-Machine Communication*. Cambridge: Cambridge University Press.

Suchman, Lucy. 1995. "Making Work Visible." *Communications of the ACM* 38(9): 56–64.

Suchman, Lucy. 2007. *Human-Machine Reconfigurations: Plans and Situated Actions*. Cambridge: Cambridge University Press.

Takahashi, K., and S. Yamanaka. 2006. "Induction of Pluripotent Stem Cells from Mouse Embryonic and Adult Fibroblast Cultures by Defined Factors. *Cell* 126(4): 663–676.

Taylor, Gordon Rattray. 1968. *The Biological Time Bomb*. Cleveland, OH: World.

Thompson, Charis. 2005. *Making Parents: The Ontological Choreography; Reproductive Technologies*. Cambridge, MA: MIT Press.

Throsby, Karen. 2004. *When IVF Fails: Feminism, Infertility and the Negotiation of Normality*. London: Palgrave.

Turner, Frederick Jackson. 1947. *The Frontier in American History*. New York: Henry Holt.

Turner, Frederick Jackson. 1961. *Frontier and Section: Selected Essays of Frederick Jackson Turner*. Englewood Cliffs, NJ: Prentice-Hall.

Verlinsky, Yury, and Anver Kuliev. 2005. *Atlas of Preimplantation Genetic Diagnosis*. London: CRC Press.

Waddington, Conrad H., and A. J. Waterman. 1933. "The Development In Vitro of Young Rabbit Embryos." *Journal of Anatomy* 67(3): 355–370.

Wagner, Roy. 1975. *The Invention of Culture*. Englewood Cliffs, NJ: Prentice-Hall.

Walker, Alice. 1983. *In Search of Our Mother's Gardens: Womanist Prose*. New York: Harcourt Brace Jovanovich.

Warner, Marina. 1996. *The Inner Eye: Art beyond the Visible*. London: Vintage.

Warnock, Mary. 1985. *A Question of Life: The Warnock Report on Human Fertilisation and Embryology*. Oxford: Basil Blackwell.

Weiner, Annette. 1978. "The Reproductive Model in Trobriand Society." *Mankind* 11(3): 175–186.

Wendling, Amy E. 2009. *Karl Marx on Technology and Alienation*. Houndmills, U.K.: Palgrave Macmillan.

White, Leslie. 1959. *The Evolution of Culture: The Development of Civilization to the Fall of Rome*. New York: McGraw-Hill.

Williams, Linda. 1988. "'It's Going to Work for Me': Responses to Failures of IVF." *Birth* 15(3): 131–196.

Williams, Raymond. 1990. *Television*. London: Routledge.

Winkler, Ute. 1989. "He Called Me Number 27." In Klein 1989, 90–100.

Wittig, Monique. 1969. *Les guérillères*. Paris: Les Editions de Minuit.

Wittig, Monique. 1992. *The Straight Mind*. London: Harvester Wheatsheaf.

Yanagisako, Sylvia J. 1985. "The Elementary Structure of Reproduction in Kinship and Gender Studies." Paper presented at the Annual Meeting of the American Anthropological Association, Washington, DC.

Yanagisako, Sylvia J., and Jane Collier. 1987. "Toward a Unified Analysis of Gender and Kinship." In Collier and Yanagisako 1987a, 14–52.

Young, Iris Marion. 1990. *Throwing Like a Girl and Other Essays in Feminist Philosophy and Social Theory*. Bloomington: Indiana University Press.

Yoxen, Edward. 1986. *The Gene Business: Who Should Control Biotechnology?* Oxford: Blackwell.

Zvelebil, Marek. 1994. "Plant Use in the Mesolithic and Its Role in the Transition to Farming." *Proceedings of the Prehistoric Society* 60: 35–74.

INDEX

Page numbers followed by *f* indicate a figure; those followed by *t* indicate a table.

123*t*, 279–80; stem techniques in, 129–33; at University of Illinois, 103–4. *See also* frontier idioms

Ewart, James, 322n28

Ex Ovo Omnia (Glover), 284–85

Experience of Infertility, The (Pfeffer and Woollett), 207–9

experimental embryology. *See* embryology / embryological research

Experimental Embryology (Jenkinson), 114

face work, 233

Fairburn, William, 40–41

family: definitions of, 195; normative conventions of, 206, 221, 233; pressures from, 222, 232; structures of, 183, 227, 316n17. *See also* kinship

family planning, 201

fatherless offspring (Pincogenesis), 132–43

Fausto-Sterling, Anne, 179

feminist biology, 179

Feminist International Network of Resistance to Reproductive and Genetic Engineering (FINRRAGE), 199–206, 211–12, 327nn10–11

feminist political activism: infertility experiences and, 205–19, 222; opposition to NRTS in, 199–206; on reproductive empowerment and agency, 205–6

feminist scholarship, 9; analysis of technological change in, 272–74; on biology of gender, 179; Butler on technologies of gender in, 160, 178–81, 183, 213, 242, 326n20; diversity of perspective within, 189–92, 199–200, 205–7, 327nn4–6; on double consciousness, 237–38, 329n10; on female infertility, 207–19, 222; in Firestone's new population biology, 73–77, 101, 105, 318n4; on the gendered frontier, 290–96; Haraway on engagement with science and technology in, 76–77, 81–82, 86, 96, 100–101, 265, 318n5; Haraway's cyborg manifesto in, 68–73, 181, 317n3, 332n17; of IVF and new reproductive technologies (NRTS), 184–99, 326n2; on kinship and gender technologies, 155–84, 228–42; on Lévi-Strauss's structuralist anthropology, 161–70, 324–25nn9–14; links with activism of, 199–206, 211–12, 327nn10–11; on nature-culture dichotomy, 160; on reproduction and new divisions of labor, 32, 45–48, 52, 65; Rubin on sex/gender systems in, 160–66, 170, 176–79, 324nn8–9, 324–25nn12–13; science studies in, 189; Strathern's instrumental analysis of gender and kinship in, 172–78, 235; Strathern's merographic thought experiments in, 155–60, 182–83, 227–28, 306, 323nn4–7; technological ambivalence in, 184–99, 255, 311–12, 327n6, 327n8; on technologies of sex and gender, 19–23, 25, 52; on visual culture of IVF, 244–45; on women's experiences of reproductive technology, 23, 25–26, 159, 184, 205–19, 328n16

fertility anxiety, 223–24

fertility reassurance, 225

fertility tourism, 231, 332n17

fetal photography, 219, 256, 330n18

FINRRAGE (Feminist International Network of Resistance to Reproductive and Genetic Engineering), 199–206, 211–12, 327nn10–11

Firestone, Shulamith, 20, 24, 66–67, 325n17; new population biology of, 73–77, 101, 105, 318n4; on sexual inequality, 162; on societal change, 208

Fitzgerald, Deborah, 103

"Foetal Images: The Power of Visual Culture in the Politics of Reproduction" (Petchesky), 197–99

Fortes, Meyer, 172–73

Forum against Oppression of Women, 205

Foucault, Michel, 24; on biopower and technologies of self, 15–16, 48–49, 50, 65, 273; on genealogies of normalization, 6, 34–35, 49, 315n4, 316n16; on genealogy as technics, 279, 280; on life itself, 87; on the population, 50–51; on the strangely muddled zone of technology, 273–74; on technologies of sex, 9, 19, 47–49, 51–52, 64–65, 159, 181, 245–46, 314nn9–10, 324–25n12, 330n16

Frankenstein (Shelley), 244

Freud, Sigmund, 161

"From Walking Wombs to Test-Tube Babies" (Oakley), 196–98

frontier idioms, 9, 24–26, 54, 102–11, 143–45, 221, 258–60, 312, 319nn3–4; accidents and indeterminacy in, 105–6, 117–18, 143–44; biofuturism and, 265–68; contact zones as, 259, 265–68, 300, 331–32nn10–12; ethi-

frontier idioms (*continued*)

cal contexts of, 268–75; expectation of continual progress in, 226–27, 263–64, 269–70, 295–96, 331n9; fusion of model organisms in, 125; in Gell's accounts of technology, 107–8, 143, 262; gendered spaces of, 290–96; human-tool relations in, 263–65; in the lab's hole-in-the-wall design, 18–19, 20*f*, 21*f*, 24, 26, 53–56, 260; in New World national narratives, 108–10, 134, 262–63, 320nn13–16, 330n4; as projections into the future, 109–11, 143–44, 259, 330n1, 332n1; Rapp's "moral pioneering" as, 9, 295–96, 308; visual culture of conception and, 243, 274–96. *See also* evolution of reproductive biomedicine

Frontiers of Knowledge pamphlet (ALA), 260–63, 268–69, 330n2

Fujimura, Joan H., 106, 107

Fukuyama, Francis, 22, 327n6

fusion embryos, 10–11, 24

Garfinkel, Harold, 326n20

Geertz, Clifford, 97, 170, 176, 315n4

Gell, Alfred, 107–8, 143, 150–54, 181–82, 262, 331n11

Gender and Kinship (ed. Collier and Yanagisako), 172

gender identity, 174–75; Butler's configuration of, 179–80, 213, 233–35, 242; infertility and, 208, 212–13, 216, 220, 222, 224, 237–38

Gender of the Gift, The (Strathern), 159–60, 173, 176–78

gender technology. *See* sex/gender technology

Gender Trouble (Butler), 179–81

genealogical translation, 66–67

generative relations, 24

genetic capital, 15

Genetic Interest Group (GIG), 63, 66

genetic maternity, 313n6

genomics, 21; biological tools of, 332n16; epigenetic reprogramming and gene transfer in, 266–67; Human Genome Project of, 31–32, 51, 313n5, 332n16; merographic thinking in, 157–58

germplasm, 317n20

gestational maternity, 313n6

Gilbert, Scott, 25, 118

Ginsburg, Faye, 328n2

globalization of IVF, 240, 330n15

Global Nature, Global Culture (Franklin, Lury, and Stacey), 23

Glover, Gina, 26, 260, 274–96, 311–12; *The Art of A.R.T.*, 260, 274, 281–96, 312; *Chromosome Socks*, 275–81; *Eggs Donation*, 283–84; *Ex Ovo Omnia*, 284–85; fabrics used by, 287–89; *Nigella*, 287, 288*f*; *Seeing Eggs Everywhere*, 285; *Sperm Morphology*, 283*f*; *Very Small and Far Away*, 282–83; *Yes!*, 287, 288*f*

Goffman, Erving, 326n20

Gonzalez-Santos, Sandra, 230–31

good manufacturing practice (GMP), 70, 82–83, 92, 318n9

Gordon, Ian R., 322n32

Greer, Germaine, 325n17

Griffin, Susan, 194

guérillères, Les (Wittig), 324–25n12

Guy's Hospital, London, 18; *The Art of A.R.T.* installation at, 260, 274, 281–96; assisted conception unit (ACU) at, 9, 18–19, 20*f*, 21*f*, 24, 26, 53–56, 260, 281; *Chromosome Socks* installation at, 275–81; cytology lab at, 275–78; dish model of disease at, 97–100, 294; stem cell derivation lab of, 52–56, 77–101. *See also* lab culture

Habermas, Jürgen, 22, 27, 263–64, 270, 302, 327n6, 331n6

Hacking, Ian, 279

Hagen people, the, 168–69

Haldane, J. D. S., 75, 245

Hamburger, Victor, 124

Hammond, John, 142, 322n33

Hanmer, Jalna, 201–2

Haraway, Donna, 9, 11, 13, 24, 66–67, 151, 317n1; on analogies in science, 69; on contextual engagement with science and technology, 76–77, 81–82, 86, 96, 100–101, 181, 265, 300, 318n5; cyborg politics of, 68–73, 181, 203, 317n3, 332n17; on interpretive/symbolic anthropology, 170; on scientific models, 97–100; on technological ambivalence, 185–86

Harris, Evan, 58, 59*f*

Harrison, Ross, 130–31, 135

Harstock, Nancy, 198

Heape, Walter, 56, 126–29, 131, 148, 266, 321–22nn27–31

in vitro fertilization (IVF) (*continued*)
329n13; stem cell research and, 17–19, 20*f*,
21*f*, 54–56; technologies of sex and, 19–22;
transformational role of, 14–15, 33–35, 37*f*,
49–52, 61, 64–66, 97, 222, 306; visual culture of conception in, 129–33, 229, 243–
55, 307. *See also* assisted conception unit
(ACU); condition of being after IVF
iPhone, 246–47, 266
"Is Female to Male as Nature Is to Culture?"
(Ortner), 162–66
"It's Going to Work for Me" (Williams), 217
iVF, 247*f*
"IVF — an Irrational Choice" (Koch), 217–18
IVF-stem-cell interface, 14, 18, 54–55, 97, 294,
312

Jasanoff, Sheila, 320n13
Jenkinson, J. W., 114, 122, 123, 124
Jennings, Herbert Spencer, 320n10
Johnson, Martin, 23, 35, 147
Jordanova, Ludmilla, 168

Kahn, Susan, 232
Kaplan, E. Ann, 198
Keating, Peter, 314n8
Keller, Evelyn Fox: on the biological gaze, 70,
248, 279–81; on feminist accounts of sex
and gender, 179; on gendering of science,
291–92; on making sense of life, 2–3; on
postwar reproductive bioscience, 104
Kevles, Daniel, 318n1
kinship, 4, 6–8, 26–27, 150–55; in anthropological study, 52; anxiety of the future and,
298–309; blood ties in, 16–17; disciplining
of reproduction and, 15–16, 22–23, 50–52,
65, 82–83, 313nn5–6; in evolution of tools
and techniques, 111; Foucault's account
of, 48–49, 316n17; Gell's account of, 107,
150–51; genealogical translation of, 66–67;
Haraway's account of, 71–73; hyperconventional roles in, 234–35, 329n8; IVF as model
of, 152–55; law of exogamy in, 48–49, 154,
164–65, 323n2; as mode of production, 165;
new categories of, 37, 159; ontological quest
of ART and, 231–42, 328nn3–5; reconfiguration of, 23; social aspiration in, 226–28;
Strathern's instrumental analysis of, 172–
78; Strathern's merographic thought experi-

ment with, 155–60, 182–83, 227–28, 306,
323nn4–7, 326n21; as technology, 9–10,
15, 25–29, 51, 55, 148–55, 228–31, 326n21;
Yanagisako and Collier's practice theory of,
170–72. *See also* biological relativity
kinship theory, 150–55, 298–309
Kirby, Vicki, 11, 331–32n12
Klein, Renate, 201–2, 208–12
Koch, Lene, 211–12, 217–18
Kolodny, Annette, 290–92, 296

lab culture, 52–56, 77–101, 317n20; bioartistic
rendering of, 260, 274–96, 332n18; craftsmanship in, 83–86; disciplining of reproduction in, 82–83; female sociability in, 78;
gendered divisions of labor in, 329n7; genealogies of tools and techniques in, 111–26;
hole-in-the-wall frontier in, 18–19, 20*f*, 21*f*,
24, 26, 53–56, 260; human-tool-machine
synergy in, 86–96, 318nn6–7; passaging
(propagation) process in, 79–81, 91–94;
quality control (GMP) practices in, 70,
82–83, 92, 318n9
labor of IVF, 232–42, 328nn3–5
Lamarck, Jean-Baptiste, 2
Landecker, Hannah, 25, 308, 330n19; on
biology as engineering, 134–35; on cells as
living tools, 82, 86, 130–31, 247, 267–68; on
plasticity and parthenogenesis, 139–41
laparoscopy, 118, 147
Latour, Bruno, 11, 16, 38, 77, 87, 331n11
Leenhardt, Maurice, 111
Lemonnier, Pierre, 264, 331nn8–9
Leroi-Gourhan, André, 11, 303–4, 315n8, 331n8
Lesnik-Oberstein, Karin, 225–26
Lévi-Strauss, Claude, 160, 273; critiques of
ethnocentrism of, 166, 170, 324–25nn12–13;
on free play and creativity, 108, 111, 154; on
kinship technology, 58, 181–82, 323n2; on
marriage exchange, 173–74; Ortner's reading of, 163–66, 324nn10–11; Rubin's analysis of, 161, 163–66, 170, 177, 324nn8–9,
324–25nn12–13; on social aspiration, 227;
structuralist anthropology of, 161–70, 177–
78, 324–25nn12–14
Lewin, Ellen, 328n2, 328n4
life. *See* making sense of life
Lloyd, Ian, 109–10, 320n16
Lock, Margaret, 23, 45–46

socialist feminism, 199–200. *See also* feminist scholarship

social theory, 11–13. *See also* kinship

social understanding. *See* cultural/social matrix of reproductive biomedicine

sociological models of technology, 260

Sociology of Gender, The (ed. Franklin), 23

Socrates, 300–303

Solomon, Alison, 211–12

somatic cell nuclear transfer, 37*f*

Spallone, Patricia, 196, 199–200

Spar, Debora, 22

Spemann, Hans, 279–80, 321n25; constriction experiments of, 122–26, 306; handmade microtools of, 120–22, 123*t*

Spemann micropipettes, 111, 112*f*

Spencer, Herbert, 127

sperm capacitation, 137

Sperm Morphology (Glover), 283*f*

Spillers, Hortense, 179

Spivak, Gayatri, 179

Squier, Susan, 244–46

Stacey, Jackie, 23

standardization, 52, 55–56

Stanworth, Michelle, 196–97, 206–7

Steinberg, Deborah Lynn, 196, 199–200

stem cell banking, 19, 38, 52, 55–56, 70

stem cell derivation labs. *See* lab culture

stem cell technology, 307; cell reprogramming and, 37, 54; induced pluripotent stem (iPS) cells, 3, 17–18, 37, 266, 306, 313n7, 320n12; passaging (propagation) process in, 79–81; public opinion on, 61–63, 271–72, 317n23. *See also* human embryonic stem cell (hES) research; lab culture

stem technologies, 14–15, 129–33, 306

Steptoe, Patrick, 22, 36, 118, 145–49

Stiegler, Bernard, 12–13, 44, 87, 263–64, 331n7

Stilled Lives (Chadwick), 286–87, 332n14

strategic biologization, 329n12

strategic naturalization, 159

Strathern, Marilyn, 15, 20–21, 25, 246, 273, 296, 317n22; instrumental analysis of gender and kinship of, 172–78, 235; interpretive/symbolic anthropology of, 170; on kinship thinking, 183, 229, 326n21; on Melanesian sex and gender practices, 168–69, 173–78, 325n18; merographic thought

experiment on kinship of, 155–60, 182–83, 227–28, 255, 306, 323nn4–7; on structuralist anthropology, 166–70

structural functionalism, 169, 172–73

structuralist anthropology, 161–70, 177–78, 326n19

"Structure, Sign, and Play" (Derrida), 325n13

substantialization, 16–19, 27; of biology as technology, 33; of blood, 16–17; tools as, 13, 64, 66

substitutability, 317n22

Suchman, Lucy, 331n11

Suffolk Puffs (Glover), 287, 289*f*, 290

surgical enhancement of fertility, 189

surrogacy, 189, 219

synthetic biology, 2–3, 21, 266–67, 272, 322n35

tactical biopolitics, 295

Tarkowski, Andrei, 120*t*

techne (as term), 28

technical activity, 150–51

technics, 279, 280, 331n7, 332n17; Derrida on regeneration and, 26–27, 302–7, 332n17; dialogic future of, 312

technologia (as term), 28

technological ambivalence, 8–9, 34–35, 184, 219–20, 307–12, 314n3; diversity of perspectives and, 190; feminist political activism and, 199–206, 211–12, 327nn10–11; feminist scholarship on IVF and, 184–99, 255, 326n2, 327n6, 327n8; gender identity and IVF and, 208, 212–13, 216, 220, 222, 224; toward future possibilities, 299–300; in women's encounters with IVF, 184, 206–19, 274, 328n16

technological determinism, 263

technological reproduction, 11–13. *See also* reproduction

Technologies of Procreation (Edwards et al.), 23

technology, 1–2, 26–29, 314nn9–10; cultural matrix of change and, 4–6, 9, 18–19, 22–29, 32–35, 314n8; definitions of, 28; expectation of continual progress with, 226–27, 263–64, 269–70, 295–96, 331n9; Gell's account of, 107–8, 143, 150–51, 181–82; Heidegger's account of, 11, 13–14, 66, 302; human inheritance of, 10–13, 27–28, 144; kinship identity and, 28–29, 51, 148–55, 228–42; Marx's and Engels's models of, 9,

11–14, 24, 45, 68, 181–82, 226–27, 243–44, 263–64, 303–9, 315–16nn8–11, 316n13, 331nn5–7; original goals of, 10; in Plato's *Phaedrus*, 299–307, 312; reproduction of relationships in, 153–55; of sex, 9, 19–22, 25, 32–33, 46–49, 51–52, 65–66; sociological models of, 9, 260. *See also* bioindustry; biologization of technology; frontier idioms; human embryonic stem cell (hES) research; in vitro fertilization (IVF)

telegony, 126–27, 322n28

tentative pregnancy, 238–39, 329n13

Tentative Pregnancy: Prenatal Diagnosis and the Future of Motherhood, The (Rothman), 191–95

Test-Tube Women: What Future for Motherhood? (ed. Arditti, Klein, and Minden), 191–95, 196, 199

thick genealogies, 23, 315n4

"Thinking Sex" (Rubin), 179

Thompson, Charis, 6–7, 26, 45–46, 159, 177–78; on NRTS as text for feminist theory, 186; on ontological choreography of ART, 231, 233–35, 240, 242, 255, 328n2, 328n4, 329n12; on women's experiences of IVF, 215, 217

Through the Flower (Chicago), 292

Tissue Culture and Art project, 332n18

"Tissue Culture Kings" (J. Huxley), 245

Tomorrow's Child: Reproductive Technologies in the 1990s (Birke et al.), 208–9, 328n13

tools and techniques, 3, 19; coevolution of substance and, 54, 138–41, 151, 263–64, 315n8, 322–23nn38–39; genealogies of, 116–26, 132–33, 320nn17–18; hand-tool-embryo relations and, 67, 243, 251, 254; hand-tool relations and, 9, 13–14, 40–45, 65, 89, 116–18, 182; hand tools and handiwork in, 18, 39, 42, 83, 95, 106, 305, 318nn8–9, 332n18; Haraway's account of, 72–73, 76–77, 81–82, 86, 96, 100–101, 318n5; human embryos as, 57–58, 64, 294; hybrid embryos as, 10–11, 24, 58–63; machine age of, 38–44, 64–65, 147, 244; in Marx's and Engels's models of technology, 9, 11–13, 64–65, 263, 315–16nn8–11, 316n13; in Marx's human-tool-machine relations, 40–44, 64–65, 86–91, 116, 130, 244, 318nn6–7; scientific models

as, 97–100, 279; stem technologies in, 14–15, 129–33, 306; as substantialized concepts, 13, 64, 66; of in vitro culture methods, 129–33. *See also* evolution of reproductive biomedicine; technology

"Traffic of Women: Notes on the 'Political Economy' of Sex, The" (Rubin), 48, 160–70, 324n8, 325n13

transbiology, 317n21

transférance, 307

transformational role of IVF. *See* condition of being after IVF

transgenesis, 37, 246

transgenic mice, 13

transhumanism, 246

Turner, Frederick Jackson, 110, 262–63, 290

UBINIG, 205–6, 327n12

UK Stem Cell Bank, 19

ultrasound, 219, 330n18

UN Decade for Women, 200–201

United Kingdom: biocapitalist policies of, 56–58, 240; support of stem cell research in, 61–63, 268

United States: public opinion on stem cell research in, 317n23; right-to-life movement in, 197–98, 330n18; science policy in, 102–3, 269–70, 332n13

University of Illinois, 103–4

values. *See* cultural/social matrix of reproductive biomedicine

Venter, Craig, 267

Very Small and Far Away (Glover), 282–83

virgin birth, 323n1

visual culture of conception, 1, 10, 23, 26, 229, 243–57, 307; anti-abortion movement's use of, 197–98, 330n18; bioartistic rendering of, 260, 274–96, 332n18; biological gaze in, 70, 248, 279–81, 294–95; handheld screens in, 246–47; with in vitro culture models, 129–33; Nilsson's work in, 248, 250, 330n20; optical techniques in, 115–16, 321nn23–24; in Pincus's *The Eggs of Mammals*, 140f, 141–42

Volonté de Savoir, La (Foucault), 324–25n12

Waddington, Conrad Hal, 36, 75, 131, 145

Wagner, Roy, 170

Walker, Alice, 179